普通高等教育"十一五"国家级规划教材

全国高等医药院校药学类专业第二轮实验双语教材

有机化学实验与指导

（第3版）

主　　审　陆　涛
主　　编　杜　鼎
副 主 编　张晓进　江　辰　陈　明
编　　者　（以姓氏笔画为序）
　　　　　卢　帅　江　辰　杜　鼎
　　　　　张晓进　陈　明　董　颖
　　　　　谢　程　鲍丽丽

中国健康传媒集团
中国医药科技出版社

内 容 提 要

本书是"全国高等医药院校药学类专业第二轮实验双语教材"之一。内容包括有机化学实验的一般知识、基本操作实验、基础性有机合成实验、综合性有机合成实验和设计性有机合成实验五部分；实验部分共选取了28个实验，大部分是经典的有机化学基本操作和合成实验，且经过长期的教学实践检验，每个实验后编写了实验指导，以便教学和指导学生进行实验。本书采用中英文对照，有利于学生对专业英语的学习。本书为书网融合教材，即纸质教材有机融合电子教材、教学配套资源（PPT、微课）、数字化教学服务（在线教学、在线作业、在线考试），使教学资源更加多样化、立体化。

本书可供高等医药院校药学类相关专业实验教学使用，也可供医药行业内科研、培训使用。

图书在版编目（CIP）数据

有机化学实验与指导 / 杜鼎主编 . —3 版 . —北京：中国医药科技出版社，2019.12

全国高等医药院校药学类专业第二轮实验双语教材

ISBN 978 - 7 - 5214 - 1426 - 4

Ⅰ. ①有… Ⅱ. ①杜… Ⅲ. ①有机化学 - 化学实验 - 双语教学 - 医学院校 - 教学参考资料 - 汉、英 Ⅳ. ①O62 - 33

中国版本图书馆 CIP 数据核字（2019）第 296930 号

美术编辑 陈君杞
版式设计 南博文化

出版 **中国健康传媒集团** | 中国医药科技出版社
地址 北京市海淀区文慧园北路甲 22 号
邮编 100082
电话 发行：010 - 62227427 邮购：010 - 62236938
网址 www.cmstp.com
规格 889 × 1194mm $\frac{1}{16}$
印张 13 ¾
字数 305 千字
初版 2003 年 7 月第 1 版
版次 2019 年 12 月第 3 版
印次 2022 年 11 月第 3 次印刷
印刷 三河市万龙印装有限公司
经销 全国各地新华书店
书号 ISBN 978 - 7 - 5214 - 1426 - 4
定价 **40.00 元**

获取新书信息、投稿、为图书纠错，请扫码联系我们。

教学是学校人才培养的中心环节，实验教学是这一环节的重要组成部分。"全国高等医药院校药学类专业实验双语教材"是中国药科大学坚持药学实践教学改革，突出提高学生动手能力、创新思维，通过承担教育部"世行贷款21世纪初高等教育教学改革项目"等多项教改课题，逐步建设完善的一套与药学各专业学科理论课程紧密结合的高水平双语实验教材。

本轮修订，适逢"全国高等医药院校药学类专业第五轮规划教材"及《中国药典》（2020年版）、新版《国家执业药师资格考试大纲》出版，整套教材的修订强调了与新版理论教材知识的结合，与《中国药典》（2020年版）等新颁布的法典法规结合。为更好地服务于新时期高等院校药学教育与人才培养的需要，在上一版的基础上，进一步体现了各门实验课程自身独立性、系统性和科学性，又充分考虑到各门实验课程之间的联系与衔接，主要突出了以下特点。

1. 适应医药行业对人才的要求，体现行业特色，契合新时期药学人才需求的变化，使修订后的教材符合《中国药典》（2020年版）等国家标准及新版《国家执业药师资格考试大纲》等行业最新要求。

2. 更新完善内容，打造教材精品。在上版教材基础上进一步优化、精炼和充实内容。紧密结合"全国高等医药院校药学类专业第五轮规划教材"，强调与实际需求相结合，进一步提高教材质量。

3. 为适应信息化教学的需要，本轮教材全部打造成为书网融合教材，即纸质教材与数字教材、配套教学资源、题库系统、数字化教学服务有机融合，为读者提供全免费增值服务。

4. 坚持双语体系，强调素质培养教材以实践教学为突破口，采用双语体系编写有利于加快药学教育国际接轨，提高学生的科技英语水平，进一步提升学生整体素质。

"全国高等医药院校药学类专业第二轮实验双语教材"历经15年4次建设，在各个时期广大编者的努力下，在广大使用教材师生的支持下日臻完善。本轮教材的出版，必将对推动新时期我国高等药学教育的发展产生积极而深远的影响。希望广大师生在教学实践中对本套教材提出宝贵意见，以便今后进一步修订完善，共同打造精品教材。

吴晓明

全国高等医药院校药学类专业第五轮规划教材常务编委会主任委员

2019年10月

　　《有机化学实验与指导》是依据高等医药院校药学类专业教育教学要求和药学人才培养目标要求而编写的双语类实验教材。教材于2003年首次出版发行，2006年进行第一次修订，历经十余载，受到了广大师生的普遍认可和好评。为了适应高等教育新形势下的发展需要及学科的不断发展，我们在广泛征求意见的基础上，对第二版进行修订。为了优化和精选实验教学内容，我们对书中某些章节和内容进行了调整，同时对教材中的部分图片、结构式进行了更新，对语言表述不妥之处进行了更正。

　　本书主要从基础性、综合性、设计和创新性三个不同层次进行设计编写，全部采用中英文对照的形式。第一部分介绍有机化学实验的一般知识，新增"有机化学实验废物的分类和处置"内容；第二部分强调有机化学实验的基本操作技术，新增"柱色谱"内容；第三部分通过基础性有机合成实验巩固基本操作的同时，掌握有机合成实验的基本技术和方法；第四部分利用综合性有机合成实验使学生达到融会贯通的目的；第五部分设计性有机合成实验注重培养学生的综合素质以及创新思维和能力。

　　本书由杜鼎任主编，张晓进、江辰、陈明任副主编。具体分工如下：杜鼎（第一部分），江辰（第二部分），陈明（第三部分，实验十~十六），谢程（第三部分，实验十七~二十四），张晓进（第四和第五部分），董颖、卢帅、鲍丽丽（数字化资源的制作）。全书由主编统稿。

　　本书为书网融合教材，即纸质教材有机融合电子教材、教学配套资源（PPT、微课）、数字化教学服务（在线教学、在线作业、在线考试），使教学资源更加多样化、立体化。

　　在本书编写过程中，得到了中国药科大学及其教务处、理学院和有机化学课程群全体同志的关心和支持。本书由陆涛教授任主审，唐伟方教授对本书编写也提出了很多宝贵意见，在此谨向他们表示衷心的感谢。由于编者水平所限，不妥和疏漏之处在所难免，恳请广大师生和读者批评指正。

编　者
2019年9月

Contents

第一部分　有机化学实验的一般知识

扫码"学一学"

扫码"看一看"

一、实验室规则

进行有机化学实验必须高度重视实验室的安全问题，为了确保实验的正常进行，培养学生良好的实验习惯与工作作风，要求学生必须遵守下列规则。

（1）实验前认真预习有关实验的全部内容，做好预习报告。通过预习明确实验目的要求、基本原理、操作步骤和有关的操作技术，了解实验所需的原料、试剂、仪器和装置，并充分考虑如何防止可能发生的事故和一旦发生事故时采用的处理措施。

（2）进入实验室后，要熟悉实验室概貌及其周围环境，了解实验室内水、电、煤气开关位置和放置灭火器材的地点及使用方法。要穿实验服，如头发较长要束好。

（3）实验时应保持安静，精神要集中，操作要认真。要仔细观察，养成一边进行实验，一边实事求是地做好实验记录的习惯。实验中途不得擅自离开实验室。

（4）遵从教师的指导，严格按照操作步骤进行实验。学生若有新的见解或建议，如要改变实验步骤和试剂用量等，需先征得教师同意后再实施。如果发生意外事故，应立即报告教师及时处理。

（5）在实验过程中，要保持实验室及台面整洁，废物与回收溶剂等应放到指定的地方，不得乱丢乱倒。

（6）公用仪器、原料、试剂和工具应在指定的地点使用，用后立即放回原处。严格控制原料、试剂的用量。要节约水、电、煤气。破损仪器应及时报损补充，按规定赔偿。

（7）实验完毕后必须将记录（合成实验要上交产品）交教师审阅，必须将所用的仪器清洗干净，放置整齐，进行安全检查。做好这一切后征得教师同意方可离开实验室。

（8）值日生负责门窗玻璃、桌面、地面及水槽的清洁工作，以及整理公用原料、试剂和器材，清除垃圾，检查水、电、煤气安全。

二、实验室的安全

有机化学实验室是一个有潜在危险的工作场所，有机化学实验所用原料、试剂种类繁多，经常要使用易燃溶剂（如乙醚、石油醚、乙醇、丙酮、苯、甲苯和乙酸乙酯等）、易燃易爆的气体和固体（如氢气、煤气、乙炔、金属钠和苦味酸等）、有毒化学品（如氰化钠、硝基苯、光气、氯气、苯、硫化氢和硫酸二甲酯等）和有腐蚀性的化学品（氯磺酸、浓硫酸、浓硝酸、浓盐酸、溴和强碱等）。如使用不当就有可能发生着火、中毒、烧伤、爆炸等事故。实验中所用仪器大部分是玻璃仪器，如处理不当可能会发生严重的割伤事故。此外，电器老化、煤气泄漏等如处理不当也会发生事故。因此要求实验者具有在实验室工作的基本知识并严格执行操作规程，懂得该做什么，不该做什么，同时还要掌握适当的预防措施。

（一）实验时的一般注意事项

（1）熟悉安全用具如灭火器材及急救药箱的放置地点及使用方法。

（2）实验开始前应检查仪器是否完整无损，装置是否正确稳妥，必须熟悉药品和仪器的性能和装配要点，在征得指导教师同意后开始进行实验。

（3）按照实验步骤进行实验，仔细检查所取试剂是否正确无误，严格遵守操作规程。实验进行中不得随便离开，并要经常注意反应进行的情况和装置有无漏气、破裂等。

（4）在实验室内应一直佩戴护目镜。在进行有可能发生危险的实验时，要根据具体情况采取必要的安全措施，如戴面罩、手套等。对反应中产生的有害气体要按规定处理。

（5）实验中所用的易燃、易爆、有毒物品不得随意散失、丢弃。实验室内严禁吸烟、饮食。实验结束后要将手洗干净。

（二）实验中事故的预防

1. 玻璃割伤事故的预防　玻璃割伤是有机化学实验中常见事故之一。为了避免割伤应注意以下几点。

（1）玻璃管（棒）切断时不能用力过猛，切割后断面应在火上烧熔以消除棱角。

（2）将玻璃管（棒）或温度计插入塞中时，应先检查塞孔大小是否合适，玻璃是否光滑，并涂些甘油等润滑剂，然后慢慢旋转插入。握玻璃管（棒）或温度计的手应靠近塞子，防止玻璃管折断而割伤皮肤。

2. 着火的预防　着火是有机化学实验室内特有的危险，必须充分注意，切记下列事项。

（1）实验室不准存放大量易燃物。

（2）不能用烧杯等广口容器盛装易燃物，切勿将易燃溶剂放在广口容器内（如烧杯内）直火加热。

（3）尽量防止或减少易燃物的气体外逸。当处理大量的易燃性液体时，应在通风橱中或在指定的地方进行，且室内严禁有明火。

（4）高度易燃溶剂（如乙醚）不得倒入废液缸内，应放入原瓶专门回收。

（5）使用酒精灯时应用火柴引火，不可用另外的酒精灯的火焰直接引火。

（6）用油浴作热源进行蒸馏或回流时，切勿使冷凝用水溅入热油浴中，以免使油外溅到热源上而起火。

（7）防止煤气管、阀漏气。

3. 爆炸事故的预防　在实验时也可能发生爆炸事故，应引起高度重视。为杜绝事故，应注意以下几点。

（1）常压操作时切勿在密闭系统内进行加热反应，在反应进行过程中要经常注意仪器装置的各部分有无堵塞现象。

（2）减压蒸馏时不得使用机械强度不大的仪器（如锥形瓶、平底烧瓶、薄壁玻璃仪器等），要仔细检查仪器有无破损和裂缝。

（3）使用易燃易爆的气体如氢气、乙炔等时，应保持室内空气流通，严禁明火，并防止一切火花的产生。

（4）对于易爆炸的固体如重金属乙炔化物、三硝基甲苯等，不能重压或撞击，以免引起爆炸。

（5）避免金属钠与水、卤代烷直接接触，以免因剧烈反应而发生爆炸。

（6）浓硝酸、高氯酸和过氧化氢等氧化剂与有机物接触时极易引起爆炸，使用时应特别小心，切勿看错标签，加错药品。

4. 中毒事故的预防 化学药品大多具有不同程度的毒性，产生中毒的主要原因是皮肤或呼吸道接触有毒药品所引起的，在实验中，要防止中毒，应切实做到以下几点。

（1）对有毒物品应认真操作、妥善保管。实验后的有毒残渣必须及时按要求处理，不得乱放。

（2）药品不要沾在皮肤上，尤其是剧毒品。有些有毒物质会渗入皮肤，因此使用时必须戴橡皮手套，操作后应立即洗手。切勿让有毒物质接触五官或伤口。称量任何药品都应使用工具，不得用手直接接触。

（3）使用有毒试剂或反应过程中产生有毒气体或液体的实验，应在通风橱中进行。有时也可用气体吸收装置（见图1-9）以除去反应中所生成的有毒气体。

（4）对沾染过有毒物质的仪器和用具，用毕应立即处理消除其毒性。

（5）如打破水银温度计、压力计，应及时报告，尽可能设法回收水银，余留的残迹用三氯化铁溶液或硫黄粉处理。

5. 触电事故的预防 现在的有机化学实验室中，电器使用日益增多，为防止触电事故的发生，使用者必须注意。

（1）电器装置与设备的金属外壳应与地线连接，使用前应先检查其外壳是否漏电。

（2）使用电器时应防止人体与电器导电部分直接接触，不能用湿的手或手握湿物接触电插头。

（3）电器设备用毕应先关仪器电源开关，再拔去电源插头，以防发生事故。

6. 溢水事故的预防 大量溢水也是有机实验室中常见的一种事故。防止溢水应注意以下几点。

（1）经常清理水槽。

（2）废纸、玻璃、火柴梗、木屑等应扔入废物缸，不能丢入水槽中。

（3）冷凝管的冷却水不宜开得太大。

（4）停止实验后，应立即关掉冷凝水龙头。

（三）实验中事故的处理

1. 玻璃割伤的处理 受伤后要仔细观察伤口有无玻璃碎粒，取出伤口内的玻璃屑。若伤口不大可先用蒸馏水清洗，然后包扎好，或用创可贴贴紧。如伤口较大应先做止血处理（如扎止血带或按紧主血管）以防止大量出血，然后急送医疗单位。

2. 着火事故的处理 实验室如果发生着火事故，切勿惊慌失措，应沉着镇静及时采取措施，控制事故的扩大。如少量有机溶媒着火且火势很小，可立即用湿抹布、石棉布、黄沙等覆盖火源，使其隔绝空气灭火。如火势较大，首先应熄灭附近所有火源、关闭煤气、切断电源、移开附近未着火的易燃物，同时根据易燃物的性质设法灭火。

油浴和有机溶剂着火时绝对不能用水来灭火，因为这样反而会使火焰蔓延开。若衣服着火，切勿奔跑，可用不易燃的厚外衣包裹使火熄灭。较严重者应躺在地上打滚或用防火毯紧紧包住，直至火熄灭。亦可打开安全冲淋装置用大量水冲淋灭火。烧伤严重者应急送医疗单位。

下面介绍实验室中常用的两种灭火器的使用方法。

（1）二氧化碳灭火器 二氧化碳灭火器是有机实验室中最常用的一种灭火器材，用以扑灭有机物及电器设备的着火。其钢筒内装有压缩的液态二氧化碳，使用时打开开关，对准火根喷射。注意手不能握在喷二氧化碳的喇叭筒上，因喷出的二氧化碳压力突然降低，温度骤降，若手直接握在喇叭筒上易被冻伤。

（2）泡沫灭火器　电器着火不能用泡沫灭火器来灭火，因灭火液体易导电引起触电事故，而且后处理较麻烦。只在火势较大时才应用。

3. 试剂灼伤的处理

（1）酸灼伤　皮肤灼伤可立即用大量水冲洗，然后用5%碳酸氢钠溶液洗涤。眼睛灼伤可立即用生理盐水冲洗，或将干净橡皮管接上水龙头用细水流小心对准眼睛冲洗，然后再用1%碳酸氢钠溶液洗涤。

（2）碱灼伤　皮肤灼伤可先用水冲洗，再用硼酸溶液或1%醋酸溶液洗涤。眼睛灼伤立即用生理盐水洗，再用1%硼酸溶液洗。

（3）溴灼伤　应立即用酒精洗涤，再涂上甘油。亦可立即用2%硫代硫酸钠溶液洗至伤处呈白色，然后涂甘油。

4. 中毒的处理　吞下强酸中毒者，先饮大量水，然后服用氢氧化铝膏、鸡蛋白、牛奶，不要吃催吐剂。吞下强碱中毒者，先饮大量水，然后服用醋、酸果汁、鸡蛋白、牛奶，也不要吃催吐剂。吞下刺激物或其他毒物者，先服用牛奶或鸡蛋白使之冲淡缓和，再将硫酸镁（约30克）溶于一杯水中饮下催吐，有时也可用手指伸入喉部促使呕吐，然后立即送医院。将吸入气体中毒者移至室外，解开衣领及钮扣。如吸入少量氯气或溴可用碳酸氢钠溶液嗽口，严重者立即送医疗单位。

5. 烫伤的处理　皮肤接触火焰或灼热物体（如铁圈、煤气灯管、玻璃管等）会造成烧伤，先用自来水冲洗5~30分钟，并除去表面覆盖物，用干净敷料覆盖创面，严重者转送医院。

三、有机化学实验废物的分类和处置

在有机化学实验中或实验结束后往往会产生废气、废液和固体废物，为遵守国家和地方政府的环保法规，避免或减少对环境的污染和危害，可采用如下处理办法：

（1）实验室产生的废气主要包括酸雾、甲醛、苯系物、各种有机溶剂等，因此要保证实验室良好的通风；对于直接产生有毒、有害气体的实验要求在通风橱内进行，这是保证室内空气质量、保护实验人员健康安全的有效办法。

（2）对于实验室产生的液体和固体废物，要按照有害、无害分类收集于不同的容器中，对一些难处理的有害废物可送环保部分专门处理。

（3）实验室产生的废液包括化学性实验废液和一般废水。化学性实验废液主要包括多余的样品、有机溶剂、各种酸碱废液、重金属废液、实验后处理产生的废液等，必须根据其化学特性选择合适的容器进行回收，并置于通风处，容器标签必须标明废物种类、储存时间，定期处理，并做好登记。一般废水如氯化钠水溶液等可直接排入下水道，少量酸（如盐酸、硫酸、硝酸等）或碱（如氢氧化钠、氢氧化钾等）在倒入下水道之前必须中和并用水稀释。

（4）实验室产生的固体废物包括多余样品、反应产物、消耗或破损的实验用品（如玻璃器皿、滤纸等）、残留或失效的化学试剂和药品、废弃的试剂空瓶等，必须根据固体性质选择合适的容器和方法进行回收。实验过程中产生的化学固体废物（如化学试剂和药品，使用过的滤纸、硅胶、手套等）应集中收集存放于特定的化学固体废物容器中；废弃的试剂空瓶应单独统一回收，并做好登记；破损的玻璃仪器和用过的针头等利器应收集于特定的利器回收容器中；无害的固体废物如未接触化学品的纸、软木塞、橡胶管、金属制品等可倒入普通废物桶。

（5）对能与水发生剧烈反应的化学品如金属钠，处理之前需用适当方法在通风橱内进行分解。

（6）对可能致癌的物质，处理一定要格外小心，避免与皮肤接触。

（7）严禁将有害实验废弃物随意排入下水道及任何水源，严禁乱丢乱弃、堆放在走廊、过道及其他公共区域，生活垃圾和实验垃圾不得混放。

四、实验室常用仪器设备和技术

（一）玻璃仪器

1. 普通非标准磨口玻璃仪器　实验室常用的普通玻璃仪器如图 1-1 所示。

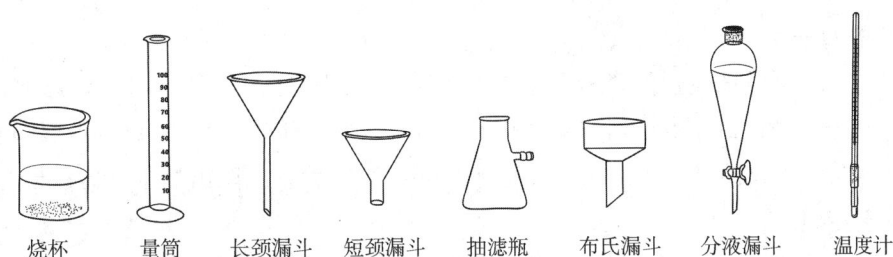

烧杯　量筒　长颈漏斗　短颈漏斗　抽滤瓶　布氏漏斗　分液漏斗　温度计

图 1-1　普通玻璃仪器

2. 标准磨口玻璃仪器　目前，有机化学实验中越来越多地使用带有标准磨口的玻璃仪器，称为标准磨口仪器。常见标准磨口玻璃仪器如图 1-2 所示。

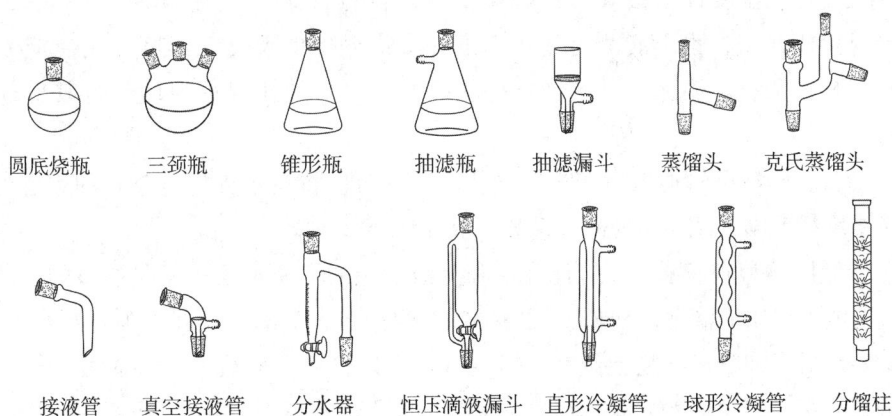

圆底烧瓶　三颈瓶　锥形瓶　抽滤瓶　抽滤漏斗　蒸馏头　克氏蒸馏头

接液管　真空接液管　分水器　恒压滴液漏斗　直形冷凝管　球形冷凝管　分馏柱

图 1-2　标准磨口玻璃仪器

由于仪器容量大小及用途不一，通常标准磨口有 10 口、14 口、19 口、24 口、29 口等。这些数字编号系指磨口最大端直径的毫米数。相同编号的内外磨口可相互连接。有时两仪器因磨口编号不同无法直接连接，则可借助于不同编号的磨口接头使之连接。

使用标准磨口玻璃仪器时应注意如下事项。

（1）磨口处必须洁净。若附有固体则磨口对接不紧密，将导致漏气。若杂质很硬，甚至损坏磨口。

（2）一般使用磨口仪器不需涂润滑剂。若反应中有强碱，则应涂润滑剂，以免磨口连接处因碱腐蚀粘牢而无法拆开。减压蒸馏时，若需真空度较高，应细心地在磨口大的一段涂上薄薄一层真空油脂。切勿涂的太多，以免污染产物。

（3）用后应拆开洗净，否则长期放置后磨口连接处常会粘牢不易拆开。如磨口处涂了润滑剂或真空油脂，清洗前应先用纸将润滑剂或真空油脂擦干净。

3. 仪器的洗涤 把仪器淋湿后，将浸湿的毛刷蘸取肥皂粉进行擦刷，除去壁上的污物后，用水将肥皂粉冲去，洗净晾干。器壁应不留污物，不现油渍。

有机化学实验反应种类繁杂，有时用肥皂粉不能达到清洗效果。这时应根据实验具体情况，选用清洗手段。如已知瓶内残渣为碱性物质时，可用稀盐酸或稀硫酸溶解；残渣为酸性物质时，可用稀氢氧化钠溶液清洗。如已知瓶内残渣溶于某种溶剂时，可用适量该溶剂洗涤。

对需要仪器清洁度更高的实验，如精制产品或有机分析等，可用洗涤剂、蒸馏水依次洗涤仪器。

4. 仪器的干燥

（1）晾干 清洁的仪器倒置，水珠易流下，干燥得快。

（2）烘干 放入烘箱的仪器应除去软木塞或橡皮塞，带有磨口玻璃塞的仪器也应拔出塞子；放置时应将仪器口向上，烘箱温度以 $110 \sim 120℃$ 为宜。取出烘干仪器前最好使烘箱内温度降至室温。

（3）吹干 如急需用少量干燥仪器，可用鼓风干燥器或电吹风吹干。

（4）有机溶剂助干燥 急用时可用有机溶剂助干，如用少量95%乙醇或丙酮荡洗，把溶剂倒到回收瓶中，然后用电吹风吹干。

5. 仪器的保养

（1）温度计 温度计水银球部位玻璃很薄，容易破损，使用时要格外小心，不能用温度计当搅拌棒使用，也不能测定超越温度计最高刻度的温度。温度计用后应使其慢慢冷却，特别是在测量高温之后，切勿立即用冷水冲洗。使用过的温度计待其冷却后洗净擦干收好。

（2）冷凝管 冷凝管通水后较重，安装冷凝管时应将夹子夹住冷凝管的重心处。洗涤冷凝管时要用长毛刷。洗净后应直立放置，便于晾干。

（3）分液漏斗和滴液漏斗 分液漏斗和滴液漏斗的活塞和盖子都是磨口的，若是非原配的，就可能不严密而滴漏，所以使用时要注意保护。各个漏斗之间也不要互相调换塞子。用后一定要在活塞和磨口间垫上纸片，以免日久难以打开。分液漏斗和滴液漏斗用后必须拔出塞子和活塞，擦净上面的润滑油，洗净后再放入烘箱烘干。

6. 仪器的选择

（1）塞子的选择 橡皮塞塞得严密，但能被某些有机溶剂溶解。此时可改用磨口玻璃塞，其优点是密封性更强，结合更紧密，防止气体挥发和外界气体进入污染，但盛放碱液的瓶子不能用磨口玻璃塞，要用橡胶塞。

（2）仪器的选择 选择仪器是根据反应物的体积、反应的条件及反应物（或生成物）的理化性质而决定。①反应瓶的大小，应该是使反应物体积不超过其容积的2/3，一般约为1/2。②回流反应一般采用圆底烧瓶和球形冷凝器；回流搅拌并需控制反应温度时采用三颈瓶。③蒸馏操作需用蒸馏瓶；减压蒸馏采用减压蒸馏瓶（克氏蒸馏头接在圆底烧瓶上）。④常压蒸馏中，被蒸馏液体体积不超过蒸馏瓶容积的 2/3；减压蒸馏中，被蒸馏液体体积不超过蒸馏瓶容积的 1/2。⑤被蒸馏物的沸点低于 130℃ 时用直形冷凝器，高于 130℃ 用空气冷凝器。⑥温度计的选择，一般是根据反应温度选用高于反应温度 10 ~ 20℃ 的温度计。水银温度计适用于测量 −30 ~ 300℃ 的物质；温度低于 −38℃ 时常用内装有机液体的低温温度计（因水银会凝固）。

（二）实验常用设备及使用方法

1. 加热

（1）水浴　水浴是最安全和方便的热源，100℃ 以下的反应或后处理大多可用水浴加热（图 1 − 3）。若将容器放在水浴锅盖上则为蒸汽加热。

（2）油浴　实验室最常用的热源为油浴（图 1 − 4）。油浴的构造也很简单，在结晶皿或陶瓷皿中加入油并安置电热丝，然后再和调压变压器连接。有时也应用电磁搅拌来保持油浴温度均匀。油浴所用的油有甘油、植物油和石蜡油（适于 150℃ 以下的加热）等。最好使用硅油，可加热至 250℃ 以上，但其价格较贵。油浴使用方便安全，容器内的反应物受热均匀，加热温度范围广。

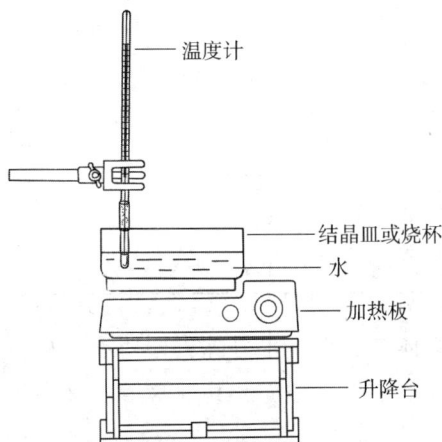

图 1 − 3　水浴加热（以加热板加热）

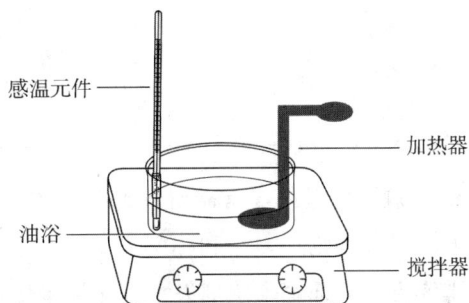

图 1 − 4　油浴加热

（3）电加热套　电加热套是一种用于加热圆底烧瓶的常用装置。它由玻璃纤维包裹电热丝编织而成，外接调压变压器以调节加热温度。它的优点是安全、方便。但一种规格加热器只适用于一定容积的烧瓶，故需配备几种尺寸的加热套。用加热套加热时必须注意温度的控制，若稍微疏忽就会使升温过高而影响反应。要避免化学药品撒入电热套内，以免电热丝烧毁甚至引起火灾。

（4）电热板　电热板常用于加热水和其他高沸点溶剂组成的溶液和反应混合物，特别适用于加热平底容器内的溶液（图 1 − 5）。低沸点易燃性溶剂，如乙醚、石油醚、丙酮、二硫化碳等，不宜用电热板加热。

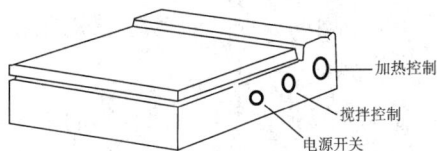

图 1 − 5　电热板（带磁力搅拌）

（5）沙浴　当要求加热温度较高时，可采用沙浴。温度可达 350℃。沙浴一般由铁盘装入干燥的细沙制成，把反应器半埋在沙中加热。沙浴特别适用于加热沸点在 200℃ 以上的液体。沙浴传热慢、散热快，所以温度上升慢，且不易控制。因此反应瓶底下的沙层要薄一些，沙浴中应插入温度计，并使温度计水银球靠近反应瓶。

（6）红外灯　红外灯适用于加热较低温度的反应，亦比较安全。

2. 冷却　低于室温的反应可用水浴、冰水浴、冰盐浴进行冷却降温。液氮或干冰和溶剂的混合物则适用于极低温度下进行的反应。在搅拌下将液氮慢慢倒入有机溶剂中直至形成油膏状即为所需冷却剂，在使用时可随时添加液氮以保持冷却温度。干冰和有机溶剂亦可配制成冷却剂，将干冰碎块加入溶剂中即可。操作时应经常添加干冰以保持冷却效果。常用的冷却剂见表 1-1。

表 1-1　常用冷却剂的组成及冷却温度

冷却剂	温度，℃
碎冰（或冰-水）	0
碎冰（3份）-氯化钠（1份）	-20
干冰-四氯化碳	-32
液氮-氯苯	-45
干冰-乙醇	-72
干冰-丙酮	-78
液氮-甲苯	-95
干冰-乙醚	-100
液氮-乙醚	-116
液氮-异戊烷	-160
液氮	-196

3. 干燥　实验中经常需要将附在气体、液体或固体内的少量水分除去即所谓干燥。干燥的方法可分为物理方法和化学方法。加热干燥、真空干燥、冷冻、共沸蒸馏、吸附等为物理干燥方法，而用干燥剂去水为化学干燥方法。

（1）气体的干燥　要除去气体中的水，可使其通过充满无水氯化钙或固体氢氧化钾的干燥塔，或者通过装有浓硫酸的洗瓶。为了防止空气中的潮气进入反应系统中，在空气的可能入口处需要装上填了干燥剂的干燥管。常用的干燥剂为无水氯化钙。它容易吸收水分，但吸水后会结成块状将干燥管堵塞。故每次用过后的干燥管应保存在干燥器中防止吸潮。如管中氯化钙已潮解，则需重新装管。

（2）液体的干燥　液体中存在的少量水分，可直接加入干燥剂除去，还可用分子筛或用分馏、共沸蒸馏等方法除去。

1）干燥剂去水　干燥剂去水的原理是和水形成水合物或者形成新的化合物。其中有两种。

①与水可逆地结合成水合物的干燥剂：无水硫酸钙与水形成半分子水的水合物$CaSO_4 \cdot \frac{1}{2}H_2O$，吸水量小，但作用快。含有蓝色指示剂的无水硫酸钙用于干燥管中，吸水后变为粉红色。

无水氯化钙与水形成六水化合物 $CaCl_2 \cdot 6H_2O$，作用快，效果好，为实验室常用的干燥剂。无水氯化钙能与羧酸、胺类、醇类等反应或形成复合物，因此这些化合物不能用无水氯化钙进行干燥。

无水硫酸钠属中性干燥剂，作用慢，它能与水形成 10 个结晶水的水合物 $Na_2SO_4 \cdot 10H_2O$。无水硫酸钠因性质稳定和吸水能力强，为实验室中常用的干燥剂。

无水硫酸镁属弱酸性干燥剂。它能与水形成 7 个结晶水的水合物 $MgSO_4 \cdot 7H_2O$。吸水速度和强度都比无水硫酸钙和无水氯化钙小。吸水能力也较无水硫酸钠差，它的优点是不与有机物起反应。有机化合物如酯、醛、腈和酰胺等均可用它进行干燥。

采用干燥剂不可能将气体或液体中的水分完全除去，因为水在干燥剂与被干燥液体之间存在着平衡。加热虽然可以加快干燥速度，但远不如水合物释放出水的速度快。因此干燥通常在室温下进行。蒸馏前应将干燥剂除去。

②与水作用生成新化合物的干燥剂：如五氧化二磷、氧化钙和金属钠等。五氧化二磷利用它与水生成磷酸而去水，作用快，干燥效力高，但价格较贵，常用于干燥烷烃、卤烃、溴液、芳香卤化物、醚和腈等，但不适用于醇、酮、有机酸和有机碱等物质的干燥。氧化钙为碱性干燥剂，与水作用生成水溶性的氢氧化钙，对热稳定，不挥发，价格低，常用于干燥低分子量的醇或吸湿性很强的有机碱。金属钠常用压钠机压成钠丝用于苯、乙醚、石油醚、四氢呋喃等溶剂作最后的干燥。各类有机物常用的干燥剂见表 1-2。

表 1-2　各类有机物常用的干燥剂

化合物	干燥剂
烃	$CaCl_2$、Na、P_2O_5
卤代烃	$CaCl_2$、$MgSO_4$、Na_2SO_4、P_2O_5
醇	K_2CO_3、$MgSO_4$、CaO、Na_2SO_4
醚	$CaCl_2$、Na、P_2O_5
醛	$MgSO_4$、Na_2SO_4
酮	K_2CO_3、$CaCl_2$、$MgSO_4$、Na_2SO_4
酸、酚	$MgSO_4$、Na_2SO_4
酯	$MgSO_4$、Na_2SO_4、K_2CO_3
胺	KOH、$NaOH$、K_2CO_3、CaO
硝基化合物	$CaCl_2$、$MgSO_4$、Na_2SO_4

2）分子筛去水　分子筛是一种含水硅铝酸盐的晶体，把它加热至一定的温度，水分子就可被脱去，而晶体内部就形成许多孔穴。在用分子筛干燥有机溶剂时，水分子就可进入这些孔穴而达到干燥的目的（水分子的直径为 3Å，分子直径最小的有机化合物甲烷的分子直径为 4.9Å）。吸附了水分子的分子筛可加热至 350℃ 以上使水分子解吸，然后重新使用。新的分子筛使用前必须先活化脱水（温度为 550±10℃，常压下加热 2 小时，待温度降至 200℃ 后立即取出存放入干燥器内备用）。如果有机溶剂含水较多，应先用其他干燥剂先脱水，剩下微量的水分再用分子筛脱水。

3）分馏及共沸去水　采用分馏和生成共沸混合物的方法可除去少量水分。分馏及共沸混合物去水的原理及装置见实验五及实验二十二。

（3）固体的干燥　精制后的固体化合物需要经过干燥才能进行产量计算、含量测定、元素分析以及各种波谱分析。少量固体可放在表面皿或蒸发皿中自然干燥，一些见光不易分解的固体可用红外灯烘干。实验室最常用的干燥固体的方法是用干燥器。将需干燥的固体放在开口的容器中，置于干燥器的多孔磁板上。干燥器底部可放入无水氯化钙、硅胶、五氧化二磷、浓硫酸或固体氢氧化钾等干燥剂，必要时抽真空以增加干燥的效果（质量不好的真空干燥器在抽真空时会破裂，所以新的真空干燥器需用铁丝网罩好，用真空泵抽气3小时，确保质量可靠后再使用）（图1-6）。

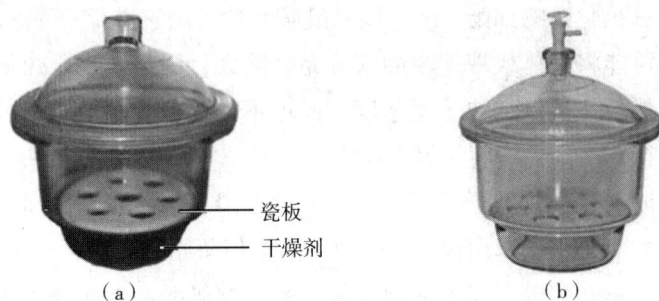

图1-6 干燥器

(a) 普通干燥器；(b) 真空干燥器

4. 搅拌 搅拌是有机制备实验常用的基本操作，其目的是为了使反应物均匀混合，反应体系的热量容易散发和传导，从而使反应体系的温度更加均匀，促进反应的进行。

搅拌的方法主要分为人工搅拌、磁力搅拌搅拌和电动（机械）搅拌三种。由于有机化学反应一般时间较长，因此制备实验一般采取后两种方法。

（1）磁力搅拌器 这种搅拌器通过搅拌器内磁场的不断旋转带动容器内软铁搅拌子随之旋转，从而达到搅拌的目的。在控制转速的同时进行加热（图1-7）。

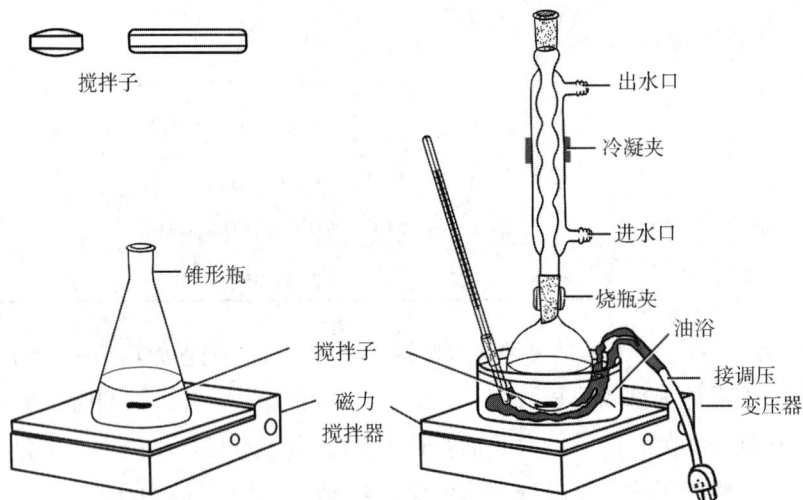

图1-7 磁力搅拌器及搅拌子

（2）电动搅拌器 电动搅拌器也称为机械搅拌器。当反应物较黏稠或进行大量反应时经常采用电动搅拌。使用此种搅拌器时应注意接上地线，不能超负荷。要经常保持电动搅拌器的清洁，防潮、防腐蚀，并要经常保持轴承转动润滑。在装配机械搅拌时，可采用简单的橡皮管密封或液封管（图1-8）。搅拌棒与玻璃管或液封管应配得合适，既不太松又不太紧，使搅拌棒能在中间自由地转动。

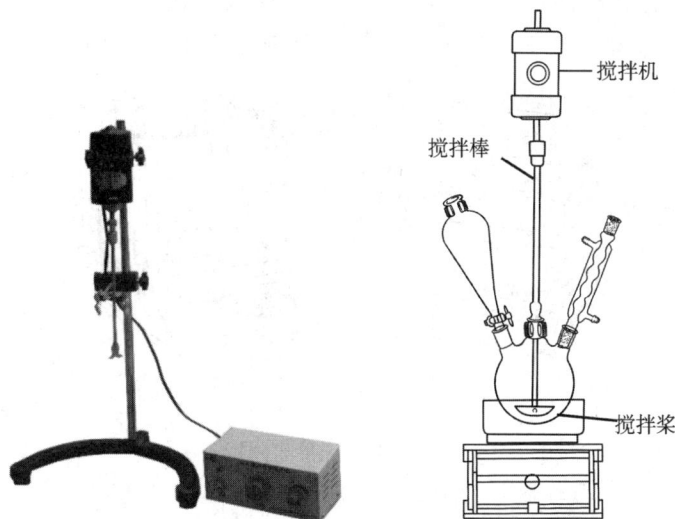

图 1 - 8　电动搅拌器和装有电动搅拌的反应装置

5. 有害气体的吸收　有些化学反应会产生一些挥发性的有毒或刺激性物质，这些反应必须在通风良好的通风橱内操作，此外，反应中产生的有毒或刺激性水溶性气体（如氯化氢、溴化氢、二氧化硫和氨等）可用图 1 - 9 所示的装置来吸收。图中倒置的漏斗和吸收液面应有一小段距离，避免气体被吸收后整个系统产生负压将吸收液倒吸入反应瓶中。

6. 溶剂脱除（旋转蒸发仪）　有机化学实验中常常需要除去溶剂（浓缩）。常压蒸馏可以除去溶剂，但只适用于沸点较低的一些溶剂，如乙醚、丙酮、三氯甲烷等。沸点较高的溶剂一般用减压浓缩除去。此法不但速度快，而且蒸馏时温度低可避免产物分解或颜色变深。减压浓缩常用的设备是旋转蒸发仪（图 1 - 10），这种仪器使用方便，效率高，可以连续进料，除去溶剂后的产物均匀地聚集在瓶的底部。旋转蒸发仪运转时蒸馏瓶应始终浸在热浴的浅表层内。这样在浓缩过程中溶液不会爆沸，同时可加快蒸发速度。

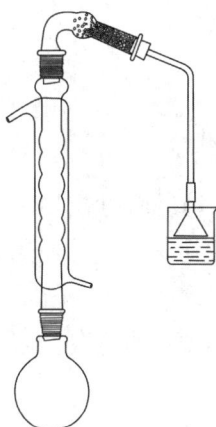

图 1 - 9　有害气体吸收装置　　　　图 1 - 10　旋转蒸发仪

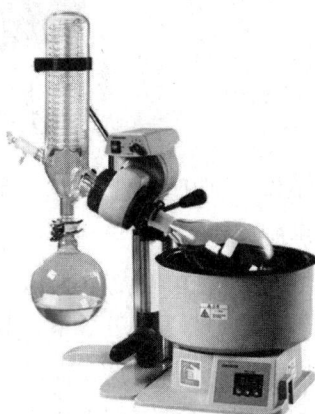

7. 称量方法　有机合成反应必须准确称量所用试剂和反应物的量。对于已知密度的液体，最方便的称量方法是用移液管、注射器或量筒量取并转移。而对于一些液体和所有固体，往往采用电子天平进行称量。对于质量大于 0.5 g（500mg）的样品，能够精确称量到

0.01g（10mg）的电子天平即可满足要求当反应规模很小时，有必要采用能精确到0.001g（1mg）的带防尘罩的电子天平（图1-11a）或分析天平（精确到0.0001g）（图1-11b）。

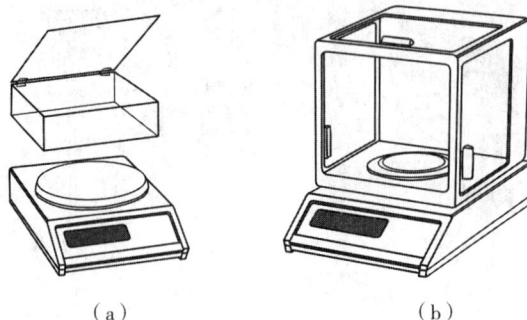

图1-11 电子天平和分析天平

（a）带防尘罩的电子天平；（b）带防尘罩的分析天平

目前使用的电子天平一般都设有皮重装置，在称量样品质量时可从将一张纸或者其他容器的重量去皮清零，然后加入样品即可称量其自身质量。注意，称量时不要超过天平的最大量程。

8. 循环水真空泵 循环水真空泵又叫水环式真空泵，是一种实验室常用的抽真空泵，具有体积小、耐腐蚀、污染小、移动方便等优点（图1-12）。使用循环水真空泵时应注意以下几点。

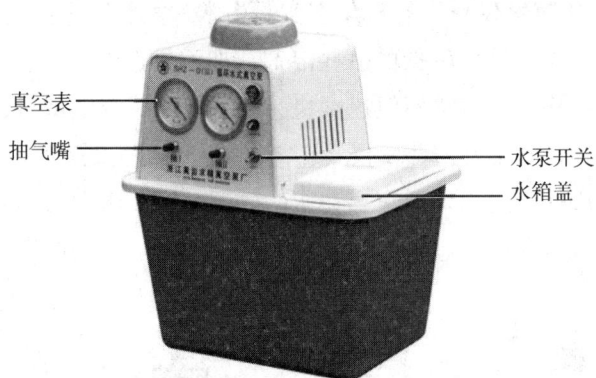

图1-12 循环水真空泵

（1）准备工作。打开水箱盖加水，水面即将升至水箱后面的溢水嘴下高度时停止加水。重复开机可不再加水。每星期至少更换一次水，如水质污染严重，使用频率高，则须缩短更换水的时间，保持水箱中的水质清洁。

（2）抽真空作业。接通电源，关闭循环开关，将需要抽真空的装置通过耐压管与本机抽气嘴相连，打开水泵电源开关，即可开始抽真空作业。

（3）当本机需要长时间连续作业时，水箱内的水温将会升高，影响真空度，此时，可将进水软管与水源（自来水）接通，溢水嘴作排水出口，适当控制自来水量，即可保持水箱内水温不升，使真空度稳定。

（4）当需要为反应装置提供冷却循环水时，在前面第三条操作的基础上，将需要冷却装置的进水、出水管分别接到本机后部的循环水出水嘴、进水嘴上，调节循环水开关至ON位置，即可实现循环冷却水供应。

9. 油泵 油泵的效能，通常决定于油泵的机械结构及泵油的好坏。一般使用精炼的高沸点矿物油作泵油。减压蒸馏的整个系统既要畅通又要密封，连接各种仪器应尽量靠近。所以在实验室内可用一个小推车装载包括油泵在内的减压蒸馏系统，这样既便于移动，又不占用实验台面。

10. 气体钢瓶 实验室中常用的气体钢瓶有氧、氢、乙炔、氯气、二氧化硫、氨气及光气等，这些气体有的易燃、易爆，有的有毒。不同气体钢瓶上涂着不同的颜色（表1-3）。钢瓶需存放在阴凉处，竖立并用框架或围栏固定，防止撞击或倾倒，最好不放在实验室内，不用时必须装上帽盖。

表1-3 气体钢瓶的颜色

气体类别	瓶身颜色
氮	黑
氯	草绿
氨	黄
氧	天蓝
氢	深绿
二氧化碳	黑

氧及乙炔瓶阀上必须保持没有油脂性物质。钢瓶上的氢气表及氧气表不得互换。开启瓶阀时必须先小渐大，调节好压力后再使用。气体钢瓶周围严禁烟火，如遇火情应立即关闭钢瓶阀门。如钢瓶发热，则可用冷水将瓶冷却。

五、常用有机溶剂及纯化

（一）乙醚（$C_2H_5OC_2H_5$）

MW 74.1，bp 34.5℃，d_4^{20} 0.71。乙醚沸点低，极易挥发，高度易燃，有爆炸性！使用乙醚时严禁明火。乙醚几乎能和所有的有机溶剂任意混合，在水中的溶解度约10%。乙醚久置易产生过氧化物，蒸馏久置的乙醚时切忌蒸干，以免因过氧化物引起爆炸。乙醚应贮存于密闭容器中并放阴凉处。

（1）过氧化物的检验 取少量乙醚，加等体积的2%碘化钾水溶液和几滴稀硫酸，振摇，再加1滴淀粉试液，呈紫蓝色即表示有过氧化物存在。

（2）过氧化物的除去 用酸性硫酸亚铁溶液（110ml 水，6ml 浓硫酸，60g 硫酸亚铁）洗涤乙醚可除去过氧化物。然后用水洗涤，用无水氯化钙干燥，蒸馏得纯乙醚。

（3）无水乙醚的制备 将100ml 乙醚放在干燥锥形瓶中，加入20~25g 无水氯化钙，加塞放置1天以上，并间断摇动，然后蒸馏收集33~37℃馏分。用压钠机将1g 金属钠直接压成钠丝放入盛乙醚的瓶中，用带有氯化钙干燥管的木塞塞住，或在木塞中插一末端拉成毛细管的玻璃管。这样既可防止潮气侵入，又可使产生的气体逸出。放置至无气泡发生即可使用。若钠丝表面已变黄变粗，须再蒸一次，然后再压入钠丝。

（二）乙醇（C_2H_5OH）

MW 46.1，bp 78.5℃，d_4^{15} 0.78。乙醇为具有酒味的无色透明液体，易燃，能与水任意混合，对人体的毒性较低，许多极性和极性较小的有机化合物能溶解在乙醇中，因此乙醇是重结晶有机化合物的良好溶剂。乙醇能与水形成共沸物（bp 78.2℃），用一般的分馏法不能完全除去其中的水。市售乙醇的含量为 95%。

1. 无水乙醇的制备（含量为 99.5%）　在 250ml 圆底烧瓶中，放入 45g 生石灰、100ml（95%）乙醇，装上回流冷凝器（上接一无水氯化钙干燥管），在水浴上回流 2~3 小时，然后改为蒸馏装置蒸馏，弃去少量前馏分后收集得无水乙醇。

2. 绝对乙醇的制备（含量为 99.95%）

（1）用金属钠制备　在 250ml 圆底烧瓶中，将 2g 金属钠加入 100ml 纯度至少是 99% 的乙醇中，加几粒沸石，装上球形冷凝器（上接一个无水氯化钙干燥管），回流 30 分钟。再改成蒸馏装置蒸馏，收集得绝对乙醇。若要制备纯度更高的绝对乙醇，则可在回流 30 分钟后，加入 4g 邻苯二甲酸二乙酯，再回流 10 分钟，然后改成蒸馏装置蒸馏，收集产品即得。

（2）用金属镁制备　装置同上，在 250ml 圆底烧瓶中加入 0.6g 干燥镁条（或镁屑）和 10ml 99.5% 乙醇。在水浴上微热后移去热源，立即投入几小粒碘粒加速反应进行（注意不要摇动）。不久碘粒周围即发生反应（如反应太慢可加热或补加碘粒），慢慢扩大，最后可达到相当激烈的程度。当全部镁条反应完毕后，加入 100ml 99.5% 乙醇和几粒沸石，回流 1 小时，以下操作同（1）。

（三）丙酮（CH_3COCH_3）

MW 58.1，bp 56.5℃，d_4^{20} 0.788。丙酮易燃，溶于水，与多种有机溶剂能任意混合。丙酮对有机化合物有较好的溶解度，是精制有机物质的良好溶剂。丙酮可用无水硫酸钙或无水碳酸钾干燥去水。

工业丙酮常含有醛或其他还原性杂质。加入少量高锰酸钾回流可将杂质除去。若高锰酸钾紫色很快褪去，再加入少量高锰酸钾继续回流，直至紫色不褪为止。然后将丙酮蒸出，用无水硫酸钙或无水碳酸钾干燥，过滤，蒸馏即得较纯的丙酮。

（四）甲苯（$CH_3C_6H_5$）

MW 92.1，bp 111℃，d_4^{20} 0.86。甲苯为易燃无色液体，它的毒性较苯小。甲苯几乎不溶于水，它也能与水形成共沸混合物（bp 85℃）。共沸混合物中约含 20% 的水，因此甲苯的去水量相当大，加上它本身又是一个较好的溶剂，因此在实验中经常用甲苯除去反应中生成的水。

普通甲苯中可能含有少量甲基噻吩。除去甲基噻吩是在 1000ml 甲苯中加入 100ml 浓硫酸、摇荡约 30 分钟（温度不要超过 30℃），除去酸层，甲苯层用水洗至中性。用无水氯化钙干燥，过滤，蒸馏，即可得纯品。

（五）苯（C_6H_6）

MW 78.1，bp 80℃，d_4^{20} 0.87。苯是无色透明的液体，易燃，与水不混溶。苯是非极性溶剂，常用来提取、重结晶和层析有机化合物。苯和水能形成共沸混合物（bp 69℃，含水量为 9%），故常利用苯的这种性质来除去反应中生成的水。苯蒸气有毒，长期接触会引起慢性中毒，主要表现为破坏人体造血功能。

工业苯常含有少量噻吩和水，不能用分馏方法除去。

（1）噻吩的检验　取 1ml 苯加入 2ml 溶有 2mg 吲哚醌的浓硫酸溶液，振荡片刻，若酸层呈墨绿色或蓝色，即表示有噻吩存在。

（2）噻吩和水的除去　将苯和 1/10 体积的浓硫酸振摇，使噻吩形成噻吩–2–磺酸，重复几次，直到检验无噻吩为止。然后分去酸层，苯层用水洗涤至中性，用无水氯化钙干燥后蒸馏，收集 80℃馏分。再压入金属钠丝即成无噻吩无水的苯。

（六）甲醇（CH₃OH）

MW 32.1，bp 64.6℃，d_4^{20} 0.79。甲醇为无色透明的易燃性液体，它与水及许多极性溶剂任意混合，是实验中常用的良好溶剂。甲醇剧毒，饮用后引起眼盲甚至死亡。甲醇与水不形成共沸物，可直接用高效分馏法制备无水甲醇，或用镁处理后制备无水甲醇（参考无水乙醇的制备）。

（七）乙酸乙酯（CH₃COOC₂H₅）

MW 88.1，bp 77.2℃，d_4^{20} 0.90。乙酸乙酯为无色易燃液体，能与多数有机溶剂混合，100ml 水中能溶解 8.6g 乙酸乙酯。乙酸乙酯与水的共沸物沸点为 70.38℃。乙酸乙酯是许多有机化合物的良好溶剂，它能与胺类起反应，精制这些胺类化合物时不能用乙酸乙酯作溶剂。

不纯的乙酸乙酯常含少量的乙酸和乙醇，可依次用 5％碳酸钠溶液洗、水洗。然后用无水硫酸钠或无水硫酸镁干燥，蒸馏即得较纯的乙酸乙酯。

（八）二甲亚砜（C₂H₆SO）

MW 78.1，bp 189℃，d_4^{20} 1.10。二甲亚砜是高极性的非质子溶剂，能与水互溶，广泛用于有机反应和光谱分析中的溶剂。二甲亚砜易吸潮，常压蒸馏时会分解。如要制备无水二甲亚砜，可以用活性氧化铝、氧化钡或硫酸钙干燥过夜，滤去干燥剂后减压蒸馏收集 75～76℃/12mmHg 或 85～87℃/20mmHg 馏分，放入分子筛储存待用。

（九）三氯甲烷（CHCl₃）

MW 119.4，bp 61.7℃，d_4^{20} 1.48。三氯甲烷为无色透明液体，微溶于水，蒸气不燃烧。三氯甲烷能溶解许多有机化合物，实验中可用它萃取和精制有机化合物。三氯甲烷能与水形成共沸物，沸点为 61℃。

三氯甲烷不能和碱性试剂或溶液接触，因碱能使三氯甲烷分解为二氯卡宾，有时这种分解反应很剧烈。一般不用三氯甲烷作胺类的溶剂，也不能用三氯甲烷来提取强碱性物质。三氯甲烷具有毒性，大量接触后会引起肝肾损伤和心律不齐。三氯甲烷暴露在日光和空气中会慢慢氧化为剧毒的光气。一般三氯甲烷中均加入 0.5～1％乙醇作为稳定剂。

除去三氯甲烷中的乙醇可用其体积一半的水洗涤 5～6 次，然后用无水氯化钙干燥，再蒸馏。三氯甲烷纯品要放置于暗处。三氯甲烷不能用金属钠干燥，因为会发生爆炸。

（十）二氯甲烷（CH₂Cl₂）

MW 84.9，bp 40℃，d_4^{20} 1.32。二氯甲烷不易燃，与水不溶。它是许多有机化合物的优良溶剂，因沸点低，可在低温下浓缩。二氯甲烷是氯代甲烷中毒性最低的一种溶剂，如有可能可用它来代替三氯甲烷。

用水、碳酸钠溶液洗涤不纯的二氯甲烷，然后用无水氯化钙干燥，分馏后可得较纯的二氯甲烷。

（十一）石油醚

石油醚是低分子量烷烃类的混合物。市售石油醚按其沸程可分为 30～60℃、60～90℃

和 90～120℃ 三种规格。石油醚中含有少量不饱和烃，因这些不饱和烃的沸点与烷烃相近，因此用蒸馏法不能将它们分离除去。

石油醚的精制通常是用其体积 1/10 的浓硫酸将石油醚洗涤二至三次，再用 10% 的硫酸加入高锰酸钾配成的饱和溶液洗涤，直至水层中的紫色不再消失为止。然后再用水洗，经无水氯化钙干燥后蒸馏。如要绝对干燥的石油醚则可压入钠丝（参考无水乙醚的制备）。

（十二）正己烷（C_6H_{14}）

MW 86.2，bp 69℃，d_4^{20} 0.66。正己烷为无色透明液体，易燃，不溶于水。常用正己烷来提取，精制和层析有机化合物。

正己烷中的主要杂质是烯烃和芳香族化合物，可按下述方法将这些杂质除去。即将正己烷与浓硫酸的混合液进行搅拌，分去浓硫酸后再用 0.1mol/L 高锰酸钾溶液和 10% 硫酸溶液进行搅拌，分出上层正己烷液层，用水洗涤至中性，用无水氯化钙干燥。干燥后的正己烷再经蒸馏，馏出液中压入金属钠丝除去微量的水分，即得到纯的无水正己烷。

（十三）环己烷（C_6H_{12}）

MW 84.2，bp 80.7℃，d_4^{20} 0.778。环己烷是无色透明液体，易燃，不溶于水，它能与多种有机溶剂混溶。环己烷中主要杂质是苯和一些不饱和烃，可用冷的浓硫酸和浓硝酸混合液洗涤数次除去。分去酸层后的环己烷用水洗涤至中性，无水氯化钙干燥后分馏，再压入金属钠丝除去微量水分成为无水环己烷。

（十四）四氢呋喃（THF，C_4H_8O）

MW 72.1，bp 66℃，n_D^{20} 0.89。四氢呋喃为可燃性无色液体，可与水或其他有机溶剂任意混合，是有机反应的良好溶剂。四氢呋喃含水，久贮后可能含有过氧化物，在加碱处理或蒸馏近干时会引起爆炸。

（1）过氧化物的检验　将四氢呋喃加入到等体积的 2% 碘化钾溶液和淀粉溶液中，再加入几滴酸摇匀，如呈蓝或紫色，表示有过氧化物存在。

（2）无水四氢呋喃的制备　用氢化铝锂在隔绝潮气下回流（通常 1000ml 约用 2～4g 氢化铝锂）除去其中的水和过氧化物。处理过的四氢呋喃中加入钠丝和二苯酮，应出现深蓝色的二苯酮钠，且加热回流蓝色不褪。在氮气保护下蒸馏，收集 66℃ 的馏分。

在处理四氢呋喃时，应先取少量进行试验，待确定其只含有少量水分和过氧化物后，才可进行大量的处理。如果四氢呋喃含水量较多，则可将固体氢氧化钾或其浓溶液与四氢呋喃回流加热，此时四氢呋喃溶液将出现红色难溶性树脂状物质，然后蒸出四氢呋喃再作处理。

（十五）吡啶（C_5H_5N）

MW 79.1，bp 115℃，d_4^{20} 0.98。吡啶吸水力强，能与水、醇和醚任意混合。吡啶与粒状氢氧化钾（钠）一起回流，然后隔绝潮气蒸出即得无水吡啶。

（十六）乙腈（CH_3CN）

MW 41.1，bp 82℃，d_4^{20} 0.787。乙腈为易燃性液体，能与水混合。乙腈是许多有机物的良好溶剂。乙腈可用 5% 五氧化二磷一起蒸馏而精制。

（十七）N,N-二甲基甲酰胺（DMF，C_3H_7NO）

MW 73.1，bp 153℃，d_4^{20} 0.95。N,N-二甲基甲酰胺是可燃性液体，能与水任意混合。

它对许多有机物的溶解度均较大，但很少用于有机物质的精制。吸入过多的 DMF 蒸气后会引起恶心呕吐。DMF 和其蒸气易通过皮肤被吸收。

N,N – 二甲基甲酰胺含有少量水分，在常压蒸馏时部分 DMF 会分解，若有酸或碱存在，分解加快。因此最好用硫酸钙、硫酸镁、氧化钡、硅胶或分子筛干燥后，减压蒸馏收集 76℃/36mmHg 馏分。如含水较多，可加入 1/10 体积的苯，在常压 80℃ 以下蒸去水和苯，然后用硫酸镁或氧化钡干燥，再进行减压蒸馏。

（十八）　二氧六环（$C_4H_8O_2$）

MW 88.1，bp 101℃/750mmHg，d_4^{20} 1.03。二氧六环中常含有少量乙醛，缩醛和水，通常用下面的方法精制。

在 500ml 二氧六环中加入 7ml 浓盐酸和 50ml 水，在通风橱中加热回流 12 小时，回流时缓慢地将氮气通入溶液以除去乙醛。待溶液冷却后加入粒状氢氧化钾直至不再溶解。分去水层，有机层再加入粒状氢氧化钾振摇除去痕量水。将有机层放入干燥的圆底烧瓶中，加入金属钠回流 10 ~ 12 小时，使金属钠最终保持光亮，假如不是这样，可以再加入金属钠以同样方式处理。最后蒸馏收集 101℃/750mmHg 馏分。

六、钠的使用及处理

钠的熔点 97.8℃，密度 0.97g/cm³。钠是比较软的金属，具有较低的熔融温度。金属钠非常活泼，在空气中极易氧化。能与水剧烈作用，放出大量热量，放出的热量能点燃释放出来的氢气发出爆鸣声。因此处理金属钠时必须非常仔细，必须绝对避免与水接触。

（一）　钠的储存

新鲜切割的金属钠易与空气的中的潮气和氧作用，在金属表面形成由氧化物和氢氧化物组成的氧化层，金属表面立即失去光泽呈暗灰色。为防止生成厚厚的氧化层，必须将钠储存于高沸点的惰性溶剂中。

（二）　钠的切割和称量

在 50ml 烧杯中加入 25ml 无水二甲苯，将盛有二甲苯的烧杯在台天平上称量。用镊子取出块状钠放于培养皿上，用手纸揩去溶剂油，用小刀切去表面的硬皮，得到表面具有银亮光泽的钠，迅速将其放入盛有二甲苯的烧杯中。待钠快要到达所需的重量时，可切小块钠加入，直至达到所需重量的钠。然后将多余的钠放回到储存瓶中。

（三）　钠的后处理

称好金属钠后，在切割钠的培养皿中放入乙醇分解残余的钠屑。将擦钠的纸和小刀放入烧杯中，倒入少量乙醇，待作用完后才能倒入废液缸中。切勿将钠皮等直接倒入废液缸中，以免引起燃烧爆炸事故。

七、实验前准备及实验记录和报告

（一）　实验前准备

为了保证实验顺利和安全地进行，每个学生在进入实验室之前需要做到如下几点。

（1）认真做好实验预习工作，包括检索试剂和产物的理化常数，了解这些物质的安全风险和操作时的注意事项；认真阅读实验目的、原理、仪器和实验操作等。

（2）在进行实验之前，指导教师会提供关于实验的具体细节和注意事项，因此，一定要认真听讲并做好记录。

（3）做实验时必须准备一本记录本，以便及时记录实验过程中的一些现象和结果等。

（二）实验记录和报告

1. 实验记录　一个完整的化学实验应该包括完整详细的实验记录。实验记录应注意如下几点。

（1）记录内容必须完整（包括实验的现象和时间等），保证任何人都可以按照你的记录重复实验。

（2）实验记录不得随意涂改。如果需要修改记录，可以划掉并写入正确内容，说明原因并签字。使用橡皮擦或者修正液进行修改是不被认可的。

（3）不得抄袭书本或者他人的实验记录。

2. 产率的计算　有机化学反应中，理论产量是指根据反应方程式，原料全部转化成产物的数量。实际产量是指实验中实际分离得到的纯净产物的数量。由于反应不完全、发生副反应及操作上的损失等原因，实际产量低于理论产量。产率是用实际产量和理论产量比值的百分数来表示的。

$$产率（\%）= \frac{实际产量}{理论产量} \times 100\%$$

为了提高产率，往往增加其中某一反应物的用量。究竟使哪种反应物过量，要根据这些反应物的价格、反应完成后是否容易除去或回收等情况来决定。计算理论产量时应以用量少的反应物为基准。例如：

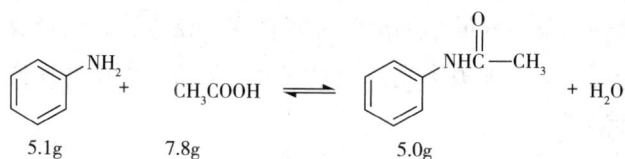

苯胺：5.1g ＝ 0.055mol

冰醋酸：7.8g ＝ 0.13mol（过量）

乙酰苯胺摩尔质量：135g/mol

理论产量：135×0.055 ＝ 7.43g

实际产量：5.0g

$$产率\% = \frac{5}{135 \times 0.055} \times 100\% = 67.3\%$$

3. 实验报告格式

实验名称＿＿＿＿＿＿

一、实验目的要求

二、实验原理

三、主要试剂及产物的物理常数

名称	分子量	性状	折光率	相对密度	熔点	沸点	溶解度

四、主要试剂用量及规格

五、仪器装置

六、操作步骤及现象

七、实验产品性状、外观及物理常数

八、产率计算

九、讨论

Part I General Knowledge of Organic Chemistry Experiments

Laboratory work is an integral and essential part of any chemistry course. Chemistry is an experimental science-the compounds and reactions that are met in a lecture or classroom work have been discovered by experimental observations. Organic compounds exist as gases, liquids, or solids with characteristic odors and other physical properties. They are synthesized, purified, and then transformed by reactions to other compounds. The purpose of experimental organic chemistry is to provide an occasion to observe the reality of organic compounds and reactions as well as techniques that are used in experimental organic chemistry and in other areas where organic compounds are treated with.

I. General Laboratory Rules

To ensure the laboratory experiments go smoothly, and cultivate the good experiment attitude, habit and work style for the students, they should abide by the following rules:

(1) Preview all the experiment content seriously and prepare the pre-lab reports before you are actually carrying out an experiment. Clarify the experiment purpose, principle, experimental procedures and related operation techniques through the preview. Find out the materials and reagents, apparatus and equipment needed in the experiment. Full consideration should be given to the precaution of accident and to the settlement of the accident happened in any case.

(2) After entering the laboratory, you should be familiar with the general situation of the laboratory and its surrounding environment, and understand the position of water, electricity and gas switches in the laboratory, as well as the location and use of fire extinguishing equipment. Wear lab clothes. Hair should be tied up if it is longer.

(3) Keep quiet, concentrate the mind, and perform the experiment attentively. Record all experimental observations and data in the notebook as they are obtained. The students are not allowed to leave the laboratory without permission.

(4) Follow the tutor's direction. Perform the experiment strictly according to the experimental

procedures. Any new opinion or suggestion, such as changing the procedure or reagent quantity, could be carried out after the tutor's approval. In case accident happened, report to the tutor at once for prompt settlement.

(5) Keep the laboratory and the benches clean and tide. The residue and recycle solvent should be put at the marked place without random disposing.

(6) The public instruments, materials and reagents and tools should be used at the appointed place, put it back after using. Strictly control the materials and reagents quantity. In case the instruments damaged, report for replacing and compensate according to the rules.

(7) Records (the product of a synthesis experiment should be submitted) must be submitted to the teacher for review after the experiment is completed. After the experiment, all the instruments used should be cleaned and put in order for safety check. With everything done and the tutor's permission, students can leave the laboratory.

(8) Students on duty are in charge of the cleaning of the windows, benches, floor and sink; the arranging of public materials, reagents and instruments; the cleaning the rubbish and the final checking of the water, electricity and gas.

II. Laboratory Safety

In any laboratory course, the most important thing is to have familiarity with the fundamentals of laboratory safety in detail. Any chemistry laboratory, particularly an organic chemistry laboratory, can be a dangerous workplace. It contains flammable liquids, fragile glassware, and corrosive or poisonous chemicals. Nevertheless, if proper precautions are taken and safe procedures are followed, it is no more dangerous. Understanding what to do and what not to do will serve well in minimizing that danger for you. Avoiding accidents is always a good practice. Remember that if you have a serious accident it will not be reversible. You won't get a second chance!

You should never undertake any unauthorized experiments. Again, the chances of an accident are high, particularly with an experiment, which has not been completely checked to reduce the hazard.

1. Fires

It is great importance to stress caution with the fire in laboratory. Because an organic chemistry laboratory course deals with flammable organic solvents at all times, the danger of fire is always present. Because of this danger, DO NOT SMOKE IN THE LABORATORY. Exercise a great deal of caution when you light matches or use any open flame. Always check to see if your neighbors on either side, across the bench and behind you are using flammable solvents. If so, either delay your use of a flame or move to a safe location. Many flammable organic substances (e. g. ether) have rather dense vapors that may travel for some distance down a bench. These vapors present a fire danger, and you should be careful, since the source of those vapors may be located at a great distance from you. Do not use the bench sinks to dispose of flammable solvents. If your bench has a trough running along it, only water should be poured into it. The trough is designed to carry the water from condenser hoses and aspirators, not to carry flammable materials.

For your own protection in case of a fire, you should find out immediately the location of the nearest fire extinguisher, the fire shower, and fire blanket. You should learn how to operate these safety devices, particularly the fire extinguisher. Your instructor can demonstrate the operation of the extinguisher.

If you have a fire, the best advice is to get away from it and let the instructor or laboratory assistant take care of it. Don't panic! Time spent in thought before action is never wasted. If it is a small fire, it usually can be extinguished quickly by placing an asbestos pad or a wet towel over the small fire. It is a good practice to have an asbestos pad or a wet towel handy whenever you are using a flame. If this method does not take care of the fire and if help from an experienced person is not readily available, then extinguish the fire yourself with a fire extinguisher.

Should your clothing catch on fire, so not run, but rather walk purposefully toward the nearest fire blanket or fire shower station. Running will fan the flames and intensify them. Wrapping yourself in the fire blanket will smother the flames quickly.

2. Eye safety

First and foremost, always wear approved safety glasses or goggles. This sort of eye protection must be worn whenever you are in the laboratory. Even if you are not actually carrying out an experiment, the person near you might have an accident, which could endanger your eyes, so eye protection is essential. Even dishwashing may be hazardous. Cases are known where a person had been cleaning glassware only to have an undetected piece of reactive material explodes, sending fragments into the person's eyes. To avoid this sort of accident it is wise to wear your safety glasses at all times.

If there are eyewash fountains in your laboratory, you should learn the location of the one nearest to you. In case any chemical enters your eyes, proceed immediately to the eyewash fountain and flush your eyes and face with large amounts of water. If an eyewash fountain is not available, the laboratory will usually have at least one sink fitted with a piece of flexible hose. When the water is turned on, this hose may be aimed upward and directly into the face, thus working much like an eyewash fountain.

3. Food in the laboratory

Because all chemicals are toxic to some extent, you should avoid accidental ingestion of toxic substances by never eating or drinking anything in the laboratory. There is always the possibility that whatever you are eating or drinking may become contaminated with a potentially hazardous material.

4. Shoes

You should always wear shoes in the laboratory. For that matter, even open-toed shoes or sandals offer inadequate protection against spilled chemicals or broken glass.

5. Organic solvents: their hazards

The first major thing to remember about organic solvents is that many are flammable and will burn if they are exposed to an open flame or a match. The second major thing to remember is that many are toxic. For example, many chlorocarbon solvents, when accumulated in the body, cause liver deterioration similar to the cirrhosis caused by the excessive use of ethanol. Constant and excessive exposure to benzene may cause a form of leukemia. Many other solvents, such as chloroform and ether, are good anesthetics and will put you to sleep if you breathe too much of them. Later they cause nausea. Pyridine causes temporary impotence. In other words, organic solvents are just as dangerous as corrosive chemicals, such as sulfuric acid, but manifest their hazardous nature in other, more subtle, ways. Minimize your direct exposure to solvents, and treat them with respect. The laboratory room should be well-ventilated, and normal cautious handling of solvents should not cause any health problem. However, if you are trying to evaporate a solution in an open flask you should perform the evaporation in the hood. Excess solvents should be discarded in a hood sink or in a container specifically intended for waste solvents, rather than down the drain at the laboratory bench.

If you should wish to check the odor of a substance, you should be careful not to inhale very much of the material. The technique for smelling flowers is not advisable here; you could inhale dangerous amounts of the compound. Rather, a technique for smelling minute amounts of a substance is used. You should pass a stopper moistened with the substance (if it is a liquid) under your nose. Alternatively, you may hold the substance away from you and waft the vapors toward you with your hand. But you should never hold your nose over the container and inhale deeply.

6. Use of flame

Even though organic solvents are frequently flammable (e. g. hexane, ether, dioxane, methanol, acetone, petroleum ether), there are certain laboratory procedures for which a flame may be used. Most often these procedures will involve dealing with an aqueous solution. In fact, as a general rule a flame should be used only to heat aqueous solutions. Most organic solvents boil well below the boiling point of water ($100\,^{\circ}\!C$), and a water bath may be used to heat these solvents. Most of commonly used organic solvents will burn. Ether, pentane, and hexane are especially dangerous since, in combination with the correct amount of air, they will explode.

Some common sense rules apply to the use of a flame in the presence of flammable solvents. Again, it should be stressed that you should check to see if anyone nearby is using flammable solvents before you light any open flame. If someone is using such a solvent, move to a safer location before you ignite your flame. Remember! if the solvent boils below $80 \sim 85\,^{\circ}\!C$, use a water bath for heating. The drainage troughs or sinks should never be used to dispose of flammable organic solvents. They will vaporize if they are low-boiling and may encounter a flame further down the bench on their way to the sink. If it is not prudent to use a flame at your bench, move to a safer location for your operations.

7. Use of glassware and explosion-proof

When you first receive laboratory equipment, examine the glassware closely for small cracks, chips, or other imperfections that might weaken it. It is particularly important to check round-bottomed flasks and condensers carefully. Cracks in a round-bottomed flask may cause it to break during use, spilling quantities of potentially dangerous and flammable chemicals. Cracks at the ring seals of condensers where the inner tube and the water jacket are joined may allow water to drain into a flask containing reagents, which may react violently with water. Replace any such imperfect glassware immediately. Take the time to properly store your equipment in your locker or drawer. Carelessly stored glassware may become cracked as a result of opening and closing drawers. Develop the habit of examining your glassware before each use.

The apparatus should be assembled correctly. The whole system should not be made tight in the process of normal distillation and reflux. Distillation to dryness is also dangerous because of the possible presence of peroxides or other explosive materials in the dry residue in the flask. A fierce explosion or combustion can be produced when some organic compounds come into contact with oxidizers.

8. First aid:cuts,minor burns,and acid/base burns

If any chemical enters your eyes, immediately irrigate the eyes with large amounts of water. Slightly warm water, if it is available, is preferable. Be sure that the eyelids are kept open. Continue flushing the eyes in this manner for 15 minutes.

In case of a cut,wash the wound well with water,unless you are especially instructed to do otherwise. If necessary,apply pressure to the wound to stop the flow of blood.

Minor burns caused by flames or contact with hot objects may be soothed by immediately immersing the burned area into cold water or ice for about five minutes. Severe burns must be examined and treated by a physician.

In the case of chemical burns,the chemical should be neutralized. For acid burns,the application of a dilute solution of sodium bicarbonate is recommended. For burns by alkali,the application of a dilute solution of a weak acid,such as a 2% acetic acid solution or a 1% boric acid solution, will neutralize the alkali. Most well-equipped laboratories will always have these safety solutions available in containers which are clearly marked FOR ACID BURNS and FOR BASE BURNS. You should learn the location of these safety solutions. After application of either sodium bicarbonate or dilute acid solution,flush the affected area with water for 10 to 15 minutes.

III. Disposal of Laboratory Waste

Experimental operations always generate different kinds of gas, liquid and solid waste. Waste disposal has been one of the major environmental issues of modern society. Special measures should be taken to observe national regulations and local organic lab regulations of waste disposal. The handling of such wastes in the lab can be done in the following ways:

(1)Laboratory exhaust gas mainly includes acid fog,formaldehyde,benzene series,various organic solvents,etc. ,so it is necessary to ensure good ventilation in the laboratory; for the direct production of toxic and harmful gases,experiments should be carried out in the fume hood,which is an effective way to ensure indoor air quality and protect the health and safety of laboratory personnel.

(2)All wastes generated in the lab can be classified into solid or liquid waste,and hazardous or nonhazardous waste. They should be disposed of properly. Some hard-to-handle hazardous waste should be delivered to the environmental department for special treatment.

(3)The waste liquid produced in the laboratory includes chemical experimental waste liquid and general waste water. Chemical experimental wastewater mainly includes superfluous samples,organic solvents,various acid and alkali wastewater,heavy metal wastewater and wastewater from experimental work-up,etc. It must be recovered by selecting appropriate containers according to their chemical characteristics and placed in ventilation places. The label of the container must indicate the type of wastes, storage time, regular treatment, and so on. Do a good job of registration. General wastewater such as water for instrument cleaning and sodium chloride aqueous solution can be discharged directly into the sewer. Small amounts of acids such as hydrochloric, sulfuric, and nitric, or bases such as sodium or potassium hydroxide, should be neutralized first and diluted with large amounts of water before flushing down the drain.

(4) The solid waste produced in laboratory includes superfluous samples, reaction products, consumed or damaged experimental materials (such as glassware, filter paper, etc.), residual or invalid chemicals, empty bottles of chemicals, etc. It must be recovered by selecting appropriate containers and methods according to solid properties. Chemical solid waste (such as chemical reagents, filter paper, silica gel, gloves, etc.) produced during the experiment should be collected and stored in specific chemical solid waste containers; waste chemical empty bottles should be recycled separately and registered; damaged glassware and used needles and other sharp materials should be collected in a special container. Harmless solid waste, such as paper, cork, rubber pipe, metal products, etc., which are not exposed to chemicals, can be poured into ordinary waste barrels.

(5) Chemicals such as sodium that can react violently with water should be decomposed in a suitable way in a hood before disposal.

(6) Some carcinogens and substances suspected of causing cancer must handed with great care, avoiding contact with your body.

(7) It is strictly forbidden to discharge harmful experimental wastes into sewers and any water source at will. It is forbidden to litter, pile up in corridors, corridors and other public areas. Domestic and experimental wastes should not be mixed up.

IV. Common Apparatus and Techniques

This section introduces the basic experimental techniques and associated glassware and apparatus that are commonly used in the organic chemistry laboratory. In some instances, only the practical aspects of a particular technique are discussed in this chapter, whereas the theoretical principles underlying it are presented in later chapters.

1. Glassware

(1) Common glassware

Common glassware in laboratories are shown in Figure 1 − 1.

(2) Standard-taper glassware

Your laboratory kit probably contains standard-taper glassware with ground-glass joints; this equipment is safe and convenient to use. Although standard-taper glassware has greatly simplified the task of assembling the apparatus required for numerous routine laboratory operations, it is expensive, so handle it carefully.

A pair of standard-taper joints is depicted above. Regardless of the manufacturer, a given size of a male standard-taper joint will fit a female joint of the same size. The joints are tapered to ensure a snug fit and a tight seal.

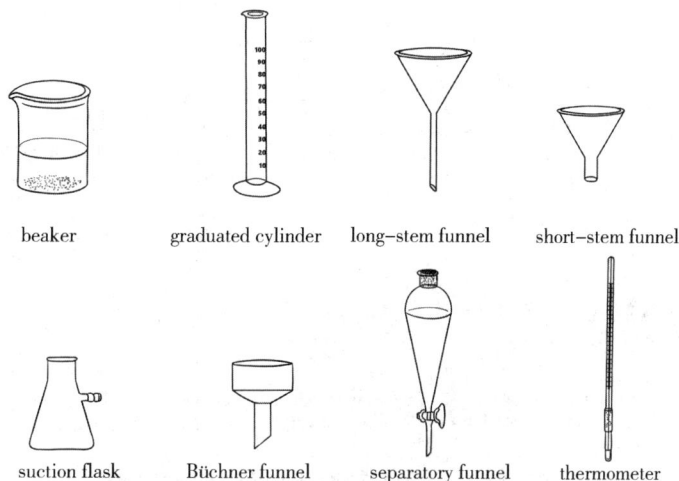

beaker　　　graduated cylinder　long-stem funnel　short-stem funnel

suction flask　　Büchner funnel　　separatory funnel　　thermometer

Figure 1 – 1　Some common glassware

When using glassware with standard-taper ground-glass joints, you must be sure that the joints are properly lubricated so that they do not freeze and become difficult, if not impossible, to separate. Lubrication is accomplished by spreading a thin layer of joint grease around the outside of the upper half of the male joint, mating the two joints, and then rotating them gently together to cover the surfaces of the joints with a thin coating of lubricant. Applying the correct amount of grease to the joints is important. If you use too much, the contents of the flask, including your product, may become contaminated; if too little lubricant is used, the joints may freeze. As soon as you have completed the experiment, disassemble the glassware to lessen the likelihood that the ground-glass joints will stick. If the pieces do not separate easily, the best way to pull them apart is to grasp the two pieces as close to the joint as possible and try to loosen the joint with a slight twisting motion.

Sometimes the pieces of glass will still not separate. In these cases there are a few other tricks that can be tried. These include the following options: ①Tap the joint gently with the wooden handle of a spatula, and then try pulling the joint apart as described earlier. ②Heat the joint in hot water or a steam bath before attempting to separate the pieces. ③As a last resort, heat the joint gently in the yellow portion of the flame of a Bunsen burner. Heat the joint slowly and carefully until the outer joint breaks away from the inner section. Wrap a cloth towel around the hot joint to avoid burning yourself, and pull the joint apart as described earlier.

The common pieces of standard-taper glassware with ground-glass miniscale procedures are shown in Figure 1 – 2.

（3）Precautions and cleaning glassware

The major rule in handling and using laboratory glassware is never applied undue pressure or strain to any piece of glassware. Strained glassware may break at the moment the strain is induced, when it is heated, or even upon standing for a period of time. When setting up a glassware apparatus for a particular experiment, be sure that the glassware is properly positioned and supported so that strain does not develop.

Sometimes it is necessary to insert thermometers or glass tubes into rubber or cork stoppers or rubber tubing. Either makes the hole slightly larger or use a smaller piece of glass. A useful aid for

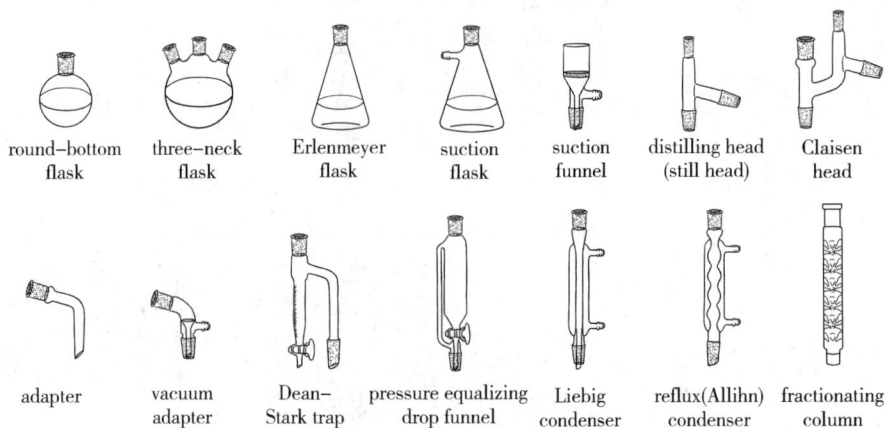

round-bottom flask   three-neck flask   Erlenmeyer flask   suction flask   suction funnel   distilling head (still head)   Claisen head

adapter   vacuum adapter   Dean-Stark trap   pressure equalizing drop funnel   Liebig condenser   reflux(Allihn) condenser   fractionating column

Figure 1 – 2　Selected standard-taper glassware

minimizing the hazard of this procedure is to lubricate the glass tube with a little water containing soap or glycerol prior to insertion into stoppers or tubing. Always grasp the glass piece as close as possible to the rubber or cork part when trying to insert it. It is also wise to wrap a towel around the glass tube and the rubber or cork stopper while inserting the tube. This usually prevents a serious cut in the event the glass happens to break.

Glassware should be thoroughly cleaned immediately after use. Residues from chemical reactions may attack the surface of the glass, and cleaning becomes more difficult the longer you wait. Before washing glassware, it is good practice to wipe off any lubricant or grease from standard-taper ground-glass joints with a towel or tissue moistened with a solvent such as hexane or dichloromethane. This prevents the grease from being transferred during washing to inner surfaces of the glassware, where it may be difficult to remove. Most chemical residues can be removed by washing the glassware using a brush, special laboratory soap, and water. Stubborn residues may sometimes remain in your glassware. Often these may be removed by carefully scraping the glassware with a bent spatula in the presence of soap and water or acetone. If this technique fails, more powerful cleaning solutions may be required, but these must be used with great care, as they are highly corrosive. Do not allow these solutions to come into contact with your skin or clothing; they will cause severe burns and produce holes in your clothing. Chromic acid, which is made from concentrated sulfuric acid and chromic anhydride or potassium dichromate, is sometimes an effective cleaning agent, but since it is a strong oxidizing acid, it must be used with great care. When handling chromic acid, *always wear latex gloves* and pour it carefully into the glassware to be cleaned. After the glassware is clean, pour the chromic acid solution into a specially designated bottle, not into the sink.

（4）Drying glassware

The common methods of drying glassware are as follows.

1）Air dry　In order to let water drops down, the glassware can be left upside down on a drying rack.

2）Oven dry　The glassware can be dried quickly by placing them in an oven. For complete drying, glass should be left in an oven at $110 \sim 120\ ℃$ for several hours. Besides, an air flow drier or hair drier also can be used.

3）Blow dry   If a small amount of drying equipment is urgently needed, it can be dried by air dryer or electric dryer.

4）Organic solvent dry   When wet glassware must be dried quickly for immediate use, it may be rinsed with small amounts of hydrophilic organic solvents such as 95% ethanol or acetone, which must be drained into an assigned bottle after use. Then, use a hair drier to evaporate the solvent afterwards.

（5）Maintenance of glassware

1）Thermometer   The glass in the mercury sphere of thermometer is very thin and easy to be damaged, so we should be careful when using it. We should not use thermometer as stirring rod or measure the temperature beyond the maximum scale of thermometer. The thermometer should be cooled slowly after use, especially after measuring high temperature. Do not rinse it with cold water immediately. The used thermometer is washed and wiped after cooling.

2）Condenser   The condenser is heavier after water is passed through. When installing the condenser, the clamp should be clamped at the center of gravity of the condenser. Use a long brush when washing condensers. After washing, it should be upright and inverted to facilitate drying.

3）Seperatory funnel and dripping funnel   The pistons and caps of the separatory funnel and the dripping funnel are all abrasive. If they are not original, they may not be tight and drip. Therefore, attention should be paid to protecting them when they are used. Do not exchange stoppers between funnels. Paper must be padded between the piston and the grinding orifice after use so as not to be difficult to open for a long time. After using the separatory funnel and dripping funnel, the stopper and piston must be pulled out, the lubricating oil on the top must be wiped off, and then washed and dried in the oven.

（6）Selection of appropriate apparatus and glassware

1）Plug selection   Rubber plug is tight, but can be dissolved by some organic solvents. At this time, grinding glass stopper can be used instead. It has advantages of stronger sealing, tighter combination, to prevent gas volatilization and external gas from entering pollution. However, grinding glass stopper cannot be used for the bottle containing alkali cannot use, instead, rubber stopper should be used.

2）The selection of glassware   It depends on the volume of reactants, reaction conditions and physicochemical properties of reactants（or products）.

A. The size of the reaction bottle should be so that the volume of the reactant does not exceed 2/3 of its volume, generally 1/2.

B. The reflux reaction usually uses round bottom flask and spherical condenser, while the reflux stirring and the reaction temperature need to be controlled by three-neck flask.

C. Distillation operations need distillation bottles; vacuum distillation uses vacuum distillation bottles（Claisen distillation head connected to round bottom flask）.

D. In atmospheric distillation, the volume of the distilled liquid does not exceed 2/3 of the volume of the distillation bottle; in vacuum distillation, the volume of the distilled liquid does not exceed 1/2 of the volume of the distillation bottle.

E. Straight condenser is used when the boiling point of the distillate is lower than 130℃, and air condenser is used when the boiling point of the distillate is higher than 130℃.

F. The selection of thermometer is generally based on the reaction temperature, which is higher than 10 ~ 20℃. Mercury thermometer is suitable for measuring substances at-30 ~ 300℃. Low temperature thermometers with organic liquids are commonly used when the temperature is below-38℃ (because mercury solidifies).

2. Apparatus and techniques

(1) Heating techniques

Heating is an important laboratory technique that serves a variety of purposes. For example, many chemical reactions require heating to proceed at a reasonable rate. Heating is also used to purify liquids by distillation, to remove volatile solvents during the work-up of a reaction and to dissolve solids when purifying solid products by recrystallization.

Two general rules regarding heating are noted here. ①Whatever device is being used to heat a liquid or solid, you must arrange the apparatus so that the heating source can be rapidly removed from the apparatus to prevent accidents. This normally means that the heating source is mounted on a ring clamp or a lab jack, either of which allows for quick removal of the device if necessary. ②As a rule, the safest way to heat organic solvents is with a flameless heat source and in a hood; this minimizes the chance of fire and avoids filling the room with solvent vapors.

Heating with electrical devices is generally the method of choice in the organic laboratory, since it is much safer than using open flames. These devices differ, however, in the medium used to transfer heat from the element to the experimental apparatus. For example, air and oil are the common used heat transfer agents respectively.

1) Water bath   The water bath is used when temperatures no higher than about 100℃ are desired (Figure 1 – 3). The water is contained in a wide-mouthed vessel such as a beaker or crystallizing dish, and preferably is heated with an electrical hot plate. Alternatively, a Bunsen burner can be used, in which case the bath is supported on a ring clamp bearing a wire mesh for diffusing the flame. You may find it helpful to cover the open portions of the bath with aluminum foil to minimize the loss of water through evaporation.

2) Oil bath   Electrically heated oil baths, which typically contain either mineral oil or silicone oil, are commonly employed in the laboratory (Figure 1 – 4). The usable range of an oil bath is 100 ~ 250℃. The temperature of the bath can easily be determined by inserting a thermometer in the liquid, and a given bath temperature may be obtained and accurately maintained by careful adjustment of the variable transformer. Although heat is transferred uniformly to the surface of the flask in the bath and there are no hot spots, there typically will be a temperature gradient of about 100℃ between the bath and the contents of the flask.

Some inconveniences are also encountered using oil baths. If the volume of heating liquid is fairly large, it may take a while to reach the desired bath temperature. The maximum temperature that may be safely attained in an oil bath is limited by the type of heating liquid being used. Silicone oils are more expensive but are generally preferable to mineral oils because they can be heated to 200 to 275℃ without reaching the flash point. Mineral oil should not be heated above about 200℃, because it will begin to smoke, and there is the potential danger of flash ignition of the vapors. Water must not be present in mineral and silicone oils, since at temperatures of about 100℃, the water will boil. If water drops are present in the oil, the heating fluid should be changed, and the container should be cleaned and dried before refilling.

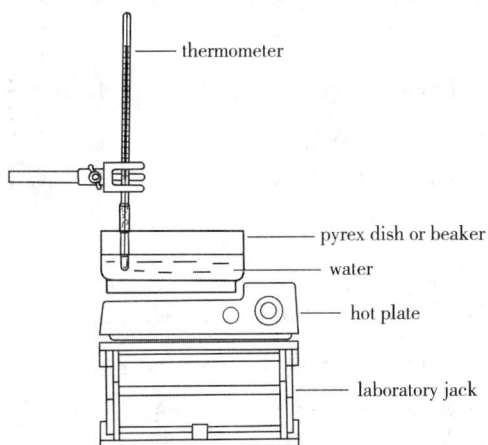

Figure 1-3 Water bath
(heated by hot plate)

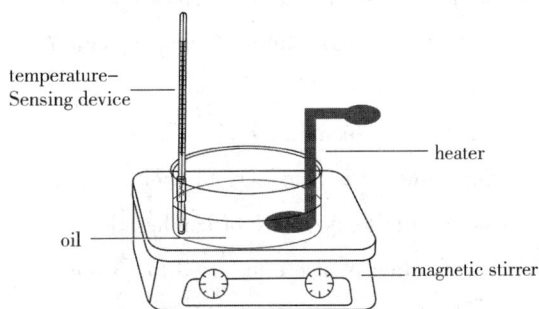

Figure 1-4 Electrically heated oil bath

3) Heat mantle A widely used device for heating round-bottom flasks is a heating mantle. The mantle is typically fashioned either from a blanket of spun fiberglass partially covered with a flexible or rigid cover or from a ceramic core contained in an aluminum housing. In either case, heat is provided by an electrical resistance coil embedded in the fiberglass or ceramic core, so when using these devices it is important not to spill liquid on them. The mantle may be equipped with a thermocouple so that its internal temperature can be monitored, but this is seldom done in undergraduate laboratories.

There are some drawbacks to using heating mantles. It is difficult to obtain a given temperature or maintain a constant temperature. Heating mantles have a high heat capacity, so if it becomes necessary to discontinue heating suddenly (for example, if a reaction begins to get out of control), the heating mantle must be removed immediately from below the flask to allow the flask to cool, either on its own or by means of a cooling bath; it is not sufficient simply to lower the voltage or turn off the electricity. After the mantle is removed, the electricity should be turned off at the transformer.

4) Hot plate When flat-bottom containers such as beakers or Erlenmeyer flasks must be heated, stirring hot plates (Figure 1-5), which are hot plates with built-in magnetic stirrers, are convenient heat sources; round-bottom flasks

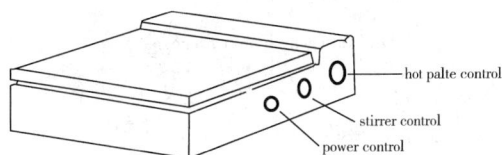

Figure 1-5 Stirring hot plate

cannot be heated effectively with hot plates. The flat upper surface of the hot plate is heated by electrical resistance coils to a temperature that is controlled by a built-in voltage regulator, which is varied by turning a knob on the front of the unit. A hot plate generally should be limited to heating liquids such as water, mineral or silicone oil, and nonflammable organic solvents such as chloroform and dichloromethane. Under no circumstances should a hot plate be used to boil highly flammable organic solvents, since the vapors may ignite as they billow onto the surface of the hot plate or the electrical resistance coils inside the hot plate. Furthermore, many hot plates use a relay that turns the electricity on and off to maintain the desired temperature, and these relays are often not explosion-proof and may produce sparks that can ignite fires.

5) Sand bath　When a heatingtemperature is required to get higher than those listed above, one can often use a sand bath. Its highest operating temperature is 350℃.

6) Infrared lamp　Infrared lamp is suitable for the lower heating temperature. It is a relatively safe heating method.

（2）Cooling techniques

Sometimes it is necessary to cool a reaction mixture either to avoid undesired side reactions or to moderate the temperature of exothermic reactions that could become dangerously hot and uncontrollable. Cooling is also often used to maximize the recovery of solid products during purification by recrystallization or to lower the temperature of hot reaction mixtures so that work-up procedures can be performed.

The most common cooling medium in the undergraduate laboratory is an ice-water bath. Liquid water is a more efficient heat transfer medium than ice, because it covers the entire surface area of the vessel with which it is in contact. Consequently, when preparing this type of bath, do not use ice alone. Finally, stirring an ice-water bath is useful for maintaining a constant temperature throughout the bath.

An ice-water bath has an equilibrium temperature of 0℃. For lower temperatures, an ice-salt bath can be prepared by mixing ice and sodium chloride in a proportion of about 3∶1 to generate a temperature of approximately-20℃. As the ice melts, more ice and salt must be added to maintain this temperature. Still lower temperatures are possible using combinations of organic liquids and either dry ice (solid carbon dioxide) or liquid nitrogen. Composition and cooling temperature of common coolants are listed in Table 1 − 1.

Table 1 − 1　Composition and Cooling Temperature of Common Coolants

Coolant	Temperature (℃)
Crushed ice (or ice-water)	0
Crushed ice-NaCl (3∶1)	− 20
Dry ice-CCl$_4$	− 32
Liquid nitrogen-chlorobenzene	− 45
Dry ice-ethanol	− 72
Dry ice-acetone	− 78
Liquid nitrogen-toluene	− 95
Dry ice-diethyl ether	− 100
Liquid nitrogen-diethyl ether	− 116
Liquid nitrogen-isopentane	− 160
Liquid nitrogen	− 196

（3）Drying techniques

1）Drying agents and desiccants　Drying a reagent, solvent, or product will be encountered at some stage of nearly every reaction performed in the organic chemistry laboratory. The techniques of drying solids and liquids are described in this and the following sections.

Most organic liquids are distilled at the end of the purification process, and any residual moisture that is present may react with the compound during the distillation; water may also cool or steam-distil with the liquid and contaminate the distillate. In order to remove these small traces of moisture before distillation, drying agents, sometimes called desiccants, are used. There are two general requirements for a drying agent: ①neither it nor its hydrolysis product may react chemically with the organic liquid being dried, and ②it must be completely and easily removed from the dry liquid. A drying agent should also be efficient so that the water is removed by the desiccant in a reasonably short period of time.

Some commonly used drying agents and their properties are listed in Table 1 – 2. These desiccants function in one of two ways: ①the drying agent interacts reversibly with water by the process of adsorption or absorption; or ②it reacts irreversibly with water by serving as an acid or a base.

With drying agents that function by reversible hydration, a certain amount of water will remain in the organic liquid in equilibrium with the hydrated drying agent. The lesser the amount of water left at equilibrium, the greater the efficiency of the desiccant. A drying agent that forms a hydrate must be completely removed by gravity filtration or by decantation before the dried liquid is distilled, since most hydrates decompose with loss of water at temperatures above $30 \sim 40℃$. Drying agents that remove water by an irreversible chemical reaction are very efficient, but they are generally more expensive than other types of drying agents. Such drying agents are sometimes more difficult to handle and are normally used to remove small quantities of water from reagents or solvents prior to a chemical reaction. For example, phosphorus pentoxide, P_2O_5, removes water by reacting vigorously with it to form phosphoric acid. Desiccants such as calcium hydride（CaH_2）and sodium（Na）metal also react vigorously with water. When CaH_2 or Na metal is used as a drying agent, hydrogen gas is evolved, and appropriate precautions must be taken to vent the hydrogen and prevent buildup of this highly flammable gas.

Of the drying agents listed in Table 1 – 2, anhydrous calcium chloride, sodium sulfate, and magnesium sulfate will generally suffice for the needs of this introductory laboratory course. Both sodium sulfate and magnesium sulfate have high capacities and absorb a large amount of water, but magnesium sulfate dries a solution more completely. Calcium chloride has a low capacity, but it is a more efficient drying agent than magnesium sulfate. Do not use an unnecessarily large quantity of drying agent when drying a liquid, since the desiccant may adsorb the desired organic product along with the water. Mechanical losses on filtration or decantation of the dried solution may also become significant. The amount of drying agent required depends upon the quantity of water present, the capacity of the drying agent, and the amount of liquid to be dried.

Table 1 – 2　Table of Common Drying Agents, Their Property and Uses

Drying Agent	Acid-Base Properties	Comments
$CaCl_2$	Weakly acidic	High capacity and fast action with reasonable efficiency; good preliminary drying agent; readily separated from dried solution because $CaCl_2$ is available as large granules; cannot be used to dry either alcohols and amines (because of compound formation) or phenols, esters, and acids (because drying agent contains some $Ca(OH)_2$)
Na_2SO_4	Neutral	Inexpensive, high capacity; relatively slow action and low efficiency; good general preliminary, drying agent; preferred physical form is that of small granules, which may be easily separated from the dry solution by decantation or filtration
$MgSO_4$	Weakly acidic	Inexpensive, high capacity, rapid drying agent with moderate efficiency; excellent preliminary drying agent; requires filtration to remove drying agent from solution
H_2SO_4	Acidic	Good for alkyl halides and aliphatic hydrocarbons; cannot be used with even such weak bases as alkenes and ethers; high efficiency
P_2O_5	Acidic	See comments under H_2SO_4; also good for ethers, aryl halides, and aromatic hydrocarbons; generally high efficiency; preliminary drying of solution recommended; dried solution can be distilled from drying agent
Na or K	Basic	Good efficiency but slow action; cannot be used on compounds sensitive to alkali metals or to base; care must be exercised in destroying excess drying agent; preliminary drying required; dried solution can be distilled from drying agent. Caution: Hydrogen gas is evolved with this drying agent
BaO or CaO	Basic	Slow action but high efficiency; good for alcohols and amines; cannot be used with compounds sensitive to base; dried solution can be distilled from drying agent
NaOH or KOH	Basic	High efficiency with solvents which have basic property cannot be used for base-sensitive substances; preliminary drying of solution is recommended; dried solution can be distilled from drying agent
Molecular Sieve 3 Å or 4 Å	Neutral	Rapid and highly efficient; preliminary drying recommended; dried solution can be distilled from drying agent if desired. Molecular sieves are aluminositicates, whose crystal structure contains a network of pores of uniform diameter; the pore sizes of sieves 3 Å and 4 Å are such that only water and other small molecules such as ammonia can pass into the sieve; water is strongly adsorbed as water of hydration; hydrated sieves can be reactivated by heating at 300 – 320 ℃ under vacuum or at atmospheric pressure

2) Drying organic solutions　When an organic solvent is shaken with water or an aqueous solution during an extraction procedure, it will contain some dissolved water. The amount of water varies with the organic solvent. Of the solvents commonly used for extraction, diethyl ether dissolves the most water. If this water is not removed prior to evaporation of the organic solvent, significant quantities of water will remain in the product and may complicate further purification. It is therefore necessary to dry the solution using a suitable drying agent, usually anhydrous sodium sulfate or magnesium sulfate.

Place the organic liquid to be dried in an Erlenmeyer flask of suitable size so that it will be no more than half-filled with liquid. Start by adding a small spatula-tip full of drying agent such as anhydrous sodium sulfate or magnesium sulfate and swirl the flask gently. Swirling increases the surface area for contact between the solid and liquid phases and generally facilitates drying. If the drying agent 'clumps' or if liquid still appears cloudy after the solid has settled to the bottom of the flask, add more drying agent and swirl again. Repeat this process until the liquid appears clear and some of the drying agent flows freely upon swirling the mixture. An amount of drying agent that covers the bottom of the flask should normally be sufficient. After drying is complete, remove the drying agent either by gravity filtration or by decantation. Rinse the drying agent once or twice with a small volume of the organic solvent and transfer the rinse solvent to the organic solution.

3) Drying solids   Solid organic compounds must be dried because the presence of water or organic solvents will affect their weight, melting point, quantitative elemental analysis, and spectra. Since proton sources must be excluded from some reactions, it is also necessary to remove all traces of moisture orprotic solvents from a solid prior to performing such a reaction.

A solid that has been recrystallized from a volatile organic solvent can usually be dried satisfactorily by allowing it to air-dry at room temperature, provided it is not hygroscopic and thus absorbs moisture from the air. After the solid is collected on a Büchner or Hirsch funnel fixed on a filter flask, it is first pressed as dry as possible with a clean spatula or cork while air continues to be pulled through the funnel and solid by use of a water aspirator or house vacuum. The solid is then spread on a piece of filter paper, which absorbs the excess solvent, or on a clean dish and allowed to stand overnight or longer.

Water is more commonly removed from organic solids using desiccators containing desiccants such as silica gel, phosphorus pentoxide, calcium chloride, or calcium sulfate (Figure 1 – 6). The desiccator may be used at atmospheric pressure or under a vacuum; however, if a vacuum is applied, the desiccator must be enclosed in a metal safety cage or wrapped with electrical or duct tape. Desiccators or tightly stoppered bottles containing one of these desiccants may also be used to store dry solids contained in small vials.

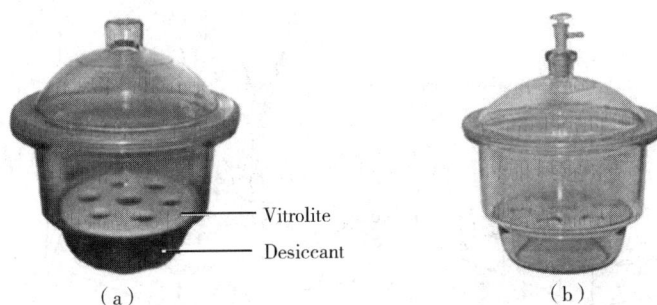

Figure 1 – 6   Ordinary desiccator and vacuum desiccator
(a) Ordinary desiccator; (b) Vacuum desiccalor

If the sample is hygroscopic or if it has been recrystallized from water or a high-boiling solvent, it must be dried in an oven operating at a temperature below the melting or decomposition point of the sample. The oven-drying process can be performed at atmospheric pressure or under vacuum. Air-sensitive solids must be dried either in an inert atmosphere, such as in nitrogen or helium, or under vacuum. Samples to be submitted for quantitative elemental analysis are normally dried to constant weight by heating them under vacuum.

(4) Swirling

Heterogeneous reaction mixtures must be stirred to distribute the reactants uniformly and facilitate the chemical reactions. Whenever the contents of a flask are being heated or cooled, stirring also ensures thermal equilibration. If a mixture is boiling, the associated turbulence is usually sufficient to provide reasonable mixing; however, stirring a boiling mixture is an alternative to using boiling stones to maintain smooth boiling action and avoid bumping, stirring is most effectively achieved using mechanical or magnetic stirring devices, but often swirling is sufficient.

The simplest means of mixing the contents of a flask is swirling, which is accomplished by manually rocking the flask with a circular motion. If a reaction mixture must be swirled, carefully loosen the clamp(s) that support the flask and attached apparatus, and swirl the contents periodically during the course of the reaction. If the entire apparatus is supported by clamps attached to a single ring stand, the clamp(s) attached to the flask do not have to be loosened. Make sure all the clamps are tight, pick up the ring stand, and gently move the entire assembly in a circular motion to swirl the contents of the flask.

1) Magnetic stirring　A very convenient mode for mixing contents of a flask is magnetic stirring. The equipment consists of a magnetic stirrer, which houses a large bar magnet that is spun by a variable-speed motor, and a stirbar (Figure 1 – 7) contained in a round-bottom flask. The metallic core of the stirbar is usually coated with a chemically inert substance such as Teflon, although glass is sometimes used for stirbars.

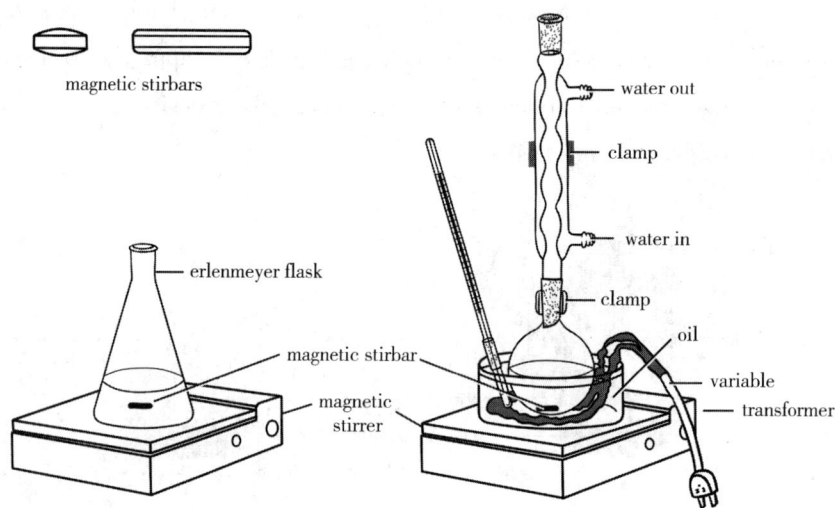

Figure 1 – 7　Magnetic stirrer and stirbars

The stirbar is normally placed in the flask before any other materials such as solvents or reagents. In the case of introducing stirbars into a flask you should not simply drop the stirbar in that may well crack or break the flask, instead, tilt the flask and let the stirbar gently slide down the side.

2) Mechanical stirring　Thick mixtures and large volumes of fluids are most efficiently mixed by using a mechanical stirrer; a typical set-up is depicted in Figure 1.8. A variable-speed, explosion-proof, electric motor drives a stirring shaft and paddle that extend into the flask containing the mixture to be stirred. The motor should have high torque, so that it has sufficient power to turn the shaft and stir highly viscous mixtures. The stirrer shaft is usually constructed of glass, and the paddle, which agitates the contents of the flask, is constructed of an inert material such as stainless steel,

Teflon or glass. A glass paddle must be used to stir reaction mixtures containing active metals such as sodium or potassium. The paddle is easily removed from the shaft to facilitate cleaning, and different-sized paddles can be used according to the size of the flask. The glass shaft and the inner bore of the standard-taper beating are ground to fit each other precisely. A cup at the top of the beating is used to hold a few drops of silicone or mineral oil, which lubricates the shaft and provides an effective seal.

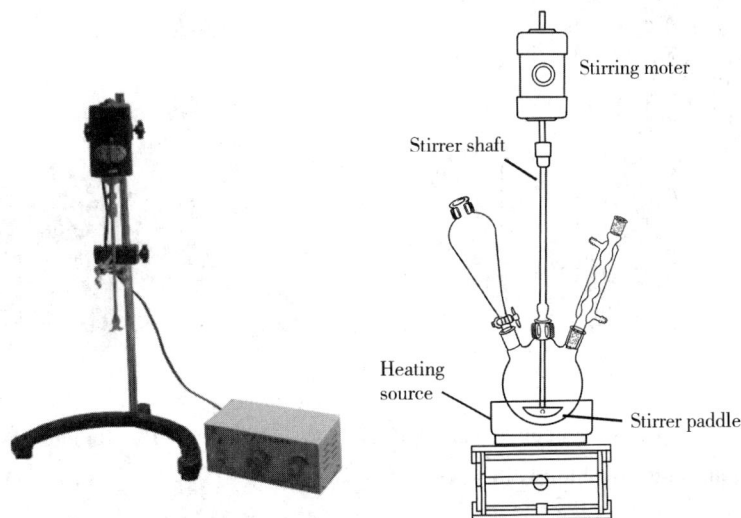

Figure 1 – 8　Mechanical stirrer and flask equipped with mechanical stirring

The stirrer shaft is connected to the motor with a short length of heavy-walled rubber tubing that is secured with twisted copper wire or a hose clamp. The motor and shaft must be carefully aligned to avoid wear on the glass surfaces of the shaft and beating and to minimize vibration of the apparatus that could result in breakage. The bearing is held in place in the flask with either a rubber band or a clamp so that it does not work loose while the motor is running. The rate of stirring is controlled by varying the speed of the motor with either a built-in or separate variable transformer.

Various operations can be performed while using mechanical stirring. For example, the flask in Figure 1 – 5 is a three-neck, standard-taper, round-bottom flask that is equipped with an addition funnel and a condenser. This apparatus could be used in cases where dropwise addition of a reagent to a stirred and heated reaction mixture is required.

(5) Gas traps

Some organic reactions release noxious gases that should not escape into the laboratory atmosphere. Such reactions should be performed in the hood, if space is available. Alternatively, a gas trap can be used.

If the gas being generated is water-soluble, the trap shown in Figure 1 – 9 may be suitable. In this example, the vapors are carried into a stemmed funnel whose rim is just above or resting on the surface of the water.

(6) Solvent removal (rotatory evaporator)

Organic chemistry experiments usually need to remove the solvents. Rotary evaporation is one of the most efficient and simplest methods of separating and removing organic solvents. Rotary evaporator operation is completed in the rotary evaporator which is shown in Figure 1 – 10. It consists of rotating evaporator driven by a motor, condenser and collector. It is usually used under decompression. Constantly rotating evaporator aims to avoid bumping. In the meanwhile, liquid is attached to the wall to form a layer of liquid film to increase the evaporation area, and thus, evaporating will be faster.

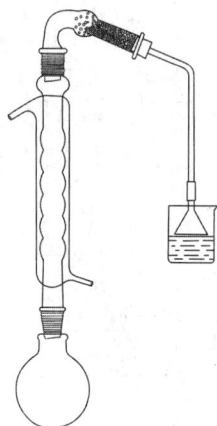

Figure 1 – 9 Gas traps for miniscale apparatus:
trapping water-soluble gas in water

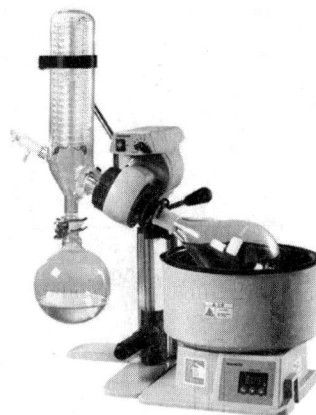

Figure 1 – 10   Rotatory evaporator

（7）Weighing methods

It will be necessary to measure quantities of reagents and reactants for the reactions you will perform. The weight of a liquid whose density is known is often most conveniently measured by transferring a known volume of the liquid to the reaction flask using a graduated pipet, a syringe or a measuring cylinder. However, for some liquids and all solids, weights are usually determined using a suitable balance. For quantities greater than 0.5g (500mg), a top-loading balance that reads accurately to the nearest 0.01g (10mg) is usually adequate. When performing reactions on the microscale, it is necessary to use a toploading balance that has a draft shield and reads to the nearest 0.001g (1mg) [Figure 1 – 11 (a)] or an analytical balance [Figure 1 – 11 (b)] that reads to the nearest 0.0001g.

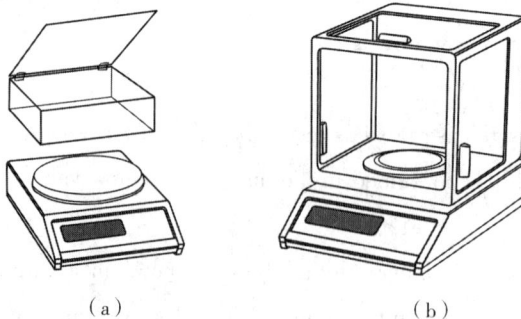

（a）   （b）

Figure 1 – 11

（a）A top-loading balance with draft shield；（b）An analytical balance with draft shield

With modern electronic balances equipped with a taring device, it is possible to subtract automatically the weight of a piece of paper or other container from the combined weight to give the weight of the sample itself directly. For example, to weigh a liquid, tare a vial and remove it from the balance. Transfer the liquid from the reagent bottle to the vial with a pipet or a graduated pipet or syringe, and reweigh the vial. Be careful to avoid getting liquid on the outside of the vial or the balance pan. Clean any spills promptly.

To weigh a solid, place a piece of glazed weighing paper on the balance pan and press the tare device: the digital readout on the balance will indicate that the paper has 'zero' weight. You should never weigh solids directly onto the balance pan. Using a microspatula, transfer the solid to be measured from its original container to the weighing paper until the reading on the balance indicates the desired weight. Do not pour the solid directly from the original bottle because spills are more likely. Carefully transfer the solid to your reaction flask or other container. You may also weigh the solid directly into the reaction vessel by first taring the flask or conical vial. Clean any spills promptly.

(8) Circulating water vacuum pump

Circulating water vacuum pump, is a commonly used vacuum pump in laboratory (Figure 1 – 12). It has the advantages of small size, corrosion resistance, small pollution and convenient movement. When using circulating water vacuum pump, we should pay attention to several points:

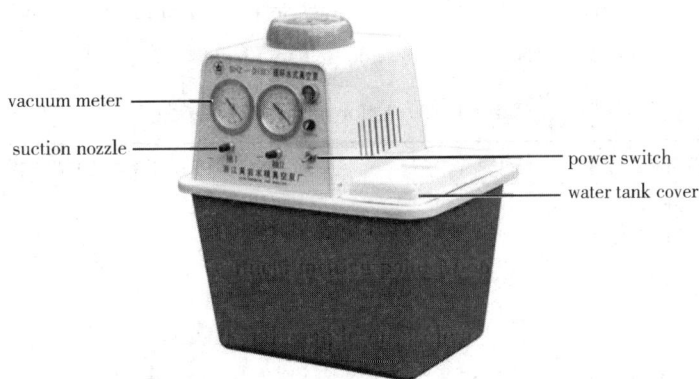

Figure 1 – 12 Circulating water vacuum pump

1) Preparation Open the water tank cover and add water. When the water level is about to rise to the height below the overflow nozzle behind the water tank, stop adding water. Repeated startup without additional water. Replacement of water at least once a week. If the water is seriously polluted and the frequency of use is high, the time for replacement of water should be shortened and the water in the water tank should be kept clean.

2) Vacuum extraction operation Turn on the power supply and turn off the circulating switch in the vacuum pumping operation. Then, connect the vacuum pumping device with the suction nozzle of the machine through the pressure tube, and turn on the power switch of the pump, so that the vacuum pumping operation can begin.

3) When the machine needs to work continuously for a long time, the water temperature in the water tank will rise, which will affect the vacuum. At this time, the drainage hose can be connected with the water source (tap water), the overflow nozzle can be used as the drainage outlet, and the tap water quantity can be properly controlled, so that the water temperature in the water tank will not rise and the vacuum degree will be stable.

4）When it is necessary to provide cooling circulating water for the reactor, on the basis of the first third operation, the inlet and outlet pipes of the cooling device are connected to the circulating water outlet and inlet nozzle of the rear part of the machine respectively, and the supply of circulating cooling water can be realized by adjusting the switch of circulating water to ON position.

（9）Vacuum oil pump

The efficiency of a vacuum oil pump usually depends on the mechanical structure of the pump and the quality of the pump oil. Refined high boiling point mineral oil is generally used as pump oil. The whole system of vacuum distillation should be unblocked and sealed, and all kinds of instruments should be connected as close as possible. So a small cart can be used to load the vacuum distillation system including the oil pump in the laboratory, which is convenient to move and does not occupy the experimental table.

（10）Gas cyclinder

Oxygen, hydrogen, acetylene, chlorine, sulfur dioxide, ammonia and phosgene are commonly used in laboratory gas cylinders. Some of these gases are flammable, explosive and some are toxic. Different colours are painted on different gas cylinders (Table 1 − 3). Cylinders should be stored in a cool place, erected and fixed with frames or fences to prevent impact or dumping, preferably not in the laboratory, caps must be installed when not in use.

Table 1 − 3　Color of gas cylinders

Gas catagory	Color of the cylinder body
nitrogen	black
chlorine	grassgreen
ammonia	yellow
oxygen	sky blue
hydrogen	dark green
carbon dioxide	black

Oxygen and acetylene bottle valves must be kept free of greasy substances. Hydrogen meters and oxygen meters used on cylinders shall not be interchangeable. When opening the bottle valve, it must be small and large first, and then use after adjusting the pressure. Fireworks are strictly prohibited around gas cylinders. In case of fire, cylinder valves should be closed immediately. If the cylinder gets hot, it can be cooled with cold water.

V. Common Organic Solvents

Ethyl Ether

Additional name(s): Ethoxyethane; ether; diethyl ether; ethyl oxide; diethyl oxide; sulfuric ether. *Molecular formula*: $C_4H_{10}O$. *Molecular weight*: 74. 12. *Elemental analysis*: C 64. 82%, H 13. 60%, O 21. 59%. *Line Formula*: $C_2H_5OC_2H_5$. *Properties*: Mobile, very volatile, highly flammable liq; Explosive! Characteristic, sweetish, pungent odor; Burning taste. Tends to form explosive peroxides under the influence of air and light, esp. when evaporation to dryness is attempted. Peroxides may be removed from ether by shaking with 5% aq ferrous sulfate soln. Addition of naphthols, polyphenols, aromatic amines, and aminophenols has been proposed for the stabilization of ethyl ether. d_4^{20} 0.7134; mp $-116.3℃$ (stable crystals); bp 34.6℃; Flash pt, closed cup: $-49℃$. Ether is slightly soluble in water and water is slightly soluble in ether. Miscible with lower aliphatic alcohols, benzene, chloroform, petr ether, other fat solvents, many oils. *Caution*: Keep away from fire; Potential symptoms of overexposure are dizziness; drowsiness; headache, excitedness and narcosis; nausea, vomiting; irritation of eyes, upper respiratory system and skin.

Ethyl Alcohol

Additional name(s): Ethanol; absolute alcohol; anhydrous alcohol; dehydrated alcohol; ethyl hydrate; ethyl 95% alcohol; alcohol. *Molecular formula*: C_2H_6O. *Molecular weight*: 46.07. *Elemental analysis*: C 52.14%, H 13.13%, O 34.73%. *Line Formula*: CH_3CH_2OH. *Properties*: Clear, colorless, very mobile, flammable liquid; pleasant odor; burning taste; absorbs water rapidly from air. d_4^{20} 0.789; bp 78.5℃; mp $-114.1℃$; Flash pt, closed cup: 13℃. Miscible with water and with many organic liquids. *Caution*: Keep tightly closed, cool, and away from flame!

Acetone

Additional name(s): 2-Propanone; dimethylformaldehyde; dimethyl ketone; beta-keto propane; pyroacetic. *Molecular formula*: C_3H_6O. *Molecular weight*: 58.08. *Elemental analysis*: C 62.04%, H 10.41%, O 27.55%. *Line Formula*: CH_3COCH_3. *Properties*: Volatile, highly flammable liquid; characteristic odor; pungent, sweetish taste. d_{25}^{25} 0.788; bp 56.5℃; mp $-94℃$. Flash pt, closed cup: $-18℃$. Miscible with water, alcohol, dimethylformamide, chloroform, ether, most oils. *Caution*: Keep away from fire! Keep away from plastic eyeglass frames, jewelry, pens and pencils, rayon stockings and other rayon garments.

Toluene

Additional name(s): Methylbenzene; phenylmethane. *Molecular formula*: C_7H_8. *Molecular weight*: 92.14. *Elemental analysis*: C 91.25%, H 8.75%. *Properties*: Flammable, refractive liq; benzene-like odor. d_4^{20} 0.866; mp $-95℃$; bp 110.6℃; Flash pt, closed cup: 4.4℃. Very slightly sol in water; miscible with alc, chloroform, ether, acetone, glacial acetic acid, carbon disulfide. *Caution*: Readily absorbed by inhalation, ingestion and somewhat by skin contact. Direct contact may cause severe dermatitis due to drying and defatting action. May present lung aspiration hazard if ingested. Potential symptoms of acute overexposure by inhalation may include local irritation; CNS excitation and depression. Low concentrations may result in transitory mild upper respiratory tract irritation, mild eye irritation, lacrimation, metallic taste, slight nausea, hilarity, lassitude, drowsiness and impaired balance. High concentrations may cause paresthesia, vision disturbances, dizziness, nausea, headache, narcosis and collapse; death from respiratory failure or sudden ventricular fibrillation. Chronic overexposure by inhalation has been associa ted with hepatotoxicity and nephrotoxicity. Syndromes following chronic inhalation involve severe muscle weakness, cardiac arrhythmias, gastrointestinal and neuropsychi atric complaints.

Benzene

Additional name(s): Benzol. *Molecular formula*: C_6H_6. *Molecular weight*: 78.11. *Elemental a-*

nalysis: C 92. 26% , H 7. 74% . *Properties*: Clear, colorless, volatile, highly flammable liquid; characteristic odor. d_4^{15} 0. 8787; bp 80. 1℃; mp 5. 5℃; Flash pt, closed cup: −11℃. Sightly sol in water. Miscible with alcohol, chloroform, ether, carbon disulfide, carbon tetrachloride, glacial acetic acid, acetone, oils. *Caution*: Keep in well-closed containers in a cool place and away from fire. Potential symptoms of overexposure by inhalation or ingestion are dizziness, headache, vomiting, visual disturbances, staggering gait, hilarity, fatigue, CNS depression, and loss of consciousness, respiratory arrest. Chronic exposure has been associated with bone marrow depression and leukemia. Direct contact may cause irritation of eyes, nose, respiratory system and skin; dermititis may develop due to defat ting action. Aspiration into the lung may lead to chemical pneumonitis.

Methanol

Additional name(s): Methyl alcohol; carbinol. *Molecular formula*: CH_4O. *Molecular weight*: 32. 04. *Elemental analysis*: C 37. 48% , H 12. 58% , O 49. 93% . *Line Formula*: CH_3OH. *Properties*: Flammable, poisonous, mobile liq. Slight alcoholic odor when pure; crude material may have a repulsive, pungent odor. Burns with a non-luminous, bluish flame. d_4^{20} 0. 7915; mp − 97. 8℃. bp 64. 7℃; Flash pt, closed cup: 12℃. Miscible with water, ethanol, ether, benzene, ketones and most other organic solvents. *Caution*: Poisoning may occur from ingestion, inhalation or percutaneous absorption. Acute Effects: Headache, fatigue, nausea, visual impairment or complete blindness (may be permanent), acidosis, convulsions, mydriasis, circulatory collapse, respiratory failure, death.

Ethyl Acetate

Additional name(s): Acetic acid ethyl ester; acetic ether. *Molecular formula*: $C_4H_8O_2$. *Molecular weight*: 88. 11. *Elemental analysis*: C 54. 53% , H 9. 15% , O 36. 32% . *Line Formula*: $CH_3COOC_2H_5$. *Properties*: Clear, volatile, flammable liq; characteristic fruity odor; pleasant taste when diluted. Slowly dec by moisture, then acquires an acid reaction. Absorbs water (up to 3. 3% w/w). d_4^{20} 0. 902; bp 77℃; mp −83℃; Flash pt 7. 2℃ (open cup). Explosive limits (% vol in air): 2. 2 to 11. 5. n_D^{20} 1. 3719. One ml dissolves in 10 ml water at 25℃; Miscible with alc, acetone, chloroform, ether. *Caution*: Keep tightly closed in a cool place and away from fire. Potential symptoms of overexposure are irritation of eyes, nose and throat, narcosis, dermatitis.

Chloroform

Additional name(s): *Molecular formula*: $CHCl_3$. *Molecular weight*: 119. 38. *Elemental analysis*: C 10. 06% , H 0. 84% , O 89. 09% . *Properties*: Highly refractive, nonflammable, heavy, very volatile, sweet-tasting liquid; characteristic odor. d_4^{20} 1. 484; bp 61 − 62℃; mp −63. 5℃. Slightly sol in water; Miscible with alcohol, benzene, ether, petr ether, carbon tetrachloride, carbon di sulfide, oils. *Caution*: Potential symptoms of overexposure are dizziness, mental dullness, nausea and disorientation; headache, fatigue; anesthesia; hepatomegaly; direct contact may cause irritation to eyes and skin.

Methylene Chloride

Additional name(s): Dichloromethane; methylene dichloride. *Molecular formula*: CH_2Cl_2. *Molecular weight*: 84. 93. *Elemental analysis*: C 14. 14% , H 2. 37% , O 83. 48% . *Properties*: Colorless liquid; vapor is not flammable and when mixed with air is not explosive. Soluble in approximately 50 parts water; miscible with alc, ether, DMF; bp 39. 8℃; mp −95℃; d_4^{20} 1. 3255. *Caution*: Potential symptoms of overexposure are fatigue, weakness, sleepiness, lightheadedness; numbness or tingle of limbs; nausea; irritation of eyes and skin.

n-Hexane

Molecular formula: C_6H_{14}. *Molecular weight*: 86. 18. *Elemental analysis*: C 83. 63%, H 16. 37%. *Line Formula*: $CH_3(CH_2)_4CH_3$. *Properties*: Colorless, very volatile liquid; faint, peculiar odor. d_4^{20} 0. 660; bp 69℃; mp − 100 to − 95℃. Insol in water; miscible with alcohol, chloroform, ether. *Caution*: Potential symptoms of overexposure are light-headedness; nausea, headache; numbness of extremities, muscle weakness; irritation of eyes and nose; dermatitis; chemical pneumonia; giddiness.

Cyclohexane

Additional name(s): Hexahydrobenzene; hexamethylene. *Molecular formula*: C_6H_{12}. *Molecular weight*: 84. 16. *Elemental analysis*: C 85. 63%, H 14. 37%. *Properties*: Flammable liq. Solvent odor. Pungent when impure. d_4^{20} 0. 7781; mp 6. 47℃; bp 80. 7℃; Flash pt, closed cup: − 18℃. Flammability limits in air 1. 3 − 8. 4% v/v. Insol in water; miscible with ethanol, ethyl ether, acetone, benzene, carbon tetrachloride. *Caution*: Potential symptoms of overexposure are irritation of eyes and respiratory system; drowsiness; dermatitis; narcosis; coma.

Tetrahydrofuran

Additional name(s): Diethylene oxide; tetramethylene. *Molecular formula*: C_4H_8O. *Molecular weight*: 72. 11. *Elemental analysis*: C 66. 63%, H 11. 18%, O 22. 19%. *Properties*: Liquid; Ether-like odor. d_4^{20} 0. 8892; mp − 108. 5℃; bp 66℃; n_D^{20} 1. 4070. Miscible with water, alcohols, ketones, esters, ethers, and hydrocarbons. *Caution*: Distil only in presence of a reducing agent, such as ferrous sulfate; peroxide explosions have occurred. Potential symptoms of overexposure are irritation of eyes and upper respiratory system; nausea, dizziness and headache; may cause skin irritation.

Pyridine

Molecular formula: C_5H_5N. *Molecular weight*: 79. 10. *Elemental analysis*: C 75. 92%, H 6. 37%, N 17. 71%. *Properties*: Flammable, colorless liq; characteristic disagreeable odor; sharp taste. d_4^{20} 0. 98272; mp − 41. 6℃; bp 115. 2℃; Flash pt, closed cup: 20℃. Miscible with water, alcohol, ether, petr ether, oils and many other organic liquids. Good solvent for many organic and inorganic compds. Weak base; forms salts with strong acids. *Caution*: Potential symptoms of overexposure are headache, nervousness, dizziness and insomnia; nausea, anorexia; frequent urination; eye irritation; dermatitis; liver and kidney damage.

Acetonitrile

Additional name(s): Methyl cyanide; cyanomethane. *Molecular formula*: C_2H_3N. *Molecular weight*: 41. 05. *Elemental analysis*: C 58. 52%, H 7. 37%, N 34. 12%. *Line Formula*: CH_3CN. *Properties*: Liquid; Ether-like odor. Poisonous! mp − 45℃; bp 81. 6℃; Flash pt 12. 8℃; d_4^{20} 0. 78745. Slightly sol in water; miscible in methanol, methyl acetate, ethyl acetate, acetone, ether, acetamide solutions, chloroform, carbon tetrachloride, ethylene chloride and many un saturated hydrocarbons. *Caution*: Potential symptoms of overexposure are asphyxia; nausea, vomiting; chest pain; weakness; stupor, convul sions. Direct contact may cause skin and eye irritation.

N, *N*-Dimethylformamide

Additional name(s): DMF; *Molecular formula*: C_3H_7NO. *Molecular weight*: 73.09. *Elemental analysis*: C 49.30%, H 9.65%, N 19.16%, O 21.89%. *Line Formula*: $HCON(CH_3)_2$. *Properties*: Colorless to very slightly yellow liquid; Faint amine odor; mp $-61℃$; bp $153℃$; d_4^{20} 0.9445; Flash pt, open cup: 67℃. Miscible with water and most common organic solvents. *Caution*: Potential symptoms of overexposu

VI. Use and Disposal of Sodium

The melting point of sodium is $97.8℃$ and the density is $0.97/cm^3$. Sodium is a soft metal with lower melting temperature. Sodium metal is very active and easy to be oxidized in air. It acts violently with water, releasing a lot of heat, which can ignite the released hydrogen and make a detonation sound. Therefore, when dealing with sodium metal, we must be very careful and absolutely avoid contact with water.

1. Storage of Sodium

Freshly cut sodium metal reacts easily with moisture and oxygen in the air, forming a group of oxides and hydroxides on the metal surface. When the oxide layer is formed, the metal surface immediately loses luster and becomes dark gray. In order to prevent the formation of thick oxide layer, sodium must be stored in inert solvents with high boiling point.

2. Cutting and Weighing of sodium

Add 25ml anhydrous xylene to 50ml beaker and weigh the beaker with xylene on the balance. Use tweezers to take out sodium blocks and place it on a culture dish. Solvent oil is wiped off with tissue. Hard skin on the surface is cut off with a knife. Sodium with silver luster is obtained. Sodium blocks are quickly put into a beaker filled with xylene. When sodium is about to reach the required weight, small pieces of sodium can be cut and added until the required weight of sodium is reached. Then put the excess sodium back into the storage bottle.

3. Disposal of Sodium

After the sodium metal is weighed, the remaining sodium chips are decomposed by ethanol in a culture dish cut with sodium. Sodium wiped paper andthe knife are put into the beaker and a small amount of ethanol is poured into the waste liquid cylinder after the action is finished. Do not directly pour the sodium into the waste liquid cylinder, in order to avoid the accident of combustion and explosion.

VII. Advance Preparation and Lab Record and Report

1. Advance preparation

In the foreword to the student, some mention was made of the importance of advance preparation in performing laboratory experiments. In this section you will find some suggestions about what specific information you should try to obtain in the course of your advance studying. Much of this information must be obtained while preparing your notebook, and so the two subjects, advance study and notebook preparation, will be developed simultaneously here.

(1) The correct approach to being successful in the laboratory is never to begin any experiment until you understand its overall purpose and the reasons for each operation that you are to do.

(2) The specific details of what you should do ahead of coming to the laboratory will be provided by your instructor.

(3) You will undoubtedly be required to maintain a laboratory notebook, which will serve as a complete, accurate, and neat record of the experimental work to be done.

(4) If there are items or techniques you don't understand, you should not be hesitant to ask questions.

(5) You should read the section entitled "Advance Preparation and Laboratory Records" right away. Although your instructor will undoubtedly have his own preferred format, much of the material here will be of help to you in learning to think constructively about laboratory experiments in advance.

2. Laboratory record and report

An important part of any laboratory experience is learning to maintain very complete records of every experiment undertaken and every datum obtained. Far too often, careless recording of data has resulted in mistakes, frustration, and lost time due to needless repetition of experiments. In cases where reports are required, proper collection and recording of data can facilitate report-writing greatly. In addition to learning good laboratory technique and the methods of carrying out basic laboratory procedures, among the many things you should learn from this laboratory course are:

(1) How to take data carefully.

(2) How to record relevant observations.

(3) How to use your time effectively.

(4) How to assess the efficiency of your experimental method.

(5) How to plan for the isolation and purification of the substance you prepare.

Because organic reactions are seldom quantitative in nature, special problems result. Frequently reagents have to be used in large excess in order to increase the amount of product obtained. In addition some of the reagents are rather expensive, which necessitates care in the amounts of these substances used. Very often many more reactions may take place than you may desire. These extra reactions, or side reactions, may form products in addition to the desired product. These are called side products. For these reasons it will be necessary to plan your experimental procedure carefully before undertaking the actual experiment.

(1) The laboratory notebook

One of the most important characteristics of successful scientists is the habit of keeping a complete and understandable record of the experimental work that has been done. Did a precipitate form? Was there a color change during the course of the reaction? At what temperature was the reaction performed and for how long did the reaction proceed? Was the reaction mixture homogeneous or heterogeneous? On what date(s) was the work performed? These are observations and data that may seem insignificant at the time but may later prove critical to the interpretation of an experimental result or to the ability of another person to reproduce your work. All of them belong in a properly kept laboratory notebook. Suggestions for such a document follow. Your instructor may specify other items to be included, but the list we give is representative of a good notebook.

When you begin the actual experiment, your notebook should always be kept nearby in order that you will be able to record in it those operations, which you perform. When working in the laboratory, the notebook serves as a place where a rough transcript of your experimental method is recorded. In it data from actual weightings, volume measurements, and determinations of physical constants, etc. , are noted. This section of your notebook should not be prepared in advance. The purpose here is not to write a recipe; rather it is to provide a record of what you did and what you observed. These observations will help you to write reports without having to resort to memory. They will also help you or other workers to repeat the experiment exactly.

When your product has been prepared and purified or, as in the case of isolation experiments, has been isolated, you should record such pertinent data as the melting point or boiling point of the substance, its density, its index of refraction, the conditions under which spectra were determined, etc.

(2)General protocol for the laboratory notebook

1)As the main criterion for what should be entered in the notebook, adopt the rule that the record should be sufficiently complete so that anyone who reads it will know exactly what you did and will be able to repeat the work in precisely the same way as it was done originally.

2)Record all experimental observations and data in the notebook as they are obtained. Include the date and, if appropriate, the time when you did the work. In a legal sense, the information entered into the notebook at the time of performance constitutes the primary record of the work, and it is important for you to follow this principle. Many patent cases have been determined on the basis of dates and times recorded in a laboratory notebook.

3)Make all entries in ink, and do not delete anything you have written in the notebook. If you make a mistake, cross it out and record the correct information. Using erasers or correction fluid to modify entries in your notebook is unacceptable scientific practice!

Do not scribble notes on odd bits of paper with the intention of later recording the information in your notebook. Such bad habits only lead to problems, since the scraps of paper are easily lost or mixed up. They are also inefficient, since transcribing the information to your notebook means that you must write it a second time. This procedure can also result in errors if you miscopy the data.

Finally, do not trust your memory with respect to observations that you have made. When the time comes to write down the information, you may have forgotten a key observation that is critical to the success of the experiment.

4)Unless instructed to do otherwise, do not copy detailed experimental procedures provided elsewhere in your notebook; this consumes valuable time. Rather, provide a specific reference the source of the detailed procedure and enter a synopsis of the written procedure that contains enough information that ①you need not refer to the source while performing the procedure and ②another chemist will be able to duplicate what you did. For example, when performing an experiment from this textbook, a reference should be given to the page number on which the procedure appears and any variation is made in the procedure should be detailed along with the reason(s) for doing so.

5) Start the description of each experiment on a new page titled with the name of the experiment. The recording of data and observations from several different procedures on the same page can lead to confusion, both for yourself and for others who may read your notebook.

(3) Calculations of the yield

A chemical equation for the overall conversion of the starting material into products is written on the assumption of simple ideal stoichiometry. Actually the ideal assumption is seldom true. Side reactions or competing reactions will also occur to give other products. For some synthetic reactions, an equilibrium state will be reached in which an appreciable amount of starting material still is present and can be recovered. Some of the reactant may also remain if it is present in excess or if the reaction was incomplete. A reaction involving an expensive reagent illustrates another need for knowledge about the extent to which a particular type of reaction converts reactants to products. In such a case it is preferable to use the method, which is the most efficient in this conversion. Thus, information about the efficiency of conversion for various reactions is of interest to the person contemplating using these reactions.

The quantitative expression for the efficiency of a reaction is given by a calculation of the yield for the reaction. The theoretical yield is the number of grams of product expected from the reaction on the basis of ideal stoichiometry, ignoring side reactions, reversibility, losses, etc.

The actual yield is simply the number of grams of desired product obtained. The percentage yield describes the efficiency of the reaction and is determined by:

$$Percentage \text{ yield} = \frac{\text{Actual yield}}{\text{Theoretical yield}} \times 100\%$$

A sample calculation, using a hypothetical value for the actual yield, can be provided using the case of the acetanilide preparation as an example:

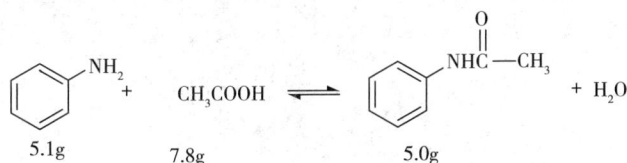

| 5.1g | 7.8g | | 5.0g | |

Aniline: 5.1g = 0.055mol

Acetic acid: 7.8g = 0.13mol (excess)

Molar quality of acetanilide: 135g/mol

Theoretical yield: $135 \times 0.055 = 7.43g$

Actual yield: 5.0g

$$Percentage \text{ yield} = \frac{5}{135 \times 0.055} \times 100\% = 67.3\%$$

（4）Laboratory reports

Various formats for reporting the results of laboratory experiments may be used. In cases where original research is being performed, these reports should include a detailed description of all of the experimental steps undertaken. Frequently the style used in scientific periodicals, such as the Journal of the American Chemical Society, is applied to the writing of laboratory reports. Your instructor is likely to have his own requirements for laboratory reports, and he should detail his requirements to you, but we provide suggested formation the sections that follow.

Experimental Report of Organic Chemistry

Experiment title

1. Experimental purpose

2. Experimental principle

3. Physical constants of materials and reagents

4. Specification of materials and reagents

5. Apparatus and equipment

6. Procedures and phenomena

7. Results

8. Yield

9. Discussion

第二部分　基本操作实验

Part II　Basic Techniques

实验一　熔点测定

扫码"学一学"

扫码"看一看"

【目的要求】

1. **掌握**　熔点测定中的误差来源与减小误差的方法；测定熔点的操作。
2. **了解**　熔点测定的意义；温度计校正方法。

【实验原理】

结晶物质的熔点是物质从固态变为液态的温度。在熔点处，固相和液相处于平衡状态。熔点测定是一种实验性的、易于实施的物理检测方法，可用于化合物的鉴定，也有助于化合物纯度和热稳定性的评价。有机化合物熔点的精确测定耗时较多。用微量法测定有机化合物熔点，操作简便，所需样品极少，所得熔点数据能满足大多数用途的要求。

微量法测得的是化合物的熔程，即结晶物质从开始熔融到全部熔融的温度范围。一般情况下，纯的结晶化合物都有固定的熔点范围，精确测定时应能观察到不超过 $0.5 \sim 1.0℃$ 的熔程。短的熔程通常提示样品为纯化合物。虽然低共熔混合物也会表现出短的熔程，但这种情形较为少见。纯化合物中混有杂质时，熔程变宽，可利用该特点进行纯化合物的鉴定。

【熔点仪】

提勒管是一种简单的熔点测定装置，如图 2 – 1（a）所示。

在大多数实验室中，提勒管已被各种使用更为方便的电子熔点仪取代。干法加热块（金属块）已被证明是替代硅油等热浴的很好的加热介质。图 2 – 2 所示的新天光 RY – 1G 熔点仪利用加热的金属块代替导热液体将热量传递到毛细管。金属块导热法清洁、无油污，还提供了自动检测熔点的可能性。Büchi M – 565 熔点仪（图 2 – 3）代表了另一类带金属块的电子熔点仪，它使用内置的 PT – 1000 铂电阻测量温度。

【实验步骤】

1. 样品准备　待测样品必须充分干燥、混匀且呈粉末状。潮湿的样品必须先干燥。粗晶和非均质样品需在研钵中研细。

将少量样品粉末放在洁净的表面皿上，将少量固体压入毛细管的开口端。此操作不应在滤纸上进行，因为滤纸的纤维可能会和化合物一起被压入毛细管中。之后，取一长约

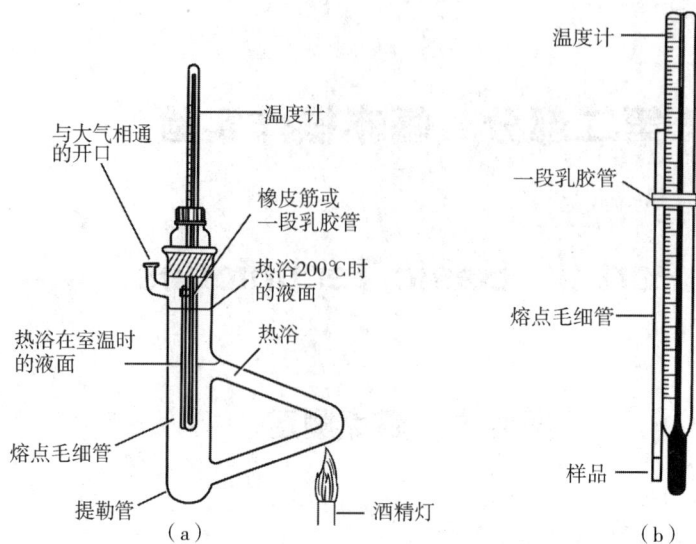

图 2－1　提勒管的组成

（a）提勒管熔点测定装置；（b）测熔点时样品与温度计的相对位置

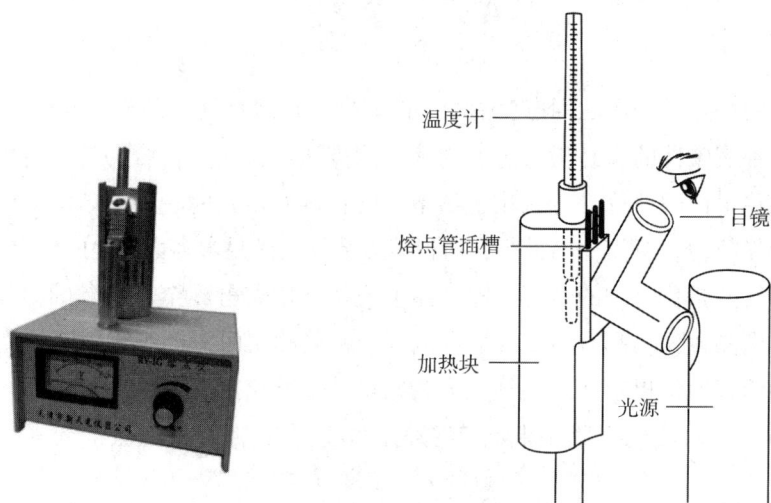

图 2－2　新天光 RY－1G 熔点仪

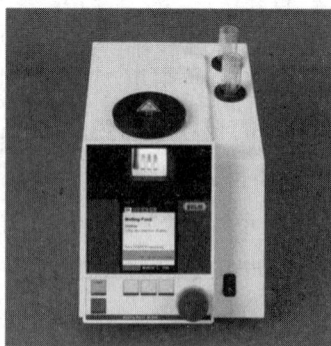

图 2－3　Büchi M－565 熔点仪

1m、直径 6~8mm 的玻璃管，将其垂直放置在工作台面或地板等坚硬表面上，让毛细管在该长玻璃管内由高到低自由跌落几次，注意毛细管的密封端应朝下。此操作可使固体样品在毛细管的封闭端填充紧密。准备好的样品在毛细管中的高度约 2~3mm。

2. 毛细管法测熔点

（1）用提勒管测熔点　用橡皮筋（或方便易得的一小段乳胶管）将熔点管固定在温度计上，使样品本身直接接近温度计的玻璃球［图2-1（b）］。橡皮筋要固定在较高的位置，保证即使热浴被加热到200℃，橡皮筋仍在热浴的上方［图2-1（a）］。完成后，将温度计放入热浴中，用温度计套管连接。提勒管一侧的开口使装置成为开放系统。切勿加热封闭系统。通过使用小型本生灯（酒精灯）加热。如果知道化合物的预估熔点，则在预估熔点15℃以前用相当快的速度（每分钟10~20℃）加热，然后减慢加热速度，使升温速率不超过每分钟2℃（非常缓慢）。记录最初观察到熔融时［初熔，图2-4（b）］的温度和剩余固体完全熔融时［终熔，图2-4（d）］的温度，并将其记录为固体的熔点。用通行的格式记录结果，例如mp 126~127℃。对同一样品进行几次平行测定。熔点的重复测定需要使用新的样品。

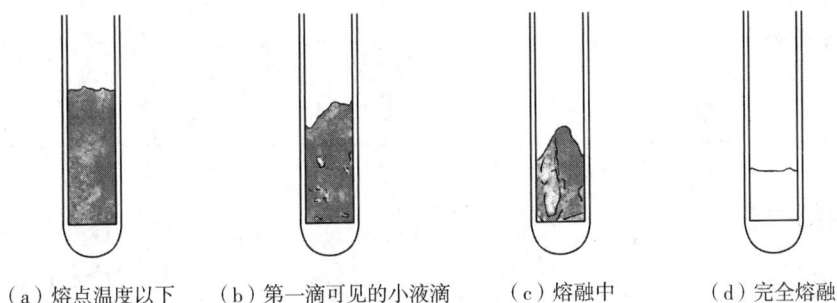

（a）熔点温度以下　　（b）第一滴可见的小液滴　　（c）熔融中　　（d）完全熔融

图2-4　受热时样品外观的变化

如果不知道化合物的预估熔点，则在整个过程中以中等速度加热样品，并确定大致的熔点。待仪器冷却后，用新样品进行更精细的测定。

（2）用RY-1G熔点仪测熔点　将含有样品的毛细管插入熔点仪目镜后面的插槽中（图2-2）。每台仪器通常有三个插槽，在熟练掌握该技术后可同时测量多个样品的熔点。打开仪器电源，调整电压值以获得适当的加热速率。合适的加热速率需要通过实验来摸索，应一边仔细观察仪器上的温度计度数一边调整。通过目镜观察仪器中的样品，目镜中的视野是被放大、且被照亮的。加热速率的要求如前所述。

（3）混合熔点　测定固体有机化合物的混合熔点时，必须将两种组分混合均匀，最好用研钵，将混合物研细混匀，也可以用玻棒或刮刀在表面皿上混合研细。

（4）实验　①从提供的已知熔点的化合物中，选一到二个化合物，用熔点管测定熔点。重复测定，直到能熟练、准确测定熔点。②从已测过熔点的化合物中，任选一个化合物，掺杂5%~10%的另一种物质。混合均匀，测定样品熔点，验证杂质对熔点的影响。③精确测定、报告由指导教师提供的未知样品的熔点。这次测定，可以作为熔点测定技术的小测验。

3. 温度计校正　使用的温度计需定期检定，以确保读数准确。根据温度计的标准测量条件，玻璃液体温度计可分为局浸式和全浸式两类。在其他浸没条件下使用温度计时，需进行校正。

温度计校正包括：在温度计的量程范围内，测量一系列温度，比较测定值与预期值之间的差别。利用测定值与预期值之间的差值可以校正温度计的读数，消除温度计的偏差。在记录本上，以温度差为横坐标，温度为纵坐标，从零到量程温度作图（温度计0℃是精确的）。这是最简单的方法，只要看一眼，就能知道偏差多少。如：温度在130℃左右时，你的温度计读数低2℃或温度在190℃时温度计读数高1.5℃。这些校正只对被校正的温度计有效，如温度计被打碎，新温度计需要重新校正。实验中所用温度计都必须校正。

为校正温度计，应仔细地测定一些标准物质的熔点，表2-1列出了一些常用标准物质及其熔点值。

表2-1 温度计校正使用的标准物质

化合物	熔点（℃）
冰-水	0
3-苯基丙酸	48.6
乙酰胺	82.3
乙酰苯胺	114
苯甲酰胺	133
水杨酸	159
4-氯乙酰苯胺	179
3,5-二硝基苯甲酸	205

【实验指导】

（一）预习要求

1. 检索和记录乙酰苯胺的化学结构式、理化常数、MSDS信息，列出参考文献或数据来源。

2. 预习熔点测定的原理，建立熔程的概念，了解物质的熔程和纯度的关系。

3. 了解熔点测定装置、测定熔点的一般步骤以及在操作中需注意的问题。

（二）注意事项

1. 当你使用煤气灯或酒精灯时，必须远离易燃溶剂；如你的头发较长，请系于脑后，远离火焰；不能烧到通煤气的橡皮管，煤气灯或酒精灯不用时应及时关掉。

2. 加热含水的石蜡油或硅油时很不安全，含水的油加热到100℃（水沸点）时，由于形成水蒸气，热油将飞溅出来，油遇明火会被点燃。实验前必须查看提勒管底部，检查是否有水滴，如有，更换浴油或更换新的提勒管，将有水的提勒管交给指导教师。

3. 石蜡油（高沸点烃的混合物）不能加热到200℃以上，特别是用煤气灯加热时，可能造成油的自燃。硅油可加热到300℃左右。

4. 对于制药行业，熔点测定的操作流程需遵循药典或指导原则的要求。

5. 防止被加热模块烫伤。防止被玻璃毛细管割伤。

6. 乙酰苯胺对水生生物有害，需按相关法规回收。

7. 避免打破温度计。测量熔点时不要取出温度计，避免温度计因温度骤降而炸裂。加热前，必须先检查温度计是否完好。

8. 如水银温度计破损，必须马上关闭加热装置，并报告老师。避免在可能有水银的地面走动。注意通风。

（三）实验说明

1. 晶体大小、晶形、升温速率和样品纯度都会影响熔点测定的准确性，热能从热浴传导到样品，热能在样品内部传导，都有时滞效应，因而晶体大小、晶形、升温速率会导致观察值与实际值不同。另外，加热太快，温度计读数将滞后于热浴温度。

2. 大多数情况下，通过仔细观察和缓慢升温（见实验步骤2），结晶物质的熔点可被简单、准确地测定，但偶尔也会观察到异常的熔融特性。大多数有机化合物在熔融前会发生晶体结构的变化，这通常是结晶溶剂被释放的结果。样品呈现出较软的，或是"湿"的外观，也可能伴随着样品在毛细管中的收缩。样品中这些类型的变化不应被解释为初熔；应等待第一滴小液滴的出现。

3. 有些化合物在熔融时发生分解，这种情况下样品的颜色通常会有明显变化。分解的产物成为样品的杂质，从而导致熔点结果偏低。如观察到样品分解，应按如下方式报告熔点，mp 183℃ d 或 mp 183℃（dec），以指示分解的发生。

4. 如化合物具有明显的挥发性，熔点的测定可伴随升华。在升华过程中，固体在熔融前会蒸发并消失。使用毛细管测熔点时，可在填充样品后通过密封毛细管的顶端来防止升华。在此情况下，可使用比正常操作更多的样品，在不远低于预期熔点的温度下测定熔点。

（四）思考题

1. 指出下列陈述正确与否。

（1）含杂质有机物熔点会较纯净物高。

（2）像纯化合物一样，共熔体有较短的熔程。

（3）如油浴的升温速率太快，测定的熔点将偏低。

（4）熔点管内样品不必装紧。

（5）用石蜡油做油浴，不能测定熔点在200℃以上固体的熔点。

2. 接近样品熔点时，热浴升温速率大约是多少？

3. 如何用混合熔点法判断两个固体样品是否可能为同一化合物？

4. 石蜡油燃烧时，释放出什么有害气体？

5. 某同学用提勒管测定一未知物的熔点，熔点记录为 mp 182℃，这个数据可信吗？解释原因。

6. 下面一组熔点数据，指出哪些是纯化合物。

（1）mp 120 ~ 122℃　　　（2）mp 147℃（dec）

（3）mp 46 ~ 60℃　　　（4）mp 162.5 ~ 163.5℃

Experiment 1　Melting Point Determination

Experimental principle

The melting point of a crystalline substance is the temperature at which it changes state from solid to liquid. At the melting point the solid and liquid phase exist in equilibrium. Melting point determination is an experimental and easily performed method of physical analysis used to find out the identity, the purity and the thermal stability of a compound. The determination of highly accurate melting points of organic compounds can be time-consuming. Fortunately, micro methods are available that are convenient, require negligible amounts of sample, and give melting-point data that are satisfactory for most purposes.

In all micro methods the melting point is actually determined as a melting range, encompassed by the temperature at which the sample is first observed to begin to melt and the temperature at which the melting process is complete. Generally, the melting point of a pure crystalline compound lies in a fixed range. When properly carried out, a range of no more than $0.5 \sim 1.0\ ℃$ should be observed. A narrow melting-point range ordinarily signals that the sample is pure, although there is a low probability that the solid is a eutectic mixture. The broadening of the melting-point range that results from introducing an impurity into a pure compound may be used to advantage for identifying a pure substance.

Melting point apparatus

A simple type of melting point apparatus is the Thiele tube, shown in Figure 2-1(a).

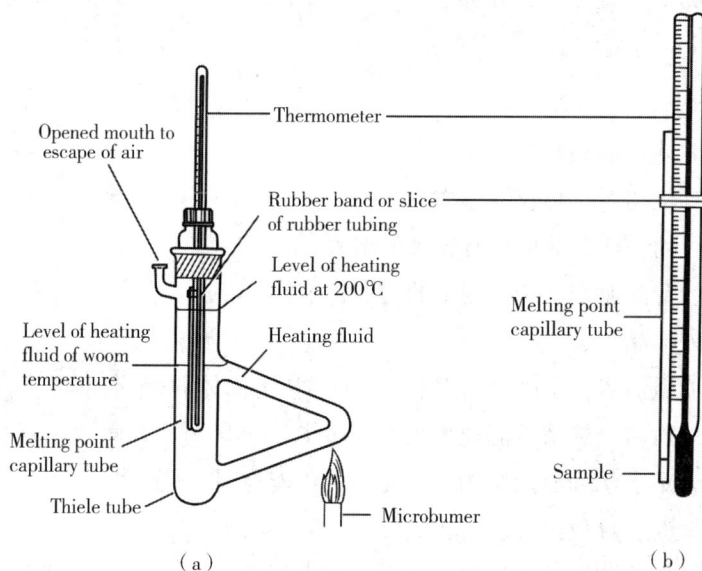

Figure 2-1   The composition of thiele melting point apparatus

(a) Thiele melting point apparatus; (b) Arrangement of sample and thermometer for determining melting point

Thiele tube has been replaced in most laboratories by various electric melting point devices, which are more convenient to use. A dry thermal block (metal block) has proven to be a good alternative to a liquid bath consisting of silicone oil. Xin Tian Guang melting point RY-1G instrument, which is showed in Figure 2-2, utilizes a heated metal block rather than a liquid for transferring the heat to the capillary tube. In addition to its clean operation, the block also offers the possibility of detecting the melting point automatically. Büchi melting point M-565 instrument (Figure 2-3) is another electric unit with a metal block, a built-in Pt-1000 resistor is used to measure the temperatures.

Experimental procedures

1. Sample preparation

The sample being investigated must be fully dry, homogeneous, and in powdered form. Moist samples must be dried first. Coarse crystalline and non-homogeneous samples are finely ground in a mortar.

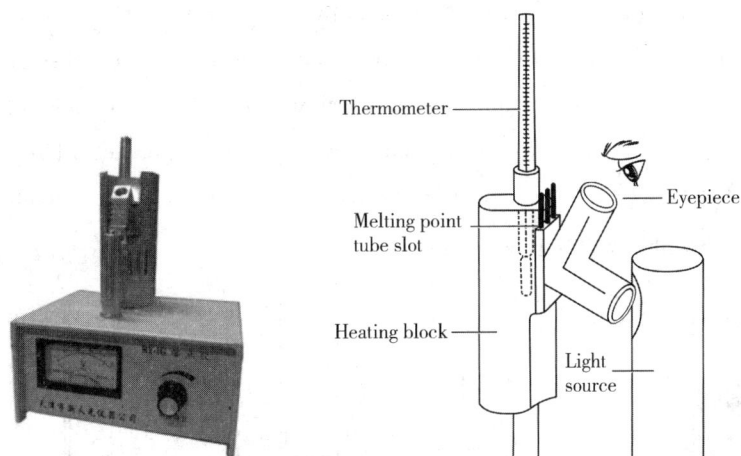

Figure 2 – 2　Xin Tian Guang melting point RY-1G instrument

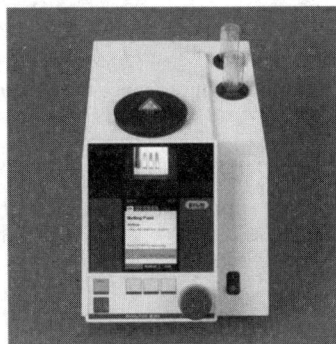

Figure 2 – 3　Büchi melting point M-565 instrument

Place a small amount of the powdered sample on a clean watch glass and press the open end of the tube into the solid to force a small amount of solid into the tube, this operation should not be performed on filter paper rather than a watch glass because fibers of paper as well as the solid may be forced into the tube. Then take a piece of 6 ~ 8mm tubing about 1m long, hold it vertically on a hard surface such as the bench top or floor, and drop the capillary tube down the larger tubing several times with the sealed end down. This packs the solid sample at the closed end of the capillary tube. The height of the prepared sample in the capillary is about 2 ~ 3mm.

2. Determination of capillary-tube melting points

Determining melting points with the Thiele tubeAttach the capillary to a thermometer by means of a small rubber band (conveniently obtained as a slice of ordinary rubber tubing). The sample itself should be directly adjacent to the bulb of the thermometer [Figure 2 – 1 (b)]. The rubber band should be positioned such that even at 200℃ it will remain above the level of the heating fluid [Figure 2 – 1 (a)]. This accomplished, place the thermometer into the heating vessel, and support it by means of a thermometer adapter. An opening on one side of the Thiele tube serves the purpose of making the apparatus an open system. *Never heat a closed system.* Raise the temperature of the heating fluid by applying heat from a small Bunsen burner (microburner). If the expected melting point of the compound is known, heat fairly rapidly (10 ~ 20℃ per minute) to 15℃ below the expected melting point, then slow the rate of heating such that the temperature increases no more than 2℃ per minute (i. e. , very slowly). Note the temperature at which melting is first observed [beginning of melting, Figure 2 −4(b)] and the temperature at which the last of the solid melts [finished melting, Figure 2 −4(d)], and record these as the melting range of the solid. Record results in a popular format, e. g. mp 126 ~ 127℃. Do several parallel determinations on the same sample. A fresh sample is necessary for a second melting point trial.

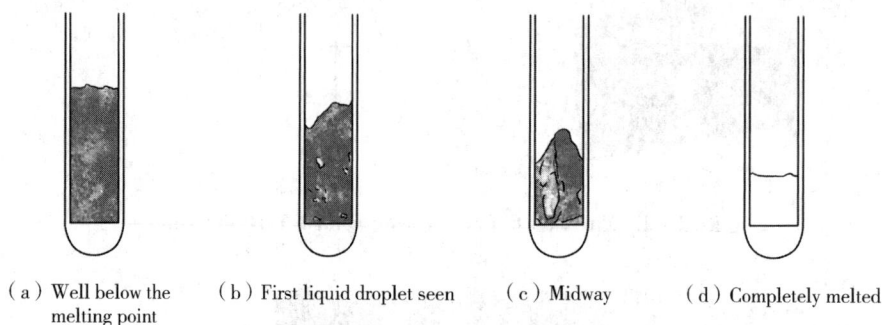

(a) Well below the   (b) First liquid droplet seen   (c) Midway   (d) Completely melted
         melting point

Figure 2 −4　Changes in the appearance of the sample when heated

If the expected melting point of the compound is not known, heat the sample at a medium rate throughout the process and determine an approximate melting point. Repeat the process with a fresh sample after allowing the apparatus to cool and perform a more careful assessment of the melting point.

Determining melting points with the RY-1G instrumentInsert the capillary tube containing the sample into a slot behind the viewfinder of a melting point apparatus (Figure 2 −2). There are usually three slots in each apparatus, and multiple melting points can be taken simultaneously after gaining experience with the technique. Turn on the apparatus and adjust the voltage value to obtain an appropriate heating rate. The rate of heating is often experimental and should be adjusted by careful monitoring of the thermometer on the apparatus. Look through the viewfinder to see a magnified view of the sample in the apparatus, which should be illuminated. The requirement of heating rate is as mentioned above.

Mixture-melting pointIn the preparation of a sample for mixture-melting point determination, it is important that the two components be thoroughly and intimately mixed. This is best accomplished by grinding them together by means of a small mortar and pestle.

Experiments①Select one or two compounds from a list of supplied compounds of know melting point. Determine the melting points (ranges) for each of these substances, using the capillary melting-point procedure. Repeat as necessary until you are able confidently and accurately to complete these measurements.

②Using one of the compounds whose melting range was determined in part (1), introduce about 5% ~ 10% of a second substance as an impurity. Thoroughly mix the two components of the mixture and determine the melting range of the sample in order to verify the anticipated effects of impurities on the melting range of a substance.

③Accurately determine and report the melting range of an unknown sample supplied by your instructor. This determination may be considered as a practical laboratory quiz pertaining to your mastery of this technique.

3. Calibration of thermometer

Thermometers used in laboratories need to be periodically calibrated to ensure accurate readings. According to the standard measurement conditions of thermometers, liquid-in-glass thermometers may be standardized for partial immersion and full immersion. For use under other conditions of immersion, a correction is necessary to obtain correct temperature readings.

Calibration of a thermometer involves the measurement of temperature at a series of known points within the range of the thermometer, and the comparison of these actual readings with expected temperatures. The difference between the actual and the expected readings provides a correction which must be applied to the actual thermometer reading in order to correct for thermometer error. Most simply, these corrections are plotted in your notebook as deviations from zero (where the thermometer is accurate) versus the temperature over the range of the thermometer. Thus at a glance you can tell, for example, that at about 130℃ your thermometer gives readings that are 2℃ too low, or that at 190℃ the readings are about 1.5℃ too high. These corrections are valid only for the thermometer used in the calibration; if the thermometer is broken, a new one must be calibrated. These corrections should then be applied to all temperature measurements taken during the course.

To calibrate a thermometer, carefully determine the melting points of a series of standard substances. A list of suitable standards is provided in Table 2－1.

Table 2－1　Standards for Thermometer Calibration

Compound	Melting Point (℃)
Ice water	0
3-Phenylpropanoic acid	48.6
Acetamide	82.3
Acetanilide	114
Benzamide	113
Salicylic acid	159
4-Chloroacetanilide	179
3,5-Dinitrobenzoic acid	205

Experimental instruction

Notes

1. If you are using a burner in this experiment, take care that no flammable solvents are nearby. If your hair is long, you should consider tying it back in order to keep it safely away from the flame. Be careful to keep the rubber tubing leading to the burner safely away from the flame. Turn off the burner when it is not actually in use.

2. Mineral and silicone oils may not be safely heated if they become contaminated with even a few drops of water. Heating these oils above 100℃ (the boiling point of water) may produce spattering of hot oil as a result of steam formation. Fire can also result as the oil comes in contact with

open flames. Examine the base of your Thiele tube for evidence of water droplets. If any are observed, either changes the oil or exchange tubes, giving the contaminated tube to your instructor.

3. Do not heat mineral oil (a mixture of high-boiling hydrocarbons) above about 200℃ because there is the possibility of spontaneous ignition, particularly when a burner is being used. Silicone oils may be heated about 300℃.

4. For the pharmaceutical industry, the processes of melting point determination should follow the requirements of Pharmacopoeia or specific guidelines.

5. Prevent scalding by heating module. Prevent cutting by glass capillary.

6. Acetanilide is harmful to aquatic organisms and needs to be disposed in accordance with regulations.

7. Avoid breaking the thermometer. When measuring melting point, do not take out the thermometer to avoid cracking caused by a sudden temperature drop. Before heating, it is necessary to check whether the thermometer is in good condition.

8. If mercury thermometer is damaged, it is necessary to close the heating device immediately, inform your instructor. Don't let anyone walk through the mercury on their way out. Keep ventilated.

Explanation

1. The observed melting point depends on a number of factors: sample size, state of subdivision of the sample, and heating rate, as well as purity and identity of the sample. The first three cause the observed melting point to differ from the actual melting point because of the time lag in heat transfer from heating fluid to sample and conduction within the sample. Furthermore, if heating is too fast, the thermometer reading will lag behind the actual temperature of the heating fluid.

2. Although in most instances the melting range of a substance may simply and accurately be determined by careful observation so long as the heating rate is slow (see part 2 of Experimental procedures), unusual melting characteristics are occasionally observed. Most organic compounds undergo a change in crystal structure just before melting, usually as a consequence of the release of solvent of crystallization. The sample takes on a softer, perhaps "wet" appearance, which may also be accompanied by shrinkage of the sample in the tube. Observance of these types of changes in the sample should not be interpreted as the beginning of melting; wait for the first tiny drop of liquid to appear.

3. Some compounds decompose on melting. When this happens, discoloration of the sample is usually evident. The decomposition products constitute impurities in the sample, and the melting point is actually lowered as a result of such decomposition. When this behavior is observed, the melting point should be reported in such a way as to denote its occurrence, for example, mp 183℃ d or mp 183℃ (dec).

4. If the compound is appreciably volatile, determination of the melting point may be accompanied by sublimation, in which the solid vaporizes and disappears before it melts. With a capillary tube, sublimation can be prevented by sealing the top end of the tube after filling. It may be possible to observe the melting point by using a larger-than-normal sample and placing it on the block at a temperature not too far below the expected melting point.

Exercises

1. Indicate which of the following statements is true (T) and which false (F).

(1) An impurity raises the melting point of an organic compound.

(2) A eutectic mixture has a sharp melting point, just as does a pure compound.

(3) If the rate of heating of the oil bath used in melting-point determination is too high, the melting point that results will likely be too low.

(4) The sample should not be packed tightly into a capillary melting-point tube.

(5) A heating bath containing mineral oil should not be used to determine the melting points of solids melting above 200℃.

2. What is the approximate rate at which the temperature of the heating bath should be increasing at the time the sample undergoes melting?

3. How does measuring a mixture melting-point help in determining the possible identity of two solid samples?

4. What toxic fumes is evolved by burning mineral oil?

5. A student used the Thiele micro melting-point technique to determine the melting point of an unknown and reported it to be 182℃. Is this value believable? Explain why or why not?

6. For the following melting points, indicate what might be concluded regarding the purity of the sample:

(1) mp 120～122℃　　　　(2) mp 147℃ (dec)

(3) mp 46～60℃　　　　(4) mp 162.5～163.5℃

实验二　沸点测定

【目的要求】

1. **掌握**　学习沸点测定的一般操作。
2. **了解**　微量沸点测定的一般原理。

【实验原理】

液体物质都有气化的趋势，气化后蒸气所产生的压力称蒸气压。液体物质的蒸气压随温度的上升而增大。当液体达到一定温度，液体的饱和蒸气压与外压相等时，液体的蒸发速度显著加快，液体中出现气泡。这个过程称为沸腾，此时的温度称为该液体的沸点。液体的沸点随外界压力改变而改变，记录沸点时，必须注明压力，如："bp 152℃ (752mm)。"在一定压力下，纯净化合物的沸点是固定的或沸程很短。沸点可用以验证液体和低熔点固体。

【实验步骤】

1. 微量沸点法　简单的微量测定仪可由内径1mm熔点管和内径4mm软玻璃管构成。用火焰将两根熔点管封口，在封口处将两根熔点管连接起来，在离接点3～4mm处将其切断，如图 2 – 5（a）所示。

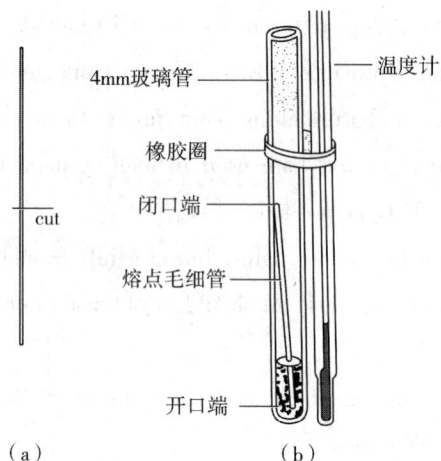

图 2 – 5 沸点测定装置

（a）毛细管制作；（b）装有温度计和毛细管的沸点测定装置

取一根内径 4mm 软质玻璃管，玻璃管的一端封口，切下一段，长度比制好的沸点管长 1cm。用橡皮圈将 4mm 玻璃管固定在温度计上，橡皮圈靠近管子顶部，管子底部位于水银球中部。用吸管滴加两滴液体到管子底部，插入沸点管，如图 2 – 4（b）所示。如果液面低于沸点管的封点，补加适量样品，将样品液面升至沸点管封点以上。

将温度计浸入加热液（提勒管或其他熔点测定仪），橡皮圈应在浴液之上。用加热器加热，控制油浴每分钟上升 5℃ 左右，直至有一连串气泡快速逸出（沸点管内空气，因受热膨胀，缓慢逸出，当温度达到沸点时，气泡逸出速度显著加快）。此时停止加热，让浴液缓慢冷却，气泡逸出速度渐渐减慢，在气泡不再冒出而液体刚要进入内管时，记录温度计读数，这就是液体沸点。

将沸点管拿出，甩掉沸点管中的液体，重新放回到样品管中，重复以上操作，在油浴温度距粗测的沸点 10～15℃ 时，控制加热速度每分钟 1～2℃。重复测定，仔细观察，几次测定的误差在 1℃ 或 2℃ 以内。

【实验指导】

（一）预习要求

1. 了解沸点测定的原理以及液体物质的沸程和纯度的关系。

2. 比较沸点测定和熔点测定在仪器装置上的异同点。

（二）注意事项

1. 挥发性有机液体易燃，加热时应十分小心。

2. 溢出的液体应用纸巾吸掉，然后按指导教师要求处理。有机液体不能接触皮肤，如皮肤沾到有机液体，应用肥皂、热水彻底清洗。

（三）思考题

判断问题 1、2 正确与否。

1. 挥发性液体加入不挥发溶质。

（1）对沸点无影响。

（2）沸点降低。

（3）沸点升高。

2. 微量沸点仪测定的沸点，是指这时的温度。

（1）气泡刚从倒置的毛细管中缓慢出来时。

（2）气泡刚从倒置的毛细管中，快速逸出。

（3）液体刚要进入倒置的毛细管中。

3. 温度达到沸点前，倒置毛细管缓慢逸出的气泡是什么？

4. 为什么测定沸点 200℃ 以上的液体，不能用石蜡油做浴液？

Experiment 2　Boiling Point Determination

Experimental principle

When the temperature of the liquid is such that the equilibrium vapor pressure of the sample equals the external pressure, the rate of evaporation increases dramatically, and bubbles form in the liquid. This is the boiling process, and the temperature associated with it is the boiling point of the liquid. As the observed boiling point is obviously directly dependent on the external pressure, in reporting boiling points it is necessary to state the external pressure, for example, "bp 152℃ (752mmHg)."

A pure liquid generally boils at a constant temperature or over a narrow temperature range, provided the total pressure in the system remains constant boiling points are useful for identification of liquids and some low-melting solids.

Experimental procedure

Micro boiling points　A simple micro boiling-point apparatus may be constructed from two 1mm capillary melting-point tubes and 4mm soft glass tubing in the following way. Seal the ends of two capillary tubes in a flame and join the tubes at the seals. Make a clean cut about 3 ~ 4mm from the joint, as shown in Figure 2 −5(a). Seal a piece of 4mm soft glass tubing at one end and cut it to a length about 1cm longer than the prepared capillary ebullition tube.

Attach the 4mm tube to a thermometer with a rubber ring, with the rubber ring near the top of the tube and the bottom of the tube even with the mercury bulb of the thermometer. Place about two drop of the liquid for which a boiling point is to be determined in the bottom of the tube by means of a capillary pipet. Introduce the capillary ebullition tube as shown in Figure 2 −5(b). If the liquid level of the sample is below the joint seal of the capillary, add enough more sample to bring it above the seal.

Immerse the thermometer and attached tubes in a heating bath (Thiele tube or other melting-point apparatus), taking care that the rubber ring is above the liquid level. Heat the oil bath at the rate of about 5℃/min until a rapid and continuous stream of bubbles comes out of the capillary ebullition tube. (A decided change from the slow evolution of bubbles caused by thermal expansion of the trapped air will be seen when the boiling temperature of the liquid is reached). Discontinue heating at this point. As the bath is allowed to cool down slowly, the rate of bubbling will decrease. At the moment the bubbling ceases entirely and the liquid begins to rise into the capillary, note the temperature of the thermometer. This is the boiling point of the liquid sample.

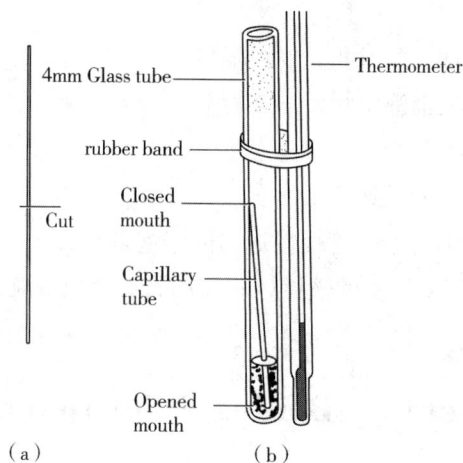

Figure 2 – 5   Micro boiling-point apparatus

（a）joining capillary tubes and cutting off one end；（b）assembling micro boiling point apparatus with correct placement of ebullition and sample tubes, and thermometer

Remove the capillary ebullition tube and expel the liquid from the small end by gentle shaking. Replace it in the sample tube and repeat the determination of the boiling point by heating the oil bath at the rate of $1 \sim 2℃/\text{min}$ when you are within $10 \sim 15℃$ of the approximate boiling point as determined in the previous experiment. With a little practice and care the observed boiling points may be reproduced to within 1 or $2℃$.

Experimental instruction

Notes

1. Volatile organic liquids are flammable, so burners should be used carefully in this experiment.

2. Spilled liquids should be carefully absorbed into a paper towel which is then discarded as directed by your instructor. Do not allow organic liquids to come into contact with your skin. If this happens, wash the affected area thoroughly with warm soap and water.

Exercises

Questions 1 and 2 may be answered by marking yes（Y）or no（N）for each part.

1. The addition of a nonvolatile solute to a volatile liquid

（1）Has no effect on the boiling point of the volatile liquid.

（2）Lowers the boiling point of the volatile liquid.

（3）Raises the boiling point of the volatile liquid.

2. The boiling point, as determined in the micro boiling point apparatus, is the temperature at the time

（1）Bubbles first emerge slowly from the inverted capillary tube.

（2）Bubbles begin to emerge rapidly from the inverted capillary tube.

（3）The liquid begins to re-enter and rise in the inverted capillary tube.

3. What are the bubbles that emerge slowly from the inverted capillary tube before the boiling temperature is reached, and why does this occur?

4. Why is mineral oil an inappropriate heating fluid for determining the boiling points of samples that exceed 200℃?

实验三　重结晶

扫码"学一学"

扫码"看一看"

【目的要求】

1. **掌握**　重结晶的基本操作方法。
2. 学习重结晶的原理，过程及其应用。

【实验原理】

　　从有机制备或由天然产物中提取得到的有机化合物常含有杂质，有机化学家致力于得到纯的有机物。重结晶是提纯固体有机化合物最常用的方法，我们应掌握这一有用的技术。

　　固体有机化合物在溶剂中的溶解度和温度密切相关，一般温度升高溶解度增大，重结晶就是利用固体物质的这一特性。如果将晶体溶解在热的溶剂中制成饱和溶液，冷却时，溶液变成过饱和而析出晶体，析出晶体的量与不同温度下，物质的溶解度差别有关。如果杂质溶于热溶剂，冷却后仍留在溶液中，而欲纯化的物质结晶析出，过滤后得纯品；或杂质在热溶剂中不溶，制成饱和溶液后，趁热过滤滤去不溶性杂质，滤液冷却析晶，则该晶体纯度亦较原晶体提高。

　　重结晶操作的一般步骤：

　　选择适当的溶剂→在溶剂沸点附近溶解待纯化固体→趁热过滤，除去不溶性杂质→冷却析晶→过滤，除去母液→洗涤，除去附着的溶液→干燥晶体

　　1. 选择溶剂　进行重结晶时，首要问题是选择合适的溶剂。理想的重结晶溶剂必须具备下列条件：①对待纯化物质和杂质，溶剂有较好的温度系数，即：待纯化物质最好在热溶剂中有较大的溶解度而在冷溶剂中几乎不溶（这可减少损失）；杂质在冷溶液中至少有中等的溶解度，冷却后仍留在溶液中，或杂质在热溶液中不溶，可趁热过滤除去。②沸点较低，干燥时，易于除去。③溶剂的沸点最好低于溶质的熔点。④不与待纯化物质发生化学反应。

　　如果化合物是已知的，文献一般有合适重结晶溶剂的资料，如果是新化合物，需要用尝试法，即可先用少量样品与溶剂进行尝试。尝试时，应记住溶解度的一般原则：极性化合物不溶于非极性溶剂而溶于极性溶剂；相反，非极性化合物溶于非极性溶剂。这些关系可概括为："相似相溶"。重结晶常用溶剂见表2－2。

表2－2　重结晶溶剂[a,b]

溶剂	沸点	凝固点[c]	水溶性	介电常数	可燃性	比重[d]
水[*,e]	100℃	0℃	—	78.54	不易燃	1.000
95%乙醇[*]	78℃		可溶	24.6	易燃	
甲醇	65℃		可溶	32.63	易燃	
石油醚[*]	可变		不溶	1.9	易燃	约0.7

续表

溶剂	沸点	凝固点[c]	水溶性	介电常数	可燃性	比重[d]
环己烷	81℃	6℃	不溶	2.02	易燃	0.779
甲苯	111℃		不溶	2.38	易燃	0.867
乙醚	35℃		微溶	4.34	易燃	0.714
四氢呋喃	65℃		可溶	7.58	易燃	
1，4-二氧六环	107℃	11℃	可溶	2.21	易燃	
二氯甲烷	41℃		不溶	9.08	不易燃	1.335
三氯甲烷	61℃		不溶	4.81	不易燃	1.492
四氯化碳	77℃		不溶	2.23	不易燃	1.594
乙酸乙酯	77℃		微溶	6.02	易燃	
丙酮	56℃		可溶	20.7	易燃	
乙酸	118℃	17℃	可溶	6.15	易燃	

a 由于毒性，苯未列出，常可以用环己烷代替苯。

b 如有其他相当的溶剂，一般不用含氯有机溶剂，如二氯甲烷，三氯甲烷和四氯化碳；如没有，小心使用，避免吸入过量含氯有机溶剂的蒸气。

c 未列出的溶剂凝固点低于0℃。

d 仅列出水不溶性溶剂的比重。

e 用尝试法寻找重结晶溶剂时，星号标记的溶剂通常应优先尝试。

2. 重结晶溶剂可按如下方法选择

在 10×75mm 试管中，放置 10~20mg 样品，加几滴溶剂，覆盖样品，如样品在室温下完全溶解，则此溶剂的溶解度太大，不适用；若样品不溶或大部分不溶，小心加热至沸，若样品仍不溶，可在加热下分批补加溶剂，如在 0.5ml 热溶剂中，大部分样品仍未溶解，则表示此溶剂的溶解度太小，不适用；如样品溶于适量的热溶剂，而在室温下微溶或不溶，将热溶液缓慢冷至室温，查看析出晶体的质量、大小、颜色和晶形。若析出晶体质量优良，则该溶剂适合重结晶使用。

（1）溶解　将待纯化样品置于适当大小的锥形瓶、烧瓶或其他合适容器中，加几毫升溶剂，加搅拌磁子或沸石，以免爆沸。用热浴加热至沸，在沸腾下，分批加入少量溶剂，直至固体全部溶解，然后通常再补加溶剂总量的 5%~10%，以避免趁热过滤时样品过早析出。有些固体溶解缓慢，因此，补加溶剂溶解时，要有一定的时间间隔。

（2）脱色　有色杂质可通过在热（不是沸腾）溶液中加入少量活性炭脱色除去，一般仅需加一小匙活性炭。杂质，特别是有色杂质吸附在炭粒表面，可过滤除去。活性炭不仅吸附杂质也吸附待纯化物质，活性炭过量，待纯化物质也被吸附，造成损失。加入活性炭后，溶液需再加热煮沸几分钟，加热时应继续搅拌或振摇，以免爆沸。

（3）趁热过滤　为除去不溶性杂质（包括尘土、活性炭），热溶液要重力过滤。如无不溶性杂质，溶液澄清，趁热过滤这一步可省略。不要用抽滤，减压下热溶剂蒸发，溶液浓缩降温，导致过早析晶。用短颈漏斗或无颈漏斗、折叠滤纸过滤，热溶液滤入另一锥形瓶（图2-6）。折叠滤纸可较快过滤，滤纸的上边应低于漏斗边沿，保持液面高度，以增加过滤面积，提高效率。注意：不能让滤液从滤纸边缘和

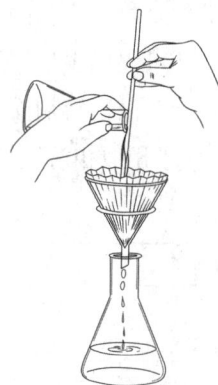

图2-6　用菊形滤纸过滤装置

漏斗间隙穿过。

折叠滤纸的方法见图 2-7，对折，再对折，折叠 2 到 3 形成 4，1 到 3 形成 5（a），然后折叠 2 到 5 形成 6，1 到 4 形成 7（b），再折叠 2 到 4 形成 8，1 到 5 形成 9（c）；现在滤纸形状如（d），注意，折叠都朝同一方向。

在折纹集中的圆心处，折时切勿重压，否则滤纸的中央在过滤时容易破裂。然后，在 1 和 9、9 和 5…之间，向相反方向折出新折纹，得折扇一样的排列（e），打开（f），再翻转（g），备用。

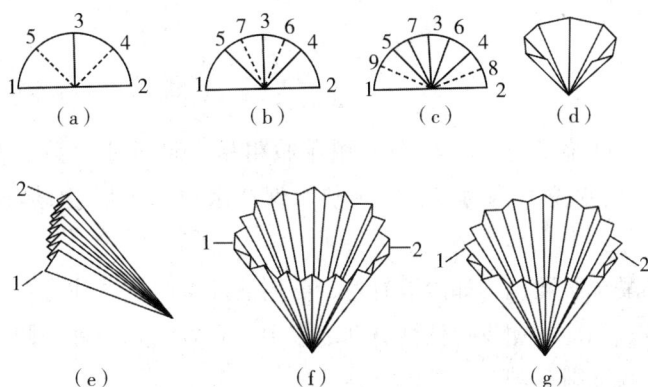

图 2-7　菊形滤纸的折叠

（4）结晶　将热滤液室温静置，缓慢冷却、析晶。如将滤液浸在冷水中迅速冷却，将得到颗粒很小的晶体，因其表面积大，极易吸附杂质。冷却时一般无需搅动，因为这样也会形成小晶体。然而，晶体太大（大于 2mm）易包藏溶液，难以干燥，干燥后含有杂质。如大晶体正在形成，可搅动，以减小晶体平均尺寸。经验越多，越易判断晶体大小是否合适。热滤液冷到室温后，再置于冰浴中冷却，以使结晶完全，减少损失。

（5）过滤　在布氏漏斗和真空装置间接一安全瓶，用水泵或真空管减压过滤结晶和溶液的混合物（图 2-8）。使用安全瓶可防止水从水泵倒吸进入抽滤瓶。滤纸应能平放在布氏漏斗内，过滤前，先用溶剂将滤纸润湿，然后减压抽气封住漏斗。用搅拌棒或刮刀帮助转移结晶，瓶内剩余晶体用滤液（母液）荡涤转移。母液一滤完，打开活塞，加少量冷的新鲜溶剂，使其恰好盖住结晶，搅动晶体，除去吸附的母液、包含的杂质。关闭活塞，除去洗涤液，并用塞子或刮刀尽量压干。

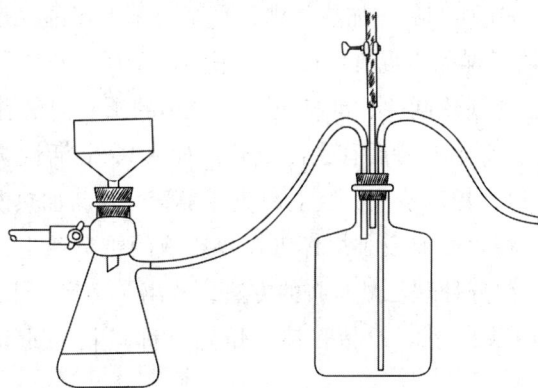

图 2-8　真空抽滤装置

（6）干燥　水泵抽气通过晶体几分钟后，大部份溶剂已去除，用刮刀将晶体转移到一干净表面皿上，放置风干几小时，彻底干燥。如需要，表面皿可放在烘箱中（烘箱温度至少比晶体熔点低20℃）、红外灯下或真空干燥器里加速干燥。

【实验步骤】

1. 样品

乙酰苯胺　　　　　　2.0g

对苯二甲酸二甲酯　1.0g

2. 步骤

（1）乙酰苯胺

1）溶解　在250ml烧杯中，加入2g乙酰苯胺粗品，60ml水，盖上表面皿，电炉上加热至沸。在烧杯上标出水位（因蒸发，需加热水保持水位），继续加热直至乙酰苯胺完全溶解。

2）脱色　纯乙酰苯胺无色，如溶液有色，需用活性炭脱色（注意：不能将活性炭加到正在沸腾的溶液中）。稍冷，加少量活性炭到溶液中，再煮沸几分钟。同时，准备漏斗、折叠滤纸和收集滤液的锥形瓶。

3）热过滤和结晶　将漏斗置于烘箱中预热，取出后，放置折叠滤纸，备好接收瓶，趁热过滤。如溶液不能一次性倾入漏斗，溶液可用热电炉（刚切断电源）保温，分批倾入。待所有的溶液过滤完后，用滤纸或倒置烧杯或松的塞子盖上锥形瓶，以防止空气中的杂质进入滤液。静置，冷至室温并不再有晶体析出。再把锥形瓶放入冰水中冷却至少15分钟，使结晶完全。

4）分离干燥　用布氏漏斗抽滤，收集晶体。用少量冷水洗涤滤饼，并用刮刀或塞子尽量将样品压干，将乙酰苯胺摊开在表面皿上，盖上滤纸防止灰尘污染，室温或红外灯下、烘箱内干燥。烘箱内温度必须比乙酰苯胺熔点低20℃以上。

5）分析　测定粗品、精品熔点，称重，按等式2-1进行计算回收率。

$$回收率 = \frac{精品重量}{粗品重量} \times 100\% \tag{2-1}$$

（2）对苯二甲酸二甲酯　在50ml圆底烧瓶中，加入1.0g对苯二甲酸二甲酯粗品、20ml 95%乙醇和沸石，装上回流冷凝管，水浴加热至沸，从冷凝管上口分批加入少量乙醇（总量不超过4~6ml），每次加完后，加热至沸，直至对苯二甲酸二甲酯完全溶解，再补加1~2ml溶剂。不要试图溶解样品中混有的砂石等不溶性杂质。记下溶剂体积，同时准备折叠滤纸、干净的锥形瓶。并预热漏斗，准备过滤。将热的沸腾溶液移出水浴（圆底烧瓶和冷凝管整体移出），稍冷，待不沸腾后移去冷凝管。加入0.2g活性炭（小心起泡，活性炭不能污染圆底烧瓶的磨口），摇动溶液，装上回流冷凝管，重新加热沸腾几分钟，用短颈漏斗和菊形滤纸趁热过滤。将表面皿或小烧杯盖在盛滤液的锥形瓶上，静置、冷却析晶。用95%乙醇代替水，按第一部分处理乙酰苯胺的方法，分离、洗涤、干燥。

分析　测定对苯二甲酸二甲酯粗品和精品熔点，称量精品重量，用式2-1计算回收率。

【实验指导】

（一）预习要求

1. 了解重结晶的原理，重结晶溶剂必须具备的条件，以及确定重结晶溶剂及其用量的方法。

2. 认识重结晶的一般操作过程和操作方法，并比较用水作溶剂和使用有机溶剂进行重结晶的异同点。

3. 查阅重结晶样品的物理性质（溶解度、熔点、色泽和晶型等）。

4. 列出乙酰苯胺和对苯二甲酸二甲酯重结晶中所需仪器的名称、规格、数量和要求。

5. 复习熔点测定的有关内容。

（二）注意事项

1. 实验中，当倾倒和转移溶液时，戴上手套或仔细操作，避免皮肤沾上溶液。有机化合物在溶液中，特别是水溶性溶剂，如乙醇、丙酮等，极易通过皮肤吸收。因此，不能用溶剂如丙酮冲洗皮肤上的有机物。实验结束后应使用热水和肥皂彻底清洗双手。

2. 不能将活性炭加到正在沸腾的溶液中，这可能造成冲料。

3. 易燃溶剂如醚、醇、烃不能放在敞口瓶里用明火加热，操作时，附近不能有明火。这些溶剂应用水浴或蒸气浴加热（或用电热丝不外露的电热板加热），如用明火，需装上回流冷凝管。过滤时应特别小心，附近不能有明火。

（三）实验说明

1. 即使首次试验就得到较好的结晶，仍需用不同溶剂试验溶质溶解性，可能会发现还有更好的溶剂，可获得较高回收率或更好的结晶。

2. 如果难于选择一种合适的溶剂，可使用混合溶剂，一种良溶剂，另一种不良溶剂。两种溶剂的比例用尝试法确定，常用混合溶剂有95%乙醇，甲苯–石油醚，乙酸–水，乙醚–乙醇和乙醚–石油醚。

3. 留一点粗品，当滤液结晶困难时，可加入晶种，诱导结晶。

4. 避免使用过量溶剂，以获得较好回收率。固体在冷溶剂中有一定的溶解度，回收率与溶解度及溶剂量有关。如大部分固体已溶解，再加溶剂，没有固体再溶解，特别仅有少量固体未溶时，溶剂量已足够。少量固体可能为不溶性杂质，可热过滤除去。

5. 如用混合溶剂，它们必须混溶。样品先溶于良溶剂，然后加不良溶剂至刚出现混浊为止，再滴加良溶剂，使其刚好澄清。通常先热过滤，然后再加不良溶剂，以免过滤时析晶。

6. 常有晶体在滤纸或漏斗表面析出，加2~3ml重结晶溶剂至接收瓶中，加热至沸，蒸气冷凝时加热漏斗，避免析晶（图2–9）。低沸点溶剂用蒸气浴加热，沸点高于90℃的溶剂可用电热油浴。

（四）思考题

1. 列出重结晶主要步骤，并简单说明每步的目的。

2. 重结晶操作的目的是获得最大回收率的精制品，解释下列操作为什么会得到相反的效果。

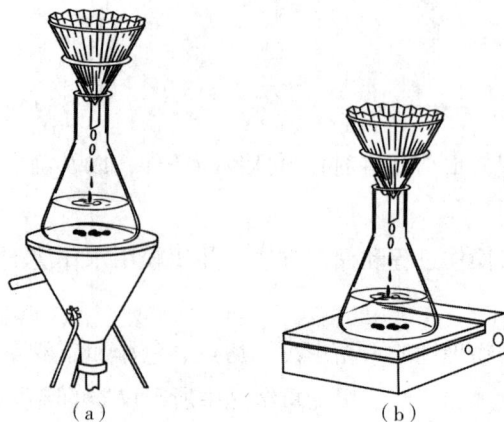

图 2-9 热过滤装置

（a）蒸汽保温；（b）加热板保温

（1）溶解时，溶剂过量。

（2）晶体干燥前，不用冷的新鲜溶剂洗涤。

（3）晶体用热的新鲜溶剂洗涤。

（4）活性炭过量。

（5）油层从热溶液中析出、固化，将其打碎，获得固体。

（6）将热溶液浸入冰水中，加速结晶。

3. 在溶剂沸腾或接近沸腾时，为什么不能加活性炭？

4. 用是（Y）或否（N）指出好的重结晶溶剂应具备下列哪些条件。

（1）溶质溶于冷溶剂。

（2）溶质与溶剂不发生化学反应。

（3）极性溶剂。

（4）沸点超过 100℃。

（5）沸点最好低于溶质的熔点。

5. 为什么析出的晶体不能太大也不能太小？

6. 真空过滤后的滤液浓缩，冷却，又有晶体析出，为什么该晶体的纯度较第一次晶体差？

7. 如何评估精品的纯度？

8. 将待结晶固体加热溶解时，为什么先加入比计算量（根据溶解度数据）略少的溶剂？然后为什么渐渐加至恰好溶解，最后再加少量溶剂？

Experiment 3　Recrystallization

Experimental principle

A compound formed in a chemical reaction or extracted from some natural source is rarely pure when initially isolated. Organic chemists devote considerable effort to the isolation of pure products. Recrystallization of solids is a valuable technique to master because it is one of the methods used most often for purification of solids.

In solution recrystallization, advantage is taken of the fact that nearly all solids are more soluble in a hot solvent than in a cold solvent. If the crystals are dissolved in a quantity of hot solvent which is insufficient to dissolve them when cold, and if that hot solution is then allowed to cool, it should be anticipated that crystals will precipitate from the cooling solution to the extent of the difference in solubility between the temperature extremes. If the impurities present in the original crystals have dissolved and remain dissolved after the solution is cooled, filtration of the crystals which have formed on cooling should then provide purified material. Or if the impurities remain undissolved in the hot solution and are filtered from it before it is allowed to cool, the crystals which subsequently form on cooling should be more pure than the original crystals.

1. Steps and techniques in recrystallization

Application of the technique of solution recrystallization involves several steps:

①selection of an appropriate solvent; ②dissolution of the solid to be purified in the solvent near or at its boiling point; ③filtration of the hot solution to remove insoluble impurities; ④crystallization from the solution as it cools; ⑤filtration of the purified crystals from the cooled supernatant solution (the "mother liquors"); ⑥washing the crystals to remove the adhering solution; ⑦drying the crystals.

(1) Selecting a solvent　A solvent must satisfy certain criteria in order to be used as a recrystallization solvent. ①Its temperature coefficients for the solute and impurities should be favorable; that is, the compound being purified should ideally be quite soluble in the hot solvent but somewhat insoluble in the cold (this will minimize losses), and the impurities should remain at least moderately soluble in the cold solvent. Another possibility here is that the impurities be insoluble in the hot solution, from which they may be filtered. ②The boiling point of the solvent should be low enough so that it can be easily removed from the crystals in the final drying step. ③It is generally preferable that the boiling point of the solvent be lower than the melting point of the solute. ④The solvent should not react chemically with the compound being purified.

If the compound has been previously studied, the chemical literature will generally give information concerning a suitable solvent. If the compound has not been studied, it will be necessary to resort to trial-and-error methods using small amounts of material. Some general solubility principles should be kept in mind if this needs to be done. Normally, polar compounds are insoluble in nonpolar solvents and soluble in polar solvents. Conversely, nonpolar compounds are more soluble in nonpolar solvents. These solubility relationships are frequently summarized with the phrase "like dissolves like." Some common solvents used in recrystallization are listed in Table 2 − 2.

The solvent, or solvent pair, to be used in the recrystallization of a substance is chosen in the following manner.

Place 10 ~ 20mg sample of the compound in a 10 × 75mm test tube and cover the solid with several drops of solvent. If the sample dissolves completely at room temperature, the solubility is too high. At the other extreme, if most of the sample remains undissolved in 0.5ml of hot solvent, the solubility is probably too low to be practiced. If the sample is soluble in the hot solvent but only slightly soluble or insoluble at room temperature, allow the hot solution to cool slowly to room temperature and compare the quantity, size, color, and form of the resulting crystals with the original solid material.

Table 2－2　Solvents for Recrystallization[a,b]

Solvent	Boiling point	Freezing Point[c]	Water Soluble	Dielectric Constant	Flammable	Specific Gravity[d]
Water ∗[e]	100℃	0℃	—	78.54	No	1.000
95% Ethanol ∗	78℃		Yes	24.6	Yes	
Methnol	65℃		Yes	32.63	Yes	
Petroleum ether ∗	Variable		No	1.9	Yes	About 0.7
Cyclohexane	81℃	6℃	No	2.02	Yes	0.779
Toluene	111℃		No	2.38	Yes	0.867
Diethyl ether	35℃		Slightly	4.34	Yes	0.714
Tetrahydrofuran	65℃		Yes	7.58	Yes	
1,4-Dioxane	107℃	11℃	Yes	2.21	Yes	
Dichloromethane	41℃		No	9.08	No	1.335
Chloroform ∗	61℃		No	4.81	No	1.492
Carbon tetrachloride	77℃		No	2.23	No	1.594
Ethyl acetate ∗	77℃		Yes	6.02	Yes	
Acetone	56℃		Yes	20.7	Yes	
Acetic acid	118℃	17℃	Yes	6.15	Yes	

a Benzene has been purposefully omitted from this list, owing to its toxicity. Cyclohexane can often be successfully substituted for it.

b As a general rule, avoid use of chlorocarbon solvents such as dichloromethane, chloroform, and carbon tetrachloride, if another equally good solvent can be found. If not, take care to avoid excessive inhalation of their vapors.

c Freezing points not lists are below 0℃.

d Only the specific gravities of water-insoluble solvents are included.

e The solvents marked with asterisks are those which should normally be employed first in a trial-and-error search for the best recrystallization solvent.

（2）Dissolution　The solid to be purified is placed in an appropriately sized Erlenmeyer flask, round bottom flask or other suitable vessel, along with a few milliliters of the desired solvent. The flask should be equipped for magnetic stirring or contain boiling stones to prevent bumping of the solution while boiling. The mixture is then heated to boiling. More solvent is added in small portions to the boiling mixture until just enough boiling solvent is present to dissolve the solid. It is generally desirable at this point to add from 5 to 10% additional solvent to prevent premature crystallization during the hot filtration, if this step appears necessary. During the dissolution of the impure solid, time should be allowed between each small addition of fresh solvent, for some solids dissolve only slowly.

（3）Decoloration　If colored impurities are present, these may often be removed by adding a small amount of decolorizing carbon to the hot (not boiling) solution. Seldom is more decolorizing carbon needed than that which can be held on the tip of a spatula. The impurities, especially colored ones, adsorb on the surface of the carbon particles and are removed during filtration. If too much carbon is used, some of the substance being purified will be adsorbed and subsequently lost in this step. After adding the carbon, the solution should be heated to boiling for a few minutes, while being continuously stirred or swirled to prevent bumping of the boiling mixture.

（4）Hot filtration　To remove insoluble impurities (including dust and decolorizing carbon, if used), the hot solution is filtered by gravity filtration. If no insoluble impurities are present and the solution is clear, this step may usually be omitted. Suction filtration is not desirable; because evaporation of the hot solvent under reduced pressure will both cool and concentrate the solution, resulting in premature crystallization. A short-stemmed or stemless glass funnel and a fluted filter paper should be used for filtration into a second Erlenmeyer flask (Figure 2 – 6). The use of fluted filter paper allows for more rapid filtration. The top of the paper should not extend above the top of the funnel.

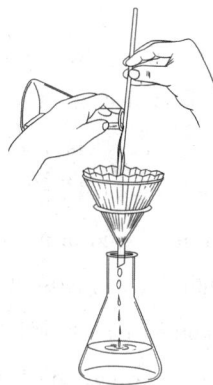

Figure 2 – 6　Executing a miniscale gravityfiltration

Be sure to pour the hot liquid on the upper portion of the filter paper in order to maximize the efficiency of the filtration. In this way the solution will come in contact with a larger area of the filter paper, and thus will be filtered more rapidly. Be careful, however, not to allow any solution to pass between the edge of the paper and the funnel.

One of several possible ways of folding a fluted filter is shown in Figure 2 – 7. Fold the paper in half, and then into quarters. Fold edge 2 into 3 to form edge 4, and then 1 into 3 to form 5 (a). Now fold 2 into 5 to form 6, and 1 into 4 to form 7 (b). Continue by folding 2 into 4 to form 8, and 1 into 5 to form 9 (c); the paper now appears as in (d). Note that all folds have been in the same direction. Do not crease the folds tightly at the center because this might weaken the paper and cause it to tear during filtration. Now make new folds in the opposite direction between 1 and 9, 9 and 5, 5 and 7, and so on, giving the paper a fanlike appearance (e). Open the paper (f) and fold each of the sections 1 and 2 in half with reverse folds to form (g). The paper is now ready to use.

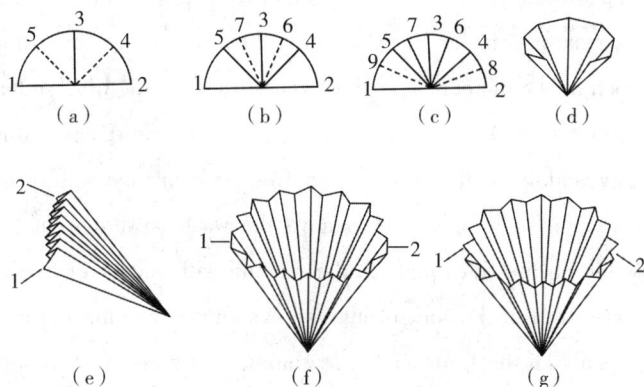

Figure 2 – 7　Folding of a fluted filter

(5) Crystallization　The hot filtrate is allowed to cool slowly by standing at room temperature. Crystallization should then result. Rapid cooling by immersion in water, for example, is undesirable because the crystals formed will tend to be quite small. Their large surface area may then facilitate adsorption of impurities from the solution. Generally the solution should not be agitated while cooling, since this will also lead to formation of small crystals. However, formation of very large crystals (larger than approximately 2mm) may cause occlusion (trapping) of solution within the crystals. Such crystals are difficult to dry and will, when dried, have deposits of impurities in them. If

large crystals seem to be forming, agitation may be used to lower the average crystal size. Judgment of proper crystal size will become easier with experience. After the hot filtrate is cooled to room temperature, it is cooled in an ice bath to complete the crystallization and reduce the loss.

（6）Filtration   The cool mixture of crystals and solution is now filtered by vacuum filtration, using a Büchner funnel and a vacuum filter flask attached to an aspirator or house vacuum line through a trap, as shown in Figure 2 – 8. The trap prevents water from the aspirator from backing up into the filter flask in case of loss of water pressure. The flask used for the trap should be a heavy-walled Erlenmeyer flask or bottle, or a second vacuum filter flask. If a filter flask is used, employ a two-holed stopper and attach to the side arm the tube leading to the aspirator. Before filtration, the filter paper, which should be of a size to lay flat on the funnel plate, should be wetted with the solvent in order to "seal" it to the funnel.

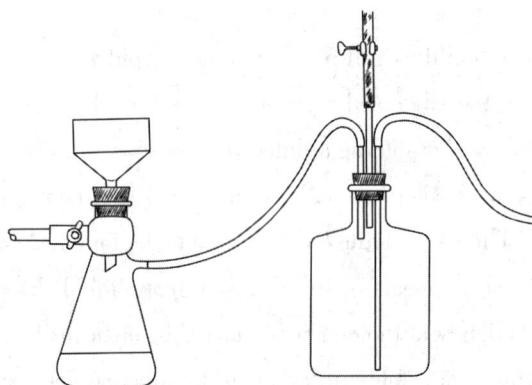

Figure 2 – 8   Apparatus for vacuum filtration

A stirring rod or spatula may be used as an aid in transferring the crystals to the funnel. The last quantity of crystals may be transferred by washing them out of the flask with some of the filtrate (mother liquor). As soon as the mother liquor has passed through the filter, release the suction by opening the screw clamp or stopcock on the trap. Wash the crystals to remove adhering mother liquor, containing impurities, by adding to the funnel cold fresh solvent just sufficient to cover the crystals. Close the trap to reapply suction and to remove the wash solvent from the crystals. Press the crystals as dry as possible on the filter plate under suction with a cork or a spatula.

Drying the crystals   Most of the solvent may be evaporated by allowing the aspirator to pull air through the mass of crystals on the funnel for a few minutes. By means of a spatula the crystals are then transferred to a clean watch glass. Complete drying is accomplished by allowing them to air-dry for a few hours. If necessary, the drying process may be accelerated by placing the watch glass in an oven (Caution: The temperature of the oven should be at least 20℃ below the melting point of the crystals), or by placing the crystals in a vacuum desiccator.

Experimental Procedure

1. Acetanilide

Dissolution   Place 2. 0g of impure acetanilide in a 250ml beaker, add 60ml of water, cover the mouth of the beaker with a watchglass, and bring the mixture to the boiling point by heating it on an electric heater. A sign indicating the water level is made on the beaker wall (some hot water should be added to keep the water level for evaporation of water). Continue heating the mixture until the acetanilide has dissolved completely.

Decoloration　Pure acetanilide is colorless, so a colored solution indicates that treatment with decolorizing carbon is necessary. Caution: Do not add decolorizing carbon to a boiling solution! Cool the solution slightly, add a microspatula-tip full of carbon, and reheat to boiling for a few minutes. Meanwhile prepare a funnel, a fluted filter (see Figure 2 – 7), and a clean flask to receive the filtrate.

Hot filtration and crystallization　Pre-heat the short-stem funnel by a water bath or an oven, then place the fluted filter in the funnel, and arrange the receiving flask to collect the hot filtrate. Without allowing the funnel or the solution to cool, pour the solution into the filter. If the solution cannot be poured into the filter in a single portion, replace it on the electric heater and continue to heat it to prevent cooling. As soon as all of the solution has been filtered. Cover the opening of the flask with a piece of filter paper, an inverted beaker, or loose-fitting cork to exclude airborne impurities from the solution, and allow the filtrate to stand undisturbed until it has cooled to room temperature and no more crystals form. To complete the crystallization, place the flask in an ice-water bath for at least 15min.

Isolation and drying　Collect the crystals on a Büchner funnel by vacuum filtration (Figure 2 – 8) and wash the filter cake with two small portions of cold water. Press the crystals as dry as possible on the funnel with a clean cork or spatula. Spread the acetanilide on a watchglass, protecting it from airborne contaminants with a piece of filter paper, and air-dry it at room temperature or in an oven. Be certain that the temperature in the oven must be lower than the melting point of acetanilide by more than 20℃.

Analysis　Determine the melting points of the crude and recrystallized acetanilide, the weight of the latter material, and calculate your percent recovery using Equation 2 – 1.

$$percent\ recovery = \frac{weight\ of\ pure\ crystals\ recovered}{weight\ of\ original\ sample} \times 100 \qquad (2-1)$$

2. Dimethyl terephthalate

Place 1.0g of impure dimethyl terephthalate, 20ml 95% ethanol and boiling stones in a 50ml round bottom flask. Fit with an upright reflux condenser, warm the mixture on awater bath until the solvent boils. Add successive small portions of ethanol through the top of the condenser (not more than 4 ~ 6ml total) and boil gently after each addition, until the dimethyl terephthalate has dissolved; then add 1 ~ 2ml more of the solvent. Do not attempt to dissolve admixed particles of sand, grit, and so on. Record the total volume of solvent used. Meanwhile prepare a fluted filter and arrange a hot funnel and a clean dry flask to receive the filtrate. Remove the boiling solution from the water bath and cool the solution slightly. Remove the condenser, add gradually 0.2g of decolorizing carbon (caution-frothing), and swirl the solution gently. Fit the reflux condenser, reheat to boiling for a few minutes and pour the hot solution into the fluted filter. Cover the mouth of the flask containing the hot filtrate with a watch glass and allow it to cool and stand undisturbed.

Continue the procedure by following the direction forCrystallization, Isolation and Drying given for acetanilide in Part 1; however, rather than water use the solvent in which you dissolved the dimethyl terephthalate.

Analysis　Determine the melting points of the crude and recrystallized dimethy terephthalate, the weight of the latter material, and calculate your percent recovery using Equation 2 – 1.

Experimental instruction

Notes

1. During the portion of this experiment when you are pouring or transferring solutions, either wear rubber gloves or be particularly careful to avoid getting these solutions on your skin. Organic compounds are much more rapidly absorbed through the skin when they are in solution, particularly in water-soluble solvents such as ethanol, acetone, and others. It is for this reason also that you should never rinse organic materials off your skin with solvents such as acetone; instead, wash your hands thoroughly with hot water and soap.

2. Do not add decolorizing carbon to a boiling solution because it may cause the mixture to boil out of the container.

3. Flammable solvent such as ether, alcohols, and hydrocarbon must never be heated in an open flask over a burner, or manipulated neat a flame. These solvents should be heated on a water or steam bathe (or an electric hot plate having no exposed hot filament). If a burner is used, the flask must be fitted with an upright reflux condenser. Take particular care to insure that no lighted burner is nearby during the filtration of the hot solution!

Explanation

1. It is a good idea to test the solubility of a solute in a variety of solvents. Even though nice crystals may form in the first solvent you try, another one might prove better if it provides either better recovery or higher-quality crystals.

2. If no single solvent provides suitable results, a mixture of two solvents can be employed, one of the solvents being a good solvent for the sample, and the other being a poor solvent for the sample. The correct proportion of the two solvents must be determined by trial and error. Some frequently used mixed solvent pairs are 95% ethanol-water, toluene-petroleum ether, acetic acid-water, diethyl ether-alcohol, and diethyl ether-petroleum ether.

3. It is good laboratory technique to save a few crystals of the impure solid; they may be needed later to induce crystallization if problems are encountered at that step.

4. A large excess of solvent must be avoided in order to maximize the recovery of purified crystals. Solids remain soluble to some extent even in cool solution, and the recovery will be reduced by an amount which depends on both this solubility and the quantity of solvent present. If near the end of the dissolution it is apparent that additional solvent is not dissolving any more of the solid, particularly when only a relatively small quantity of solid remains, enough solvent has probably been added. The remaining solid is likely to consist of insoluble impurities and may be removed in the hot filtration step.

5. When mixed solvents are used, they must, of course, be miscible. The sample is first dissolved in the solvent in which the sample is most soluble, and then small portions of the other solvent are added until a cloudiness is formed upon addition of the second solvent. Finally, more of the first

solvent is added dropwise until the solution just becomes clear again. Occasionally it is advantageous to carry out the hot filtration step before adding the second solvent to prevent crystallization during filtration.

6. Crystallization from the solution occasionally occurs in the filter paper or on the surface of the funnel. This is most conveniently avoided by adding 2 or 3ml of the recrystallization solvent to the receiving flask and heating to boiling (Figure 2 – 9). The condensing vapors will heat the funnel, preventing crystallization. For low-boiling solvents, a steam bath may be used; for solvents boiling higher than about 90℃, an electrically heated oil bath is preferable.

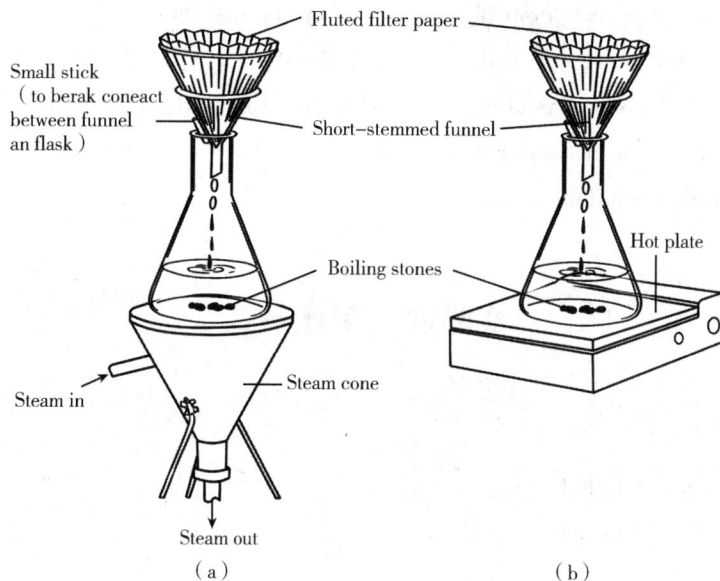

Figure 2 – 9 Miniscale hot filtration

(a) using steam cone for heating; (b) using hot plate for heating

Exercises

1. List the steps in the systematic procedure for miniscale recrystallization, briefly explaining the purpose of each step.

2. The goal of the recrystallization procedure is to obtain purified material with a maximized recovery. For each of the items listed explain why this goal would be adversely affected.

(1) In the solution step, an unnecessarily large volume of solvent is used.

(2) The crystals obtained after filtration are not washed with fresh cold solvent before drying.

(3) The crystals referred to in (2) are washed with fresh hot solvent.

(4) A large quantity of decolorizing carbon is used.

(5) Crystals are obtained by breaking up the solidified mass of an oil that originally separated from the hot solution.

(6) Crystallization is accelerated by immediately placing the flask of hot solution in an ice-water bath.

3. Why should decolorizing carbon not be added to a solvent that is at or near its boiling point?

4. By marking yes (Y) or no (N), specify which of the following criteria are met by a good solvent for a recrystallization.

（1）The solutes are soluble in the cold solvent.

（2）The solvent does not react chemically with the solutes.

（3）The solvent is polar rather than nonpolar.

（4）The boiling point of the solvent is above 100℃

（5）The boiling point of the solvent ideally is below the melting point of the solute being purified.

5. Why should the size of crystals obtained in a recrystallization be neither too large nor too small?

6. A second crop of crystals may be obtained by concentrating the vacuum filtrate and cooling. Why is this crop of crystals probably less pure than the first crop?

7. How is the purity of a recrystallized solid assessed?

8. When the solids to be crystallized are heated and dissolved, why add a solvent slightly less than the calculated amount (according to solubility data)? Then why do you add it to just dissolve, and then add a small amount of solvent?

实验四　常压蒸馏

【目的要求】

1. **掌握**　常压蒸馏的操作方法。
2. **了解**　常压蒸馏的原理及应用。

【实验原理】

蒸馏是提纯液体物质的常用方法，其基本过程是将液体加热至沸，使液体气化，然后将蒸气冷凝到另一容器中成为液体。蒸馏纯液体化合物时，蒸气从烧瓶中升起，触及温度计，再经过冷凝管，冷凝成液体，进入接受瓶。只要气液两相共存，温度将保持不变［图2－10（a）］。如蒸馏沸点相差较大的二组分液体，第一馏分蒸出时，温度保持不变。温度不变，馏出液的纯度较高。第一馏分蒸完，温度快速上升，然后第二馏分蒸出，温度又保持不变［图2－10（c）］。

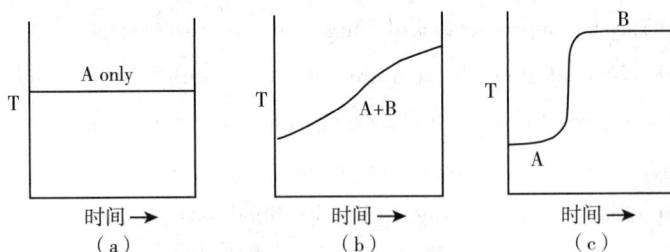

图2－10　蒸馏时三种典型的温度曲线

（a）相对较好的组分的蒸馏；（b）具有相近沸点的两组分混合物的蒸馏；

（c）沸点相差较大的两组分混合物的蒸馏，A和B能实现很好分离

沸点相差20～30℃以上，可用普通蒸馏的方法分离。当二组分沸点相差不大，或需要较高纯度时，可用分馏法提纯。

【仪器和技术】

普通蒸馏装置如图 2 – 11 所示，蒸馏瓶、冷凝管、真空接液管都需要固定。合理安装仪器装置是重要的实验技巧，它关系着实验的安全。如连接较松，蒸馏时易燃蒸气可能泄漏，泄漏的蒸气可能被附近明火点燃，发生燃烧或爆炸事故。搭建玻璃仪器装置时还应注意夹子所处的位置。初学者一般夹得过紧，这会导致不安全，因夹得越紧，越有可能产生机械应力，与夹子接触部位越易破损，既有割伤危险又可能造成易燃、腐蚀性化学物质溢出。另外，夹子安放的位置不适当，将造成仪器装置不稳。使用夹子时，夹子的倾斜方向应与所夹玻璃仪器部位平行，这样夹紧后不会产生扭转张力，既不会损坏玻璃仪器，也不会松开接点，只有当仪器连接正确，夹子的位置、方向适当时，才能将夹子夹紧。对于初学者，建议开始几个实验应请指导教师检查你的玻璃仪器是否合适，安装是否安全。从实验中获得经验，找到正确使用仪器的感觉。

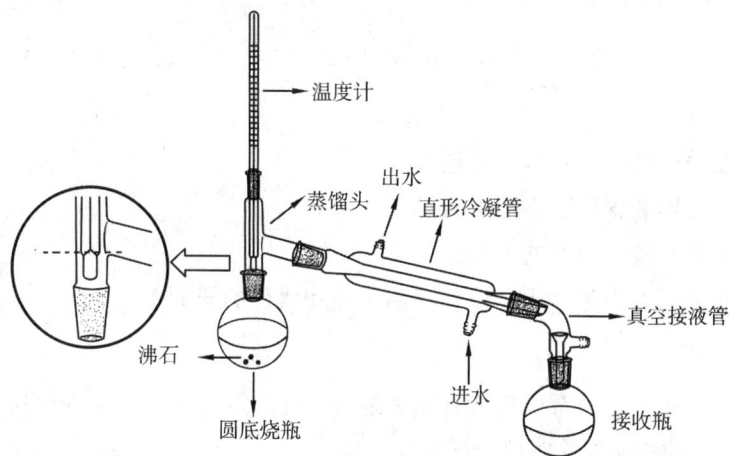

图 2 – 11　普通蒸馏装置

类似普通蒸馏这样的复杂装置，应按先下后上、先左后右的顺序进行安装。先在圆底烧瓶中加入蒸馏液和沸石，轻轻夹住圆柱部分，烧瓶要垂直，然后完全固定。调节夹子，烧瓶底部距离桌面15厘米（6英寸）左右，以便放置合适的加热器，装上蒸馏头、冷凝管，在指定位置用夹子固定。确认夹子的位置正确、倾斜方向与仪器一致后，再夹紧；微微调整，直至满意。夹子不要夹得太紧，只要使蒸馏头和冷凝管之间的接点不松脱即可。装上真空接液管，用磨口夹固定。同样，也可用磨口夹将接收瓶固定在真空接液管上，但是不能依靠磨口夹支撑较大重量。例如，250ml 或更大的瓶子，需要其他支撑，如接受液超过容积一半，100ml 接收瓶也需要其他支撑。最好将木块或升降台垫在接受瓶下。不论用哪种方法，蒸馏时接受瓶都应能很方便地移去或更换。如果用油浴或加热套加热，同样要垫升降台，调节升降台高度，以便蒸馏过程中可以移去或移入热源。蒸馏结束后，应先移去热源，停止蒸馏。

【实验步骤】

1. 样品

工业乙醇　　30ml
溴苯　　　　20ml

2. 步骤

（1）工业乙醇的蒸馏　在5ml圆底烧瓶中，加入30ml工业乙醇（通过漏斗）和2～3粒沸石，装置如图2-11所示。预测蒸出液的体积，选用适当大小的接收瓶。温度计安放的位置很重要，温度计水银球上端应和蒸馏头侧管的下限在同一水平线上。请指导教师查看你的装置后，打开冷凝水，冷凝水应从下口进入，上口流出，以保证冷凝夹层中充满水。调节中等水流，按指导教师建议的方法加热蒸馏瓶，当液体开始沸腾、蒸气到达温度计时，调节加热速度，控制蒸馏速度2～4滴/秒。当蒸馏速度调好，温度计读数恒定时，更换接受瓶，观察并记录温度计读数。继续蒸馏，定期记录馏出温度，直到蒸馏瓶内仅剩2～3ml工业酒精，停止加热。观察、记录工业酒精沸程，记下馏出液体积，完成实验后，报告指导教师。

（2）溴苯的蒸馏　在50ml圆底烧瓶中，加入20ml溴苯和2～3粒沸石，用空气冷凝管替代直形冷凝管，装置如图2-11所示，操作同工业酒精蒸馏。

【实验指导】

（一）预习要求

1. 了解常压蒸馏的原理及其应用范围。

2. 学习常压蒸馏装置的装拆顺序和操作方法。

3. 说明沸点距和液体纯度的关系。

4. 从乙醇和溴苯的物理性质比较其蒸馏仪器和操作的异同点。

（二）注意事项

1. 安装玻璃仪器前，通常要检查有无裂缝和其他缺陷，特别是检查圆底烧瓶有无星状裂缝，因为有裂缝的烧瓶加热时可能破损。

2. 正确地安装玻璃仪器可以避免仪器破损、液体溢出和蒸气泄漏。蒸馏前要确认接点紧密，装好仪器后，请指导教师检查。

3. 接受管尾部与大气相通，确保系统内外压平衡。在实验室，任何时候都不能加热密闭体系。如系统内外压不平衡，系统内物质受热膨胀，压力上升，可能导致爆炸。

4. 确认导水管安全接在冷凝管上，以防滑落而造成"水灾"。如使用加热板或油浴，当水管松脱时，水可能溅在电插头上或进入加热源，这存在潜在的危险。

5. 尽量避免吸入过多有机蒸气。

6. 蒸馏时切记不能蒸干，因为没有液体蒸发吸热，瓶内温度将迅速升高。许多液体，特别是烯和醚，可能含有过氧化物，浓缩时极具爆炸性。

（三）实验说明

1. 低沸点有机液体（如乙醚）非常易燃，实验室不能有明火。如图2-12所示，可用水浴进行加热；此外，真空接液管需连一根橡胶管于水槽处，并将接受瓶置于冰水浴中以防乙醚挥发外溢。

2. 若液体沸点超过130℃，蒸馏时要用空气冷凝管。

3. 蒸馏液体积占蒸馏瓶容积的1/3～2/3为宜。

4. 如使用煤气灯，蒸馏瓶应放在金属丝网上（最好有热分散中心）用铁圈支撑金属丝网。

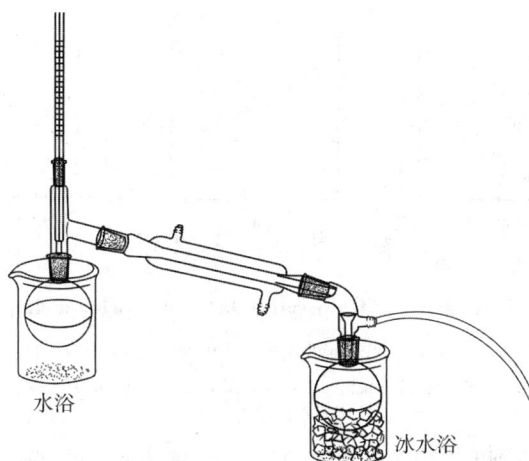

图 2－12　乙醚蒸馏装置

5. 注意冷凝管上进出水位置，进水管位置低，这样冷凝管夹层内一直充满水，水流快并没有好处，因为水压增高，可能导致橡皮管脱落。只有在必要时，才用大流量冷凝水（如蒸馏低沸点液体时）。用金属丝将橡皮管固定在冷凝管及水龙头上，这是降低橡皮管松脱危险的好方法。

6. 如液体加热后发现忘加了沸石，此时烧瓶内液体可能已经过热，必须将烧瓶内液体温度降到沸点以下，才能补加沸石，否则可能冲料。如果蒸馏中断，液体不再沸腾，沸石上小孔将充满液体。如需要继续蒸馏，原沸石已不能再用，必须另加新的沸石。

（四）思考题

1. 沸石或磁搅拌的目的是什么？

2. 普通蒸馏、分馏用冷凝管，为什么较低的引水头为进水口？

3. 温度计水银球应毗连冷凝管的出口，解释温度计水银球的位置对温度读数的影响？

（1）冷凝管出口下方。

（2）冷凝管出口上方。

4. 蒸馏液为什么要占蒸馏瓶容积的 1/3～2/3？

5. 接点严密、与大气不相通的蒸馏装置，加热蒸馏瓶中有机物时为什么有危险？

Experiment 4　Simple Distillation

Experimental principle

The most commonly used method of purifying liquids is distillation, a process that consists of vaporizing the liquid by heating and condensing the vapor in a separate vessel to yield a distillate. When a pure liquid is distilled, vapor rises from the distilling flask and comes in contact with a thermometer. The vapor then passes through a condenser which reliquefies the vapor and passes it into the receiving flask. The temperature observed during the distillation of a pure substance will remain constant throughout the distillation as long as both vapor and liquid are present in the system (see Figure 2－10a).

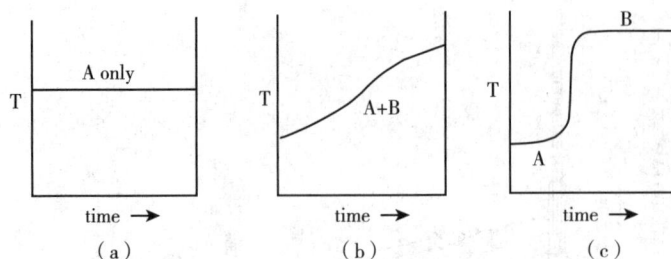

Figure 2 – 10 Three types of temperature behavior during a simple distillation

(a) a relatively pure component is being distilled; (b) a mixture of two components of similar boiling point is being distilled; (c) a mixture of two components with widely differing boiling points is being distilled. Good separation are achieved in (a) and (b).

When two components which have a large boiling point difference are distilled, one will observe that the temperature remains constant while the first component distills. If the temperature remains constant, a relatively pure substance is being distilled. After the first substance distills, the temperature of the vapors will rise, and then the second component will distill, again at a constant temperature. This is shown in Figure 2 – 10(c).

Simple distillation can sometimes be used to separate a mixture of liquids, provided the difference between the boiling points of each pure substance is greater than $20 \sim 30\ \text{℃}$. When boiling point differences are not large, and when high purity components are desired, it is necessary to do a fractional distillation.

Apparatus and technique

For a simple distillation, the apparatus shown in Figure 2 – 11 is used. The distilling flask, condenser, and vacuum adapter should be clamped.

Proper assembly of apparatus is an importantexperimental skill, which is particularly related to laboratory safety. For example, a loosely jointed distillation assembly may "leak" flammable vapors that are likely to be ignited by a nearby open fire, resulting in combustion or explosion accidents. The position of clamp should also be paid attention to. Beginners usually clamp too tightly, which is unsafe, because the tighter the clamp, the more likely it is to produce mechanical stress and the more vulnerable the contact parts with the clamp are to be damaged. This will lead to both cutting danger and possible inflammable, corrosive chemical overflow. In addition, the inappropriate placement of the clamp will cause instability of the apparatus. When using the clamp, the inclined direction of the clamp should be parallel to the position of the clamped apparatus, so that no torsional tension will occur after clamping, that is, the glass instrument will not be damaged or the contact point will not be loosened. Only when the apparatus is connected correctly and the position and direction of the clamp is appropriate, can the clamp be clamped. For beginners, it is recommended to start several experiments by asking the instructor to check whether your apparatus is suitable and safe to install. Experience is gained from the experiment to find out the feeling of using the apparatus correctly.

It is generally most efficient to put together a complex assembly from the bottom up. For example, consider assembly of the distillation apparatus shown in Figure 2 – 11.

The flask with liquid (and boiling chips!) is loosely clamped and is held in place by the column, which should be perfectly vertical and securely clamped. Adjust the clamp so that the distil-

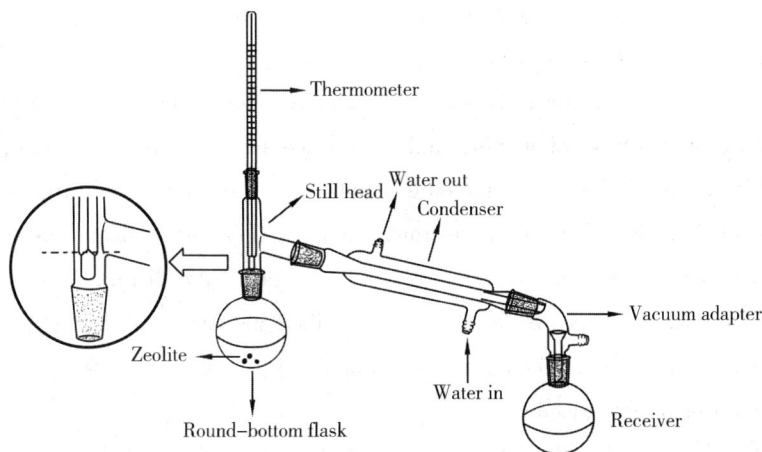

Figure 2 – 11　Typical apparatus for simple distillation

lation flask is elevated 15cm (6in.) or so above the bench to allow placement of a suitable heat source, then add the still head and thermometer. Now place the condenser in position and clamp it at the indicated position. Be sure that this clamp is properly aligned and vertically positioned before tightening it. Several minor adjustments may be needed. It is not necessary that this clamp be rigidly tight, only that it prevent the joint between the condenser and still head from slipping under normal usage. Install vacuum adapter and fix it with a grinding clamp. Similarly, the receiver flask can also be fixed on the vacuum adapter with a grinding clamp. However, you should be careful not to depend on grinding clamps to support relatively heavy weight. For example, additional support should be provided for flasks of 250ml capacity or lager, as well as 100ml flasks that may be expected to become more than half-full during the course of a distillation.

It is best if the receiving flask is supported by means of wooden blocks or laboratory jack or with a wire gauze supported by an iron ring which is attached to a ring stand. Either of these two methods will facilitate removal or change of the receiving flask during the distillation. If an oil bath or heating mantle is used for heating, it should likewise be supported by laboratory jack adjusted to such a height that the heat source can be removed from the distillation flask, by removal of the laboratory jack, to stop the distillation.

1. Materials and reagents

industrial spirit　30ml

bromobenzene　20ml

2. Procedure

(1) Distillation of industrial spirit

In a 50ml round-bottomed flask place 30ml of industrial spirit and two or three boiling chips to ensure smooth boiling. Arrange the apparatus for simple distillation according to Figure 2 – 11. Use a receiving flask of sufficient size to collect the anticipated volume of distillate. The position of the thermometer bulb is particularly important; the top of the bulb should be on a level with the bottom of the sidearm of the still head. Have your instructor check your assembly. Turn on the water tap, adjust the water flow through the condenser to a modest flow rate. Using the method of heating suggested by your instructor, begin heating the distillation flask. As soon as the liquid begins to boil and the condensing vapors have reached the thermometer bulb, regulate the heat supply so that distillation continues steadily at a rate of 2 to 4 drops per second.

As soon as the distillation rate is adjusted and the thermometer has reached a steady temperature, change the receiving flask, then note and record the head temperature. Continue the distillation, periodically recording the head temperature, until only 2 or 3ml of industrial spirit remain in the distillation flask, and then discontinue heating. Fractions (portions collected in separate flasks) are collected over narrow ranges of temperature. Note and record the distillation range of industrial spirit that you have observed. Record the volume of distilled industrial spirit that you obtain. Inform your instructor when you have completed the experiment.

(2) Distillation of bromobenzene

In a 50ml round-bottomed flask place 20ml of bromobenzene and two or three boiling chips. Using air-cooled condenser arrange the apparatus for simple distillation according to Figure 2 – 11. Continue the procedure by following the directions for distillation of industrial spirit.

Experimental instruction

Notes

1. As a general rule, always examine your glassware for cracks and other weaknesses before assembly. Look particularly for "star crack" in round-bottomed flasks because these may cause a flask to break while it is being heated.

2. Proper assembly of glassware is important in order to avoid possible breakage and spillage or the release of distillate vapors into the room. Be certain that all connections in the apparatus are tight before beginning the distillation. Have your instructor examine your set-up after it is assembled.

3. The apparatus being used is open to the atmosphere at the receiving end of the condenser. This allows for pressure equalization. At no time in the laboratory should a closed system be heated. If pressure equalization is not allowed for, material expansion within the system will result in elevated pressures and may cause the apparatus to explode.

4. Be certain that the water hoses are securely fastened to your condensers so that they will not pop off and cause a flood. If heating mantles or oil baths are used for heating in this experiment, water hoses that come loose may cause water to spray onto electrical connections or into the heating sources, either of which is potentially dangerous.

5. Avoid excessive inhalation of organic vapors at all times.

6. Distillation must always be stopped before the flask becomes completely dry. Without the absorption of heat due to vaporization, the flask temperature can rise very rapidly. Many liquids, particularly alkenes and ethers, may contain peroxides which become concentrated in highly explosive residues.

Explanation

1. Low-boiling organic liquids (for example ethyl ether) are highly flammable, so be sure that burners are not being used in the laboratory. Use flameless heating. The vapor in the collected flask should be led into a drainage tray or a ventilation hood (Figure 2 – 12).

2. When distilling materials that have boiling points in excess of 130℃, use an air-cooled condenser.

3. The size of distilling flask chosen should be such that the material to be distilled occupies between one-third and two-thirds of the bulb.

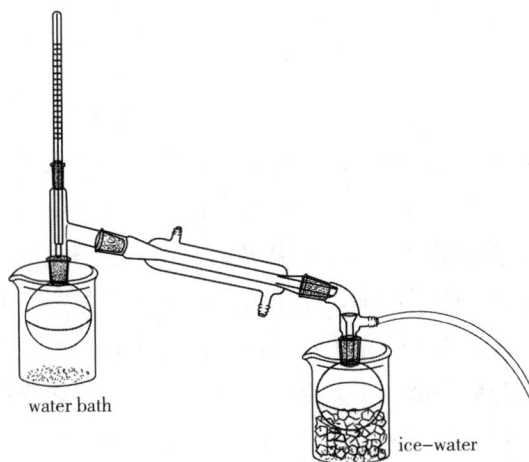

Figure 2 – 12　Miniscale apparatus for distilling ethyl ether

4. If a burner is used as a heat source, the distilling flask should rest on a piece of wire gauze (preferably one with a heat-dispersing center), which is supported on an iron ring.

5. Note the location of the "water-in" and "water out" hoses on the condenser. The tube carrying the incoming water is always attached to the lower point, which ensures that thecondenser is filled with water at all times. There is no benefit to a fast flow, and the increased pressure in the apparatus may cause a piece of rubber tubing to pop off, spraying water everywhere. Showers in the laboratory should be restricted to the emergency shower! It is good practice to wire the hoses to the condenser and to the water faucet to minimize the danger that they break loose.

6. If the boiling stone is forgotten until the liquid is hot, and possibly superheated, the flask must be cooled below the boiling point before the stone is added or the liquid may erupt. Since the pores fill with liquid as soon as boiling ceases, a stone cannot be reused, and a fresh one must be added if the distillation is interrupted.

Exercises

1. What is the purpose of the boiling chips or the magnetic stirring bar placed in a stillpot?

2. With respect to the condenser used in an apparatus for simple or fractional distillation, why should the lower rather than the upper nipple be used for the water inlet?

3. The bulb of the thermometer placed at the head of a distillation apparatus should be adjacent to the exit to the condenser. Explain the effect on the temperature reading of placement of the thermometer bulb (1) below the exit to the condenser and (2) above the exit?

4. Why should a distilling flask at the beginning of a distillation be filled to not more than two-thirds of its and filled to not less than one-third of its capacity?

5. Why is it dangerous to heat an organic compound in a distilling assembly that is closed tightly at every joint and has no vent or opening to the atmosphere?

实验五　分　馏

【目的要求】

1. **掌握**　实验室中常用的简单分馏操作。

2. **了解** 分馏的原理及其应用。

【实验原理】

简单蒸馏能满足大部分有机化合物的常规分离和提纯。但沸点相差不大的混合物或为了获得较高纯度化合物，必须采用分馏。分馏就是在蒸馏瓶和蒸馏头之间加一分馏柱（图2-13）的蒸馏。装上分馏柱且操作合理，一次蒸馏相当于连续几次的普通蒸馏。当烧瓶中的蒸气进入分馏柱时，部分冷凝成液体，向下流动。未冷凝的蒸气低沸点组分含量比冷凝液高；冷凝液中低沸点组分含量比烧瓶中液体高，沸点也较烧瓶中液体低。烧瓶中液体继续加热沸腾，新的蒸气上升至分馏柱中，与已冷凝的液体进行热交换，使其部分蒸发（新蒸气部分冷凝）。如果控制分馏柱的温度下高上低，当冷凝液向下流动时，将有部分蒸发，当蒸气上升时将有部分冷凝。未冷凝的蒸气和冷凝液蒸发形成的蒸气，在柱中越升越高，低沸点组分含量越来越高，高沸点组分含量越来越低。分馏柱中，同时不断重复这种蒸发-冷凝过程，这等于在柱内进行一系列普通蒸馏，一次次部分蒸发-部分冷凝，蒸气中易挥发组分越来越多，而向下流动的冷凝液中难挥发组分越来越多。

【仪器和技术】

分馏柱长度及类型选择取决于各组分的沸点，如各组分沸点相差15~20℃，可以用维格罗分馏柱〔图2-13（a）〕，一种带凹陷以增加分馏柱表面积的柱子。如各组分沸点相近，可以用填充柱〔图2-13（b）〕或精馏塔。填料应细碎且必须化学惰性，不与蒸馏液反应的钢丝棉也可用作填料。

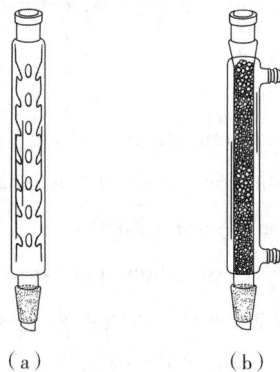

（a）	（b）	

图2-13　　　　**图2-14　分馏装置**

（a）维格罗分馏柱；（b）填充柱

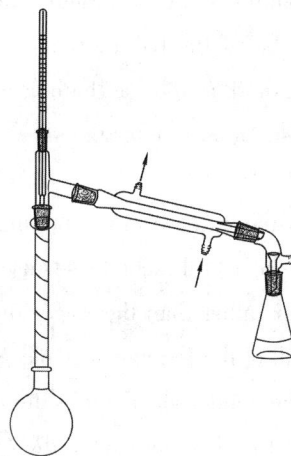

分馏装置如图2-14所示，在蒸馏瓶和蒸馏头之间有一分馏柱，其他和普通蒸馏相同。

【实验步骤】

1. 样品

环己烷　30ml

正庚烷　30ml

2. 步骤　如图2-14所示，在圆底烧瓶中，加入30ml环己烷、30ml正庚烷和2粒沸

石，安全固定分馏柱，按图2-14装好分馏装置。缓慢加热，当混合物沸腾时，仔细调节加热速度，控制蒸馏速度2ml（60滴）/分左右，第一次收集馏分如下：A瓶81~84℃，B瓶84~88℃，C瓶88~92℃，D瓶92~96℃。D馏分蒸完后，移去热源，冷却蒸馏瓶，凉干分馏柱，拆下蒸馏瓶，剩余物倾入E瓶。量出各馏分体积，结果列表（表2-3）。

表2-3　环己烷和正庚烷混合物的分馏

馏分	温度范围,℃	体积，毫升		
		第一次蒸馏	第二次蒸馏	第三次蒸馏
A	81~84			
B	84~88			
C	88~92			
D	92~96			
E	剩余物			
各馏分体积和				

如果分馏柱柱效率不足，各馏分需要再蒸馏，方法如下：将馏分A倒入圆底烧瓶，加2粒沸石，重新蒸馏，收集81~84℃馏分于A瓶；当温度升到84℃时，停止蒸馏，加入馏分B，继续蒸馏，收集馏分：A瓶81~84℃，B瓶84~88℃；当温度升到88℃时，停止蒸馏，加馏分C，继续蒸馏，收集馏分：A瓶81~84℃，B瓶84~88℃，C瓶88~92℃；当温度升到92℃时，停止蒸馏，加入馏分D，继续蒸馏，收集馏分A、B、C和D；当温度升到96℃时，停止蒸馏，加入馏分E，继续蒸馏，收集馏分A、B、C、D；当D馏分蒸完后，熄灭火焰，冷却蒸馏瓶，晾干分馏柱，拆下蒸馏瓶，剩余物倾入E瓶。量出各馏分体积，结果列表（表2-3）。如B、C、D馏分总体积大于15~20ml，按上法进行第三次蒸馏。如有必要，可进行第四次、第五次蒸馏，直至馏分A几乎全是环己烷，剩余物几乎全是正庚烷。要获得纯正庚烷，可以将剩余物E倾入小烧瓶，普通蒸馏。以各馏分温度中值为横坐标，馏出液总体积为纵坐标，绘出各次蒸馏的分馏曲线草图。在研究性实验室，蒸馏后，一般要用方便的方法分析各馏分，常用气相色谱分析各馏分。

【实验指导】

（一）预习要求

1. 理解分馏的原理和应用范围。

2. 了解常用分馏柱的种类和简单分馏操作过程。

3. 比较简单分馏和常压蒸馏的异同点。

4. 指出影响分馏效果的因素。

（二）注意事项

见实验四普通蒸馏。

（三）实验说明

1. 如使用煤气灯，烧瓶应放在有散热中心的金属网上，小火加热。将新馏分倒入蒸馏烧瓶时，应熄灭或移开火焰，因环己烷和正庚烷都有较高的蒸气压，且都易燃。

2. 为有效分馏，分馏柱保持适当的温度梯度非常重要。通常只需绝热就可保持温度梯度，在分馏柱外缠一层玻璃棉，或将镀银真空夹套套在分馏柱上，两种方法都可绝热，后者最有效。

3. 加热速度及蒸气移去的速度，显然与分馏柱温度梯度相关，如剧烈加热同时迅速移去蒸气，整个分馏柱过热，不能有效分馏（分离组分），另一方面，剧烈加热，同时顶端移去速度太慢，冷凝液聚集柱内，造成"泛流"。合理控制加热速度和"回流比"——同一时间内蒸气冷凝并回流到分馏柱的量与蒸出液量之比，一般而言，回流比越高，分馏越有效。

4. 如要记录各馏分重量而不是体积，称重带塞的接受瓶，将重量记在接受瓶标签上（皮重），最好将各接受瓶皮重也记在笔记本上，蒸馏后，称重，记下毛重，减去皮重，各馏分净重列表。如所有重量都记录在笔记本上，检查最后一行数据，如有不同表明计算有误。

5. 每次蒸馏停止后，都必须加新沸石，蒸馏完毕，瓶内剩余液体倾出，清除累积的用过沸石。

（四）思考题

1. 普通蒸馏（S）、分馏（F），哪个更适合下面工作？做上标记。

（1）由海水制备饮用水。

（2）除去对二氯苯乙醚溶液中的二氯苯。二氯苯，bp 174℃（760mmHg）；乙醚，bp 35℃（760mmHg）。

（3）从甲苯中分离出苯。苯 bp 80℃（760mmHg）；甲苯 bp 110℃（760mmHg）。

2. 分馏柱为什么必须校正到尽可能接近垂直？

3. 分离沸点相近的两组分液体时，解释为什么填充分馏柱比未填充的分馏柱有效？

4. 分馏时，如果加热太快，分离能力显著下降，根据蒸馏的一般原理解释原因。

5. 什么叫回流比？

6. 分馏柱中，顶部液体和底部液体组成有何不同（用低沸点、高沸点组分含量回答）？

7. 如果液体具有恒定的沸点，那么能否认为它是单纯物质？

8. 含水乙醇为何经过反复分馏也得不到 100% 乙醇？要制取 100% 乙醇可采用那些方法？

Experiment 5   Fractional Distillation

Experimental principle

Simple distillation works well for most routine separation and purifications of organic compounds. However, when the boiling point differences of components to be separated are not large, the technique of fractional distillation must be employed in order to obtain a good separation.

The common use of the term fractional distillation refers to a distillation operation where a fractionating column (Figure 2 – 13) has been inserted between the boiler and the vapor takeoff to the condenser. The effect of this column, when properly operated, is to give in a single distillation a separation equivalent to several successive simple distillations.

As the vapor from the distilling flask passes up through the column, some of it condenses in the column and falls back into the distilling flask. If the lower part of the distilling column is maintained at a higher temperature than the upper part of the column, the condensate will be partially revaporized as it drains down the column. The uncondensed vapor, together with that produced by revaporization of the condensate in the column, rises higher and higher in the column and undergoes a series of repeated condensations and revaporizations. This amounts to a number of simple distillations having been performed within the column, and the vapor phase produced in each step becomes richer in the more volatile component, whereas the condensate, which drains down the column, becomes richer in the less volatile component.

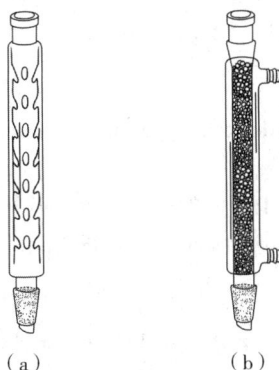

Figure 2 – 13 Fractional distillation columns

(a) Vigreux column; (b) Hempel column filled with Raschig rings

Apparatus and technique

The length and type of fractionating column required depends on the boiling points of the components to be separated. Suitable separations of components differing in boiling points by 15 to 20℃ can be accomplished by means of a Vigreux column [Figure 2 – 13(a)], a column containing indentations that increase the wall area of the column. For separations of components with closer boiling points, packed column [Figure 2 – 13(b)] or spinning band columns can be used.

The material used in a packed column should be finely divided and must be chemically insert. Small glass helices are commonly used in such columns. Steel wool may also be used providing it does not react with the components being distilled.

An apparatus for fractional distillation at atmospheric pressure or vacuum is shown in Figure 2 – 14. The principal difference between an apparatus for fractional and simple distillation is the presence of afractional distillation column between the stillpot and the stillhead.

Experimentalprocedure

1. Materials and reagents

cyclohexane   30ml

n-heptane   30ml

2. Procedure

Arrange an assembly for fractional distillation as shown in Figure 2 – 14.

Place 30ml of cyclohexane, 30ml of n-heptane in a round-bottomed flask, and two boiling chips, and fit the flask securely to the column. Heat the flask gently. As soon as the mixture starts

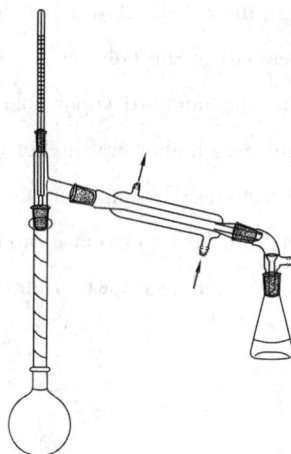

Figure 2 – 14   Miniscale apparatus for fractional distillation

to boil, regulate the heat source with particular care so that the liquid distills slowly and regularly at a rate of about 2ml (60 drops/min). In the first distillation, collect in flask A the fraction (if any) that distills between 81 and 84℃ (the 81 ~ 84℃ fraction); in flask B, the 84 ~ 88℃ fraction; in flask C, the 88 ~ 92℃ fraction; and in flask D the 92 ~ 96℃ fraction. After fraction D has distilled, remove the heat source, cool the flask, allow the column to drain, disconnect the flask, and pour the residue into E. Measure the volume of each fraction and record the results in tabular form (Table 2 – 3).

Table 2 – 3   Fractional Distillation of Cyclohexane and *n*-Heptane Mixture

Fractional	Temperature range, ℃	Volume, ml		
		1st dist'n	2nd dist'n	3rd dist'n
A	81 ~ 84			
B	84 ~ 88			
C	88 ~ 92			
D	92 ~ 96			
E	Residue			
Total volume of fractions				

If the separation efficiency of the column was not adequate, it will be necessary to redistill the different fractions. In the subsequent distillations proceed in the following way: Pour the contents of flask A into the round-bottom flask, add one or two tiny boiling chips, and redistill, collecting the 81 ~ 84℃ distillate in the same flask A. When the thermometer reaches 84℃, stop the distillation and add the contents of flask B. Continue the distillation, and collect the 81 ~ 84℃ fraction in flask A, and the 84 ~ 88℃ fraction in flask B. When the thermometer reaches 88℃, stop the distillation and add the contents of flask C. Continue the distillation and collect the 81 ~ 84℃ fraction in flask A, the 84 ~ 88℃ fraction in flask B, and the 88 ~ 92℃ fraction in flask C. When the thermometer reaches 92℃, stop the distillation and add the contents of flask D. Continue the distillation and collect the fractions A, B, C, and D. When the thermometer reaches 96℃, stop the distillation and add the contents of flask E. Continue the distillation and collect the fractions A, B, C, and D. After fraction D has distilled, extinguish the flame, cool the flask, allow the column to drain, disconnect the flask, and pour the residue into E. Measure the volume of each fraction, and record the results in tabular form.

If B, C, and D at this stage contain a total of more than 15 ~ 20ml of liquid, carry out a third distillation in the same manner. If necessary, carry out a fourth or fifth distillation, so that the fraction A will contain almost all of the cyclohexane and the residue E almost all of the *n*-heptane. To obtain almost pure *n*-heptane, E may be redistilled from a small distilling flask without a column.

Draw rough distillation graphs for each successive distillation, plotting the midpoint of the temperature range of the fractions against total volume of distillate.

In a research laboratory, it is customary to follow the progress of a distillation by some convenient analytical procedure. Gas chromatography is used commonly.

Experimental instruction

Notes

See experiment 4 simple distillation.

Explanation

1. If a burner is used as a heat source, heat the flask on a wire gauze with a heat-dispersing center, using a small flame that impinges directly below the flask. Extinguish or remove any flame when transferring fresh fractions into the round-bottom flask, since both cyclohexane and *n*-heptane have high vapor pressures and are flammable.

2. Maintenance of the proper temperature gradient in the column is a particularly important requirement for an effective fractional distillation. Frequently, this gradient can be maintain only by insulating the column with a material such as glass wool or, most effectively, with a silver-coated vacuum jacket around the outside of the column.

(1) A factor intimately related to the temperature gradient in the column is the rate of heating of the pot and the rate at which vapor is removed at the still head. If the heating is vigorous and the vapor is removed too rapidly, the whole column will heat up almost uniformly and there will be no fractionation (separation of components). On the other hand, if the pot is heated too vigorously and if vapor is removed too slowly at the top, the column will "flood" with returning condensate. Proper operation of a fractional distillation column requires judicious control of heating and "reflux ratio"— the ratio of the amount of vapor condensed and returned down the column to the amount taken off as distillate at the still head in the same time period. In general, the higher the reflux ratio, the more efficient the fractionation.

(2) If you desire to record the weight of each fraction instead of the volume, it is convenient to weigh each receiver empty, with its cork, and record this weight (called the tare) on the label of the receiver. It is good practice to record the tare of each receiver also in the notebook; when the receiver with distillate are weighed after a distillation, the gross weight is recorded, the tare subtracted, and the net weight of the fraction entered in the tabular form. If all of the weights are recorded in the notebook, you can check the figures at a later date for arithmetic errors if a discrepancy shows up.

（3）It is desirable to add a tiny fresh boiling chip each time the distillation is stopped and a new fraction introduced. At the end of the distillation series, the residual liquid in the still is poured off and the accumulated used chips are discarded.

Exercises

1. Indicate which of the two distillation techniques, simple（S）or fractional（F）, would be more suitable for the following operations by putting a check mark in the appropriate space.

（1）Preparing drinking water from sea water.

（2）Removing diethyl ether, bp 35℃（760mmHg）, from a solution containing *p*-dichlorobenzene, bp 174℃（760 mmHg）.

（3）Separating benzene, bp 80℃（760mmHg）, from toluene, bp 111℃（760mmHg）.

2. Why is it important to align the fractionating column as nearly vertical as possible?

3. Explain why a packed fractional distillation column is more efficient at separating two closely boiling liquids than an unpacked column.

4. If heat is supplied to the distillation flask too rapidly, the ability to separate two liquids by fractional distillation may be drastically reduced. In terms of the general theory of distillation presented in the discussion explain why this is so.

5. Define the term, reflux ratio.

6. How does the composition of the liquid at the top of a fractional distillation column compare with the composition of the liquid at the bottom of the column?（Answer in terms of the relative amounts of lower-boiling and higher-boiling components. ）

实验六　水蒸气蒸馏

【目的要求】

1. **掌握**　水蒸气蒸馏的仪器装置及其操作方法。
2. **了解**　水蒸气蒸馏的原理及其应用。

【实验原理】

不溶或几乎不溶于水的挥发性有机物可以用水蒸气蒸馏法分离提纯，水和有机化合物一起蒸馏的操作称为水蒸气蒸馏。当各物质不相溶时，各组分的分压（P_i）与纯物质的蒸气压（P_i^0）相等。

$$P_i = P_i^0 \tag{2-2}$$

各组分的分压与化合物在混合物中摩尔分数无关，各组分各自蒸发，相互不干扰。

根据道尔顿原理，混合物的蒸气压（P_T）等于各组分分压之和。因此，不相溶混合物的蒸气压等于各组分蒸气压之和。

$$P_T = P_a^0 + P_b^0 + \cdots P_i^0 \tag{2-3}$$

从等式可知，由于其他组分蒸气压的贡献，混合物总压力比最易挥发组分的蒸气压大，

扫码"学一学"

扫码"看一看"

混合物沸腾温度一定比组分中最低沸点还低。

水（bp 100℃）和溴苯（bp 156℃）互不相溶，通过讨论溴苯的水蒸气蒸馏，可阐明水蒸气蒸馏的主要原理。纯物质及混合物的蒸气压－温度图如图 2－15 所示。

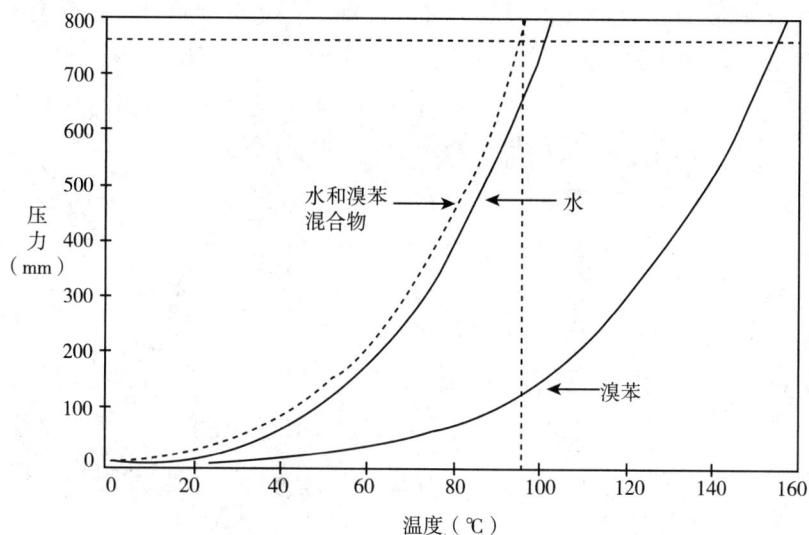

图 2－15　蒸气压－温度图

由图可知，95℃时，混合物的蒸气压等于外压，混合物应在95℃左右沸腾。这与理论预测一致，该温度低于水的沸点。由于水蒸气蒸馏的温度低于100℃，因而具有广泛用途，特别适用于对热敏感，高温会分解物质的纯化。在有机反应中，常有焦油状物生成，对从焦油状混合物中分离出有机物，水蒸气蒸馏十分有用。

水蒸气蒸馏液的组成与化合物的分子量及蒸馏温度下各组分蒸气压有关。

对于二组分混合物 A 和 B，如 A 和 B 蒸气近似理想气体，应用理想气体方程，得下面表达式：

$$P_A^0 V_A = (g_A/M_A)(RT) \qquad P_B^0 V_B = (g_B/M_B)(RT) \qquad (2-4)$$

式中 P^0 为纯液体蒸气压，V 为气体体积，g 为气相组分重量，M 为分子量，R 为气体常数，T 为绝对温度（^{0}K）。第一等式除以第二个等式得

$$\frac{P_A^0 V_A}{P_B^0 V_B} = \frac{g_A M_B (RT)}{g_B M_A (RT)} \qquad (2-5)$$

因为分子、分母中的 RT 是相同的，气体体积相同（$V_A = V_B$），等式变为

$$\frac{g_A}{g_B} = \frac{P_A^0 M_A}{P_B^0 M_B} \qquad (2-6)$$

混合物溴苯和水在 95℃时，蒸气压分别是 120mmHg 和 640mmHg（图 2－15），用式 2－6 计算蒸馏液组成：

$$\frac{g_{溴苯}}{g_{水}} = \frac{120 \times 157}{640 \times 18} = \frac{1.64}{1}$$

因而以重量计算，尽管在蒸馏温度，溴苯的蒸气压比水低很多，但蒸馏液中溴苯的含量却比水高。因为有机物分子量通常比水大得多，只要在100℃有5mmHg左右的蒸气压，就可以用水蒸气蒸馏得到良好的蒸馏效果，甚至固体也可以用水蒸气蒸馏提纯。

【仪器和技术】

从外部导入蒸气和直接在蒸馏瓶中产生蒸气是实验室常用的两种水蒸气蒸馏技术。对规模大的反应，最常用且有效的水蒸气蒸馏方法如下：在圆底烧瓶中，放置有机化合物，再装上克氏接头、蒸馏头和水冷凝管，如图 2-16 所示。

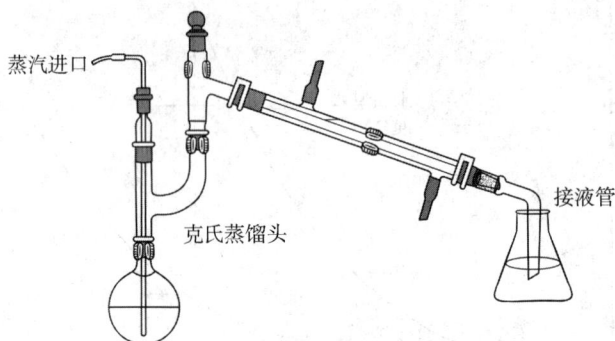

图 2-16　水蒸气蒸馏装置

水蒸气可由水蒸气发生器产生，如图 2-17 所示。在圆底烧瓶中，加入一半体积水，几粒沸石。如加热太快或导管被堵，内压将会上升，瓶上安全管可以减压。在蒸馏瓶和蒸气导管之间应安装除水器（图 2-18），除去冷凝水和蒸气中的杂质。

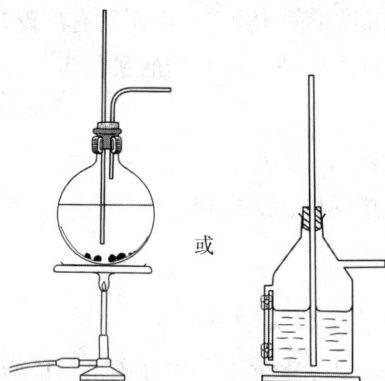

图 2-17　水蒸气发生器　　　　　　　　图 2-18　除水器

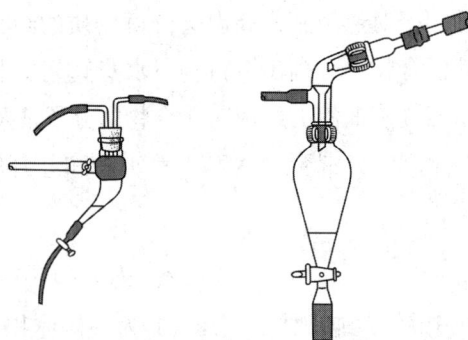

如少量水蒸气就能将混合物完全分离，可用较简单的直接蒸馏法，水和有机化合物一起放入蒸馏瓶，装置如图 2-16 所示，用塞子代替水蒸气导管，然后用煤气灯或加热套加热，收集馏出液。

【实验步骤】

1. 样品

水杨酸甲酯　　6ml

对二氯苯　　　1g

水杨酸　　　　1g

2. 步骤

（1）水杨酸甲酯的水蒸气蒸馏　根据图 2-16，在蒸馏瓶中加 6ml 水杨酸甲酯，接收瓶内加 200ml 水，牛角管水封。检查无误后通水蒸气，开始蒸馏。蒸馏过程中根据需要及时更换接收瓶，新更换的接收瓶也要预先加 200ml 水。蒸馏至再无油珠出现时结束。所有馏出液放入分液漏斗（避免振摇），静置，保留下层，上层作为废液回收处理。如需进一步精制，可用乙醚或二氯甲烷萃取，有机相用无水硫酸镁干燥后，过滤，蒸去溶剂。

（2）水蒸气蒸馏分离混合物　称 1g 对二氯苯、1g 水杨酸，先测定各样品熔点。然后在干净瓷研钵内，充分混合样品，再测定混合物熔点。

在 500ml 圆底烧瓶中放置 2g 对二氯苯和水杨酸混合样品，加少量水（瓶中水恰好能封住蒸气倒入管管口），在水蒸气发生器中加适量的水（容积的 1/2 ~ 2/3），用 250ml 锥形瓶作接收瓶，锥形瓶中加少量水（瓶中水恰好能封住牛角管管口），按图 2 - 19 装好水蒸气蒸馏装置。确认仪器已安装稳固，所有接点紧密。开始蒸馏前先将 T 形管上的螺旋夹打开，加热水蒸气发生器，当 T 形管的支管有蒸气冲出时，将夹子夹紧，让蒸气通入蒸馏瓶，同时在冷凝管内通入冷凝水，这时可以看到蒸馏瓶内混合物翻动不息，不久在冷凝管中就出现有机物质和水的混合物。调节火焰，使瓶内的混合物不致飞溅得太厉害，并控制馏出液的速度约为每分钟 2 ~ 3 滴。继续蒸馏，当馏出的蒸馏液中不再有水不溶物出现时，即可停止蒸馏，此时应先打开螺旋夹，然后停止加热。馏出液冷却过滤收集晶体，圆底瓶中残液冷却过滤收集晶体，将两种晶体分别干燥测熔点，鉴别两种晶体及其纯度。

【实验指导】

（一）预习要求

1. 了解水蒸气蒸馏的纯化原理及操作过程中的注意事项。

2. 参看实验八，了解分液漏斗的使用和保养。

3. 复习晶体的过滤收集及其干燥。

4. 复习熔点测定的操作。

（二）注意事项

1. 水蒸气蒸馏时，玻璃仪器非常烫，操作时要小心。

2. 水蒸气蒸馏结束，打开除水器放水口，取出蒸气导管。否则，蒸馏瓶中热的液体会倒流进入除水器。

（三）实验说明

1. 克氏接头能减小剧烈爆沸而将物质冲入接收瓶的可能性。它也可以用弯玻璃管代替（图 2 - 19）。

2. 水蒸气蒸馏时，蒸馏液体积不能超过蒸馏瓶容积的一半。

3. 脱水器上的螺旋夹在蒸馏前应完全打开，当水蒸气到达脱水器时，将螺旋夹夹紧。

4. 水蒸气蒸馏时，蒸馏瓶内液体有时会越来越多。如果这样，可使用加热器（如煤气灯等）加热蒸馏瓶直至瓶中的液体沸腾。使用煤气灯加热时，应用金属网分散火焰。

5. 如采用水蒸气导入法进行水蒸气蒸馏，导入水蒸气可防止爆沸，蒸馏瓶中无需加沸石。

6. 水蒸气蒸馏挥发物时，冷凝液是混浊的，共馏物冷凝后分层，出现混浊，一旦馏出液澄清，蒸馏就可以结束了。

7. 水蒸气蒸馏的物质可能在冷凝管中固化，此时应仔细观察，避免形成大块结晶，阻

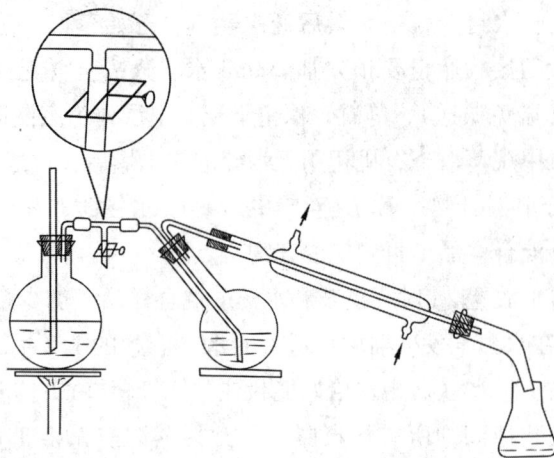

图 2-19　弯玻璃管代替克氏接头的水蒸气蒸馏装置

塞冷凝管。如大块晶体聚集冷凝管，暂时关闭冷凝水，并放掉冷凝管中水。热蒸气将熔化晶体，除去阻塞物。阻塞物一除，立即再通冷凝水。

（四）思考题

1. 指出下列各组混合物采用水蒸气蒸馏法进行分离正确与否。

（1）甲醇，bp 65℃（760mmHg），和水；甲醇与水混溶。

（2）对二氯苯，bp 174℃（760mmHg），和水；对二氯苯不溶于水。

（3）乙二醇（$HOCH_2CH_2OH$），bp 196℃（760mmHg），和水；乙二醇与水混溶。

2. 解释思考题1。

3. 为什么水蒸气蒸馏温度永远低于100℃？

4. 应用水蒸气蒸馏的化合物必须具有哪些性质？

5. 水蒸气蒸馏有哪些优点和缺点？

6. 100℃时，柠檬烯（$C_{10}H_{16}$）的蒸气压为70mmHg，如蒸馏12.6g（0.1mol）柠檬烯，需要多少水蒸气？

Experiment 6　Steam Distillation

Experimental principle

The separation and purification of volatile organic compounds that are immiscible with water or nearly so is often accomplished by steam distillation, a technique which involves the codistillation of a mixture of water and organic substances.

The partial pressure, P_i, at a given temperature of each component, i, of a mixture of immiscible, volatile substances is equal to the vapor pressure, P_i^0, of the pure compound at the same temperature (Equation 2-2) and does not depend on the mole fraction of the compound in the mixture; that is, each component of the mixture vaporizes independently of the others

$$P_i = P_i^0 \tag{2-2}$$

The total pressure, P_T, of a solution (mixture) of gases according to Dalton's law is equal to the sum of the partial pressures of the constituent gases so that the total vapor pressure of a mixture of immiscible, volatile compounds is given by Equation 2 – 3.

$$P_T = P_a^0 + P_b^0 + \cdots P_i^0 \qquad (2-3)$$

Note from this expression that the total vapor pressure of the mixture at any temperature is always greater than the vapor pressure of even the most volatile component at that temperature, owing to the contribution of the vapor pressures of the other constituents of the mixture. The boiling temperature if a mixture of immiscible compounds must then be lower than that of the lowest boiling component.

Demonstration of the principles just outlined is available from discussion of the steam distillation of a mixture of water (bp 100℃) and bromobenzene (bp 156℃) substances that are insoluble in one another. The vapor pressure versus temperature plot for a mixture of these substances, Figure 2 – 15, along with the corresponding plots for the pure liquids, shows that the mixture should boil at about 95℃, the temperature at which the total vapor pressure equals atmospheric pressure. As would be predicted from theory, this temperature is below the boiling point of water, the lowest boiling component in this example. The ability to distil a compound at the relatively low temperature of 100℃ or less by means of a steam distillation is often of great use, particularly in the purification of substances that are heat-sensitive and which would decompose at higher temperatures. It is useful also in the separation of compounds from reaction, mixtures which contain large amounts of nonvolatile resides such as the notorious "tars" so often formed during the course of an organic reaction.

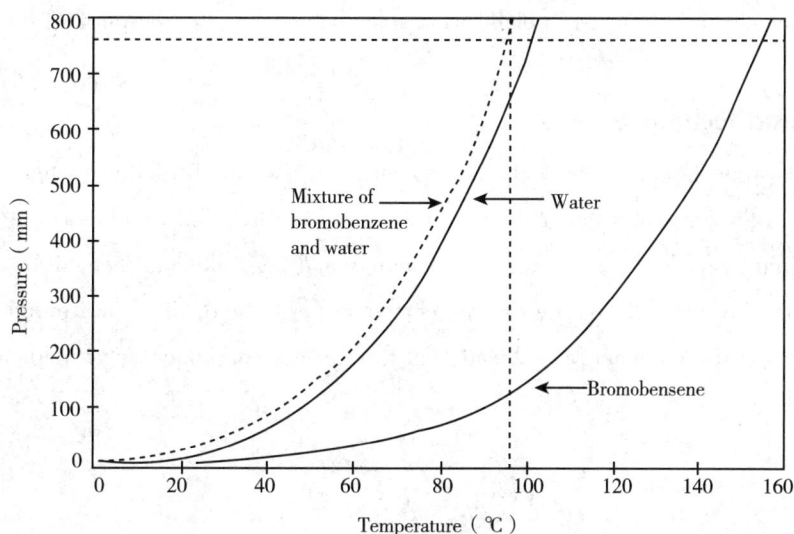

Figure 2 – 15 Vapor pressure versus temperature plots for bromobenzene,
water and a mixture of bromobenzene and water

The composition of the condensate from a steam distillation depends upon the molecular weights of the compounds being distilled and upon their respective vapor pressures at the temperature at which the mixture distils. Consider a mixture of the two immiscible components, A and B. If the vapors of A and B behave as ideal gases, the ideal gas law can be applied, and the following two expressions obtained:

$$P_A^0 V_A = (g_A/M_A)(RT) \quad and \quad P_B^0 V_B = (g_B/M_B)(RT) \qquad (2-4)$$

Where P^0 is the vapor pressure of the pure liquid, V is the volume in which the gas is con-

tained, g is the weight in grams of the component in the gas phase, M is its molecular weight, R is the universal gas constant, and T is the absolute temperature (°K). Dividing the first equation by the second, one obtains

$$\frac{P_A^0 V_A}{P_B^0 V_B} = \frac{g_A M_B (RT)}{g_B M_A (RT)} \qquad (2-5)$$

Because the RT factors in the numerator and the denominator are identical and because the volume in which the gases are contained is the same for both ($V_A = V_B$), the expression just given becomes

$$\frac{grams \quad of \quad A}{grams \quad of \quad B} = \frac{(P_A^0)(molecular \quad weight \quad of \quad A)}{(P_B^0)(molecular \quad weight \quad of \quad B)} \qquad (2-6)$$

For a mixture of bromobenzene and water, which have vapor pressures of 120 and 640mm, respectively, at 95℃ (Figure 2 – 15), the composition of the distillate would be calculated from Equation 2 – 6 as follows:

$$\frac{grams \quad of \quad bromobenzene}{grams \quad of \quad water} = \frac{120 \times 157}{640 \times 18} = \frac{1.64}{1}$$

Consequently, on the basis of weight, more bromobenzene than water is contained in the steam distillate, even though the vapor pressure of the bromobenzene is much lower at the temperature of the distillation. Because organic compounds generally have molecular weights much higher than that of water, it is possible to steam distil compounds having vapor pressures of only about 5mm at 100℃ with a fair efficiency on a weight-to-weight basis. Even solids can often be purified by steam distillation.

Apparatus and technique

The two basic techniques commonly used to carry out a steam distillation in the laboratory are differentiated on the basis of whether the steam is introduced from an external source or generated internally. For larger scale reactions, the most common and most efficient method for conducting a steam distillation involves placing the organic compound(s) to be distilled in a round-bottom flask equipped with a Claisen adapter, a stillhead, and a water-cooled condenser, as depicted in Figure 2 – 16.

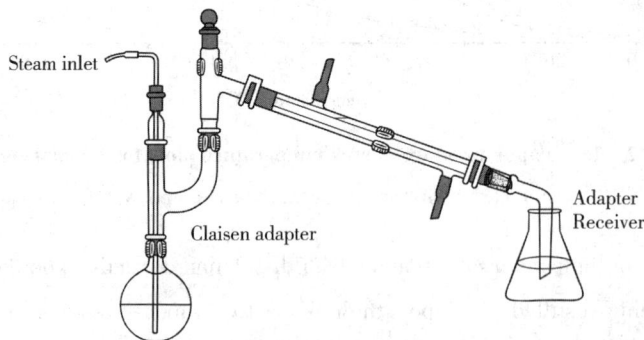

Figure 2 – 16 Apparatus for miniscale steam distillation. The steam tube is replaced with a stopper if steam is generated by direct heating

Steam may be produced externally in a generator as shown in Figure 2 – 17. The round-bottom flask is initially half-filled with water, and boiling stones are added before heating. The safety tube relieves internal pressure if steam is generated at too high a rate or the outlet tube to the apparatus becomes clogged.

A trap (Figure 2 – 18) is usually placed between the steam line and the distillation flask to permit removal of any water and/or impurities present in the steam.

If only a small amount of steam is necessary to separate a mixture completely, a simplified method involving internal steam generation may be employed. Water is added directly to the distillation flask together with the organic compounds to be separated. The flask is equipped for steam distillation by setting up the apparatus as shown in Figure 2 – 16, except that the steam inlet tube is replaced with a stopper. The flask is then heated with a Bunsen burner or heating mantle, and the distillate is collected.

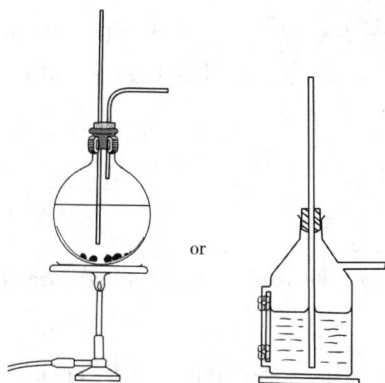

Figure 2 – 17　A steam generator

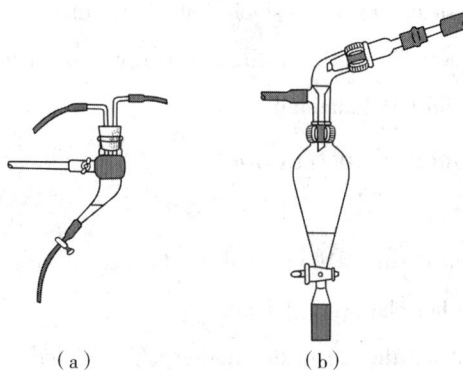

Figure 2 – 18　Water traps for use in steam distillations

(a) bent adapter trap; (b) separatory funnel trap

Experimental procedure

1. Materials and reagents

Methyl salicylate	6ml
p-dichlorobenzene	1g
salicylic acid	1g

2. Procedure

(1) Steam Distillation of methyl salicylate

An experimental device was assembled according to Figure 2 – 16. 6ml of methyl salicylate was added to the distillation bottle, 200ml of water was added to the receiving bottle. The exit of the receiver adapter was submerged in water. After checking correctly, steam was fed and the distillation was started. During the distillation process, the receiving bottle should be replaced in time as required, and the newly replaced receiving bottle should be pre-filled with 200ml of water. Distillation ends when no oil droplets appear. All distillates were put into the separatory funnel (avoid shaking), then stand a while. The lower layer was retained, and the upper layer should be recycled as waste liquid. If further purification is needed, the organic phase could be extracted with ether or dichloromethane, dried with anhydrous magnesium sulfate, filtered and distillated to remove the solvent.

（2）Separation of a Mixture by Steam Distillation

Arrange an apparatus for steam distillation as shown in Figure 2 – 16 using a 500ml round-bottom flask as the boiler and a 250ml Erlenmeyer flask as a receiver except that the steam inlet tube is replaced with a stopper. Make sure that the apparatus is supported firmly and that all stoppers and connections are tight.

Weight out 2g samples of *p*-dichlorobenzene and of salicylic acids, and determine the melting point of each sample.

In a clean porcelain mortar, thoroughly mix together the samples of *p*-dichlorobenzene and salicylic acid and determine the melting point of the mixture. Transfer the mixture to the steam distillation flask, add about 200ml of water, and heat the mixture until it boils vigorously. Continue to distill with steam until a test portion of the distillate shows that no more water-insoluble material is passing over. When the distillation is finished, save the distillate and the residue in the round-bottom flask for further examination.

Experimental instruction

Notes

1. Steam distillation involves the use of glassware that becomes very hot. Exercise care when handling hot glassware.

2. When the steam distillation is completed, the drain from the water trap must be opened and the steam inlet tube removed from the distilling flask. Otherwise, the hot liquid in the flask will "back up" into the water trap.

Explanation

1. The Claisen head helps to reduce the possibility of material being transferred to the receiving flask through excessive bumping. It may be replaced by bent glass tubes (Figure 2 – 19).

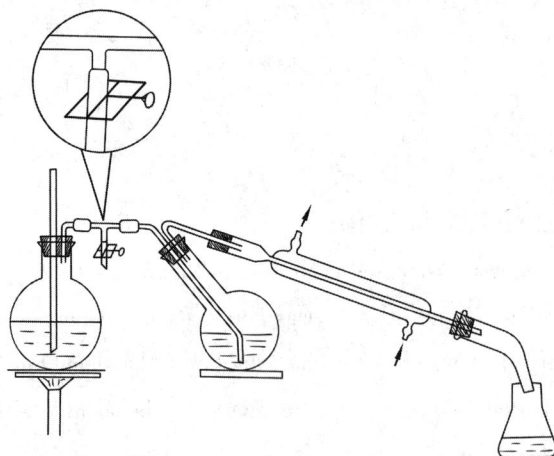

Figure 2 – 19 Steam distillation using bent glass tubes

2. The distilling flask should never be filled more than one-half full.

3. The screw clamp on the trap isopened fully before distillation. It may then be closed when the steam reaches the trap.

4. Sometimes the distilling flask may begin to fill with water during the distillation. If this happens, it may be necessary to employ a heating source such as a Bunsen burner to heat the liquid to its boiling point. The heat from the burner should be dispersed by means of a wire gauze. The entering seam helps to prevent bumping of the mixture.

5. The zeolite in the distiallation flask can be omitted if steam is introduced from an external vapor generator.

6. An ice bath can be used to increase the efficiency of the condensation of the distillate in the receiving flask.

7. The condensate will be cloudy while the steam volatile material is distilling. The substances which co-distill will separate on cooling to give this cloudiness. Once the distillate is clear, the distillation is nearly complete.

8. Since the material that distills with steam may solidify in the condenser, watch carefully to avoid the formation of a crystalline mass that may completely obstruct the condenser tube. If a large crystalline mass collects in the tube, stop the flow of water through the condenser momentarily, and drain the water from the condenser jacket. The heat from the vapors will then melt the crystals, and obstruction will be removed. As soon as this occurs, start the water again through the condenser jacket.

Exercises

1. Indicate which of the following statements is true (T) or false (F) by placing a check mark in the appropriate space.

Steam distillation would be the procedure of choice for separating mixtures of

(1) methanol, bp 65℃ (760mmHg), and water (methanol is completely miscible with water)

(2) p-dichlorobenzene, bp 174℃ (760mmHg) and water; p-dichlorobenzene is not soluble in water.

(3) Ethylene glycol ($HOCH_2CH_2OH$), bp 196℃ (760mmHg), and water; the glycol is miscible with water in all proportions.

2. Explain your answers to each part of question 1.

3. Why is the boiling point during a steam distillation always less than 100℃?

4. What properties must a substance have for steam distillation to be practical?

5. What are the advantages and disadvantages of steam distillation as a method of purification?

6. At 100℃ the vapor pressure of limonene, $C_{10}H_{16}$ is 70mm. Estimate the amount of steam required to steam distill 13. 6g (0. 1mole) of limonene.

扫码"学一学"

扫码"看一看"

实验七　减压蒸馏

【目的要求】

1. **掌握**　减压蒸馏的仪器安装和操作方法。
2. **了解**　用减压蒸馏纯化水杨酸甲酯的原理。

【实验原理】

当液体的蒸气压等于外压时，此时的温度为该液体的沸点。常压蒸馏非常方便，然而，由于许多待蒸馏化合物在低于正常沸点的温度时，就会发生分解、氧化或重排等反应。有时，杂质在高温下也能催化这些反应。而如果在低于大气压力下蒸馏，则可缓解这些问题，因为压力降低，沸点降低。这一技术就是减压蒸馏。

下面是两种估计减压对沸点影响的方法。

1. 当从一个大气压降到 25mmHg 时，高沸点化合物的沸点可由 250～300℃ 降至 100～125℃ 左右。

2. 25mmHg 以下，压力每下降一半，沸点降低 10℃ 左右。要更详尽地了解不同压力下化合物的沸点，可从文献中查阅压力 - 温度关系图或计算表，也可用物理化学介绍的 Clausius-Clapegrou 方程式的积分计算求得。

【仪器和技术】

典型的减压蒸馏装置如图 2-20 所示。待蒸馏液不能超过蒸馏瓶容积的 1/2，用油浴或其他合适的方式加热。蒸馏液液面应低于油浴液面，这样有助于防止爆沸。不能直火加热，因局部过热，易引起爆沸。油浴可用煤气灯加热，也可以用电阻丝加热。用电阻丝加热时，可用调压器控制温度。

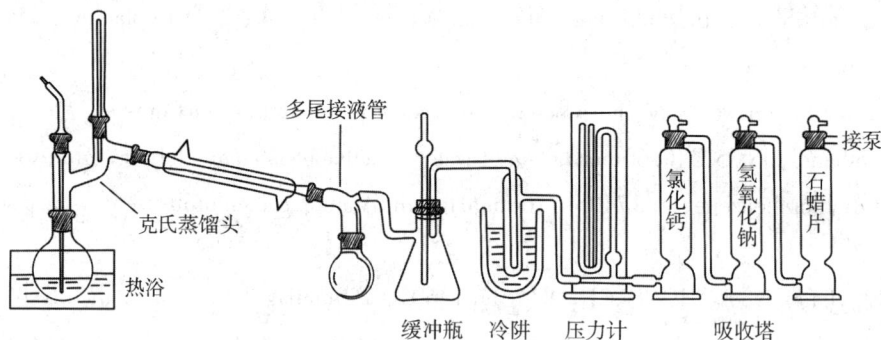

图 2-20　减压蒸馏装置（油泵抽气）

减压蒸馏时较易出现爆沸，故一般使用克氏蒸馏头，可在一定程度上可防止液体由于爆沸而冲入冷凝器。为防止蒸馏时暴沸，在克氏蒸馏头的上口插一根毛细管。毛细管下端应贴近圆底烧瓶的底部，上端连有一段橡皮管，橡皮管上夹一螺旋夹，如图 2-20 所示。螺旋夹用以调节进入空气的量和冒泡速度，保持合适的流量以提供稳定的气化中心。

此外，也可略去毛细管而直接在烧瓶中投入磁子，利用磁力搅拌保证液体受热均匀。这同样也可以有效地防止暴沸的发生。

多尾接液管与安全瓶相连。当用水泵减压水压降低时，安全瓶可防止水倒吸进入蒸馏装置。安全瓶还可用作真空支管，连接蒸馏装置、压力计，安全瓶上应有真空解压阀（活塞）。压力计可用来测量蒸馏时系统压力。

为了避免未冷凝气体污染油泵，必须用冷阱和几个不同类型的吸收塔保护油泵。冰 - 水，冰 - 盐和干冰是常用的冷阱冷却剂。根据蒸馏液的性质，选择吸收塔中的吸收剂。浓硫酸、无水氯化钙，固体氢氧化钠，粒状活性炭、石蜡片和分子筛是常用的吸收剂。

【实验步骤】

1. 样品

水杨酸甲酯（冬青油）20ml

2. 步骤

（1）检查抽气泵的效率，真空度应满足要求。

（2）按图2-20安装仪器，记住戴上防护镜！所有接收瓶都要称重，安装时在接口处涂凡士林或真空脂，封住所有接点，以防止漏气。检查固定温度计、毛细管的橡皮，确保严密不漏气。

（3）开动油泵。

（4）拧紧橡皮管上的螺旋夹，直至橡皮管几乎封闭。

（5）缓慢关闭安全瓶上的活塞。

（6）几分钟后，压力达到恒定，记录压力。如真空度不符合要求，检查所有接点是否严密。获得良好的真空度后，才能继续下面操作。

（7）缓慢打开活塞，让内外压逐渐平衡，关闭油泵，解除真空。

（8）在蒸馏瓶中用漏斗加入待蒸馏液，确证毛细管接近圆底烧瓶底部，打开油泵。此时安全瓶上的活塞应处在开启状态。真空度未达到最大，不能加热。慢慢关闭解压阀，并准备随时打开。

（9）观察毛细管中冒出的气泡，调节螺旋夹，当活塞关闭时，应有连续小气泡通过液体。

（10）当压力恒定后，开始加热蒸馏瓶。

（11）蒸馏瓶中液体沸腾后，当蒸气冷凝产生的液环逐渐上升至温度计水银球且温度计读数稳定时，收接溜出液并记录蒸馏时的温度、压力。蒸馏速度应保持1滴/秒左右，蒸馏收集101~103℃/12mmHg馏分。文献：126℃/40mmHg；115℃/20mmHg；105℃/14mmHg；101℃/12mmHg；95℃/10mmHg。

（12）当新馏分（相同压力，沸点较高）蒸出时，转动多尾接受管，更换接受瓶。

（13）蒸馏结束后，先移去加热源，让蒸馏瓶冷却，再缓慢打开螺旋夹，让系统内外压力基本平衡，然后关掉油泵、解除真空，最后移去接受瓶。

（14）实验结束后，所有玻璃仪器必须立即拆卸并清洗，以免磨口接头粘连。

【实验指导】

（一）预习要求

1. 了解减压蒸馏的原理及应用范围。

2. 指出减压蒸馏仪器装置中各部分仪器设备的名称及正确的连接顺序。

3. 了解减压蒸馏所用仪器及其安装的要求。

4. 明确操作过程中的注意事项。

（二）注意事项

1. 绝不能用有裂痕或薄壁玻璃仪器，特别是平底瓶，如锥形瓶等。即使用水泵减压，中等真空度的系统，都有几百磅的压力加在装置的外表面，薄弱点可能爆裂，急速冲进的空气粉碎玻璃，类似于爆炸。

2. 实验前仔细检查玻璃仪器，确保无裂缝。如仪器质量有问题，请教实验室管理员。

3. 实验时，必须配戴防护眼镜。

4. 当系统真空度达到最大并且稳定后才能加热。

（三）实验说明

1. 减压蒸馏时必须使用厚壁橡皮管，否则减压时橡皮管会瘪掉，如橡皮管弯折时有裂缝或能拉伸，应及时更换。

2. 减压蒸馏时，要有产生小气泡的方法，以防止液体过热或防止爆沸，传统的沸石在减压蒸馏时不起作用。减压蒸馏时常用毛细管防止爆沸，毛细管可用一节内径 6mm 的软质玻璃管拉制而成，毛细管应相当细，通过它向含丙酮的试管中吹气时，只有细小、缓慢的气泡产生。另外。如设备允许，也可在蒸馏瓶中，放一磁子（用聚四氟乙烯或玻璃包裹的柱状磁铁）代替毛细管，磁力搅拌防止爆沸。

3. 可利用压力 - 温度关系图（图 2 - 21），较精确地估计不同压力下蒸馏液体的沸点。

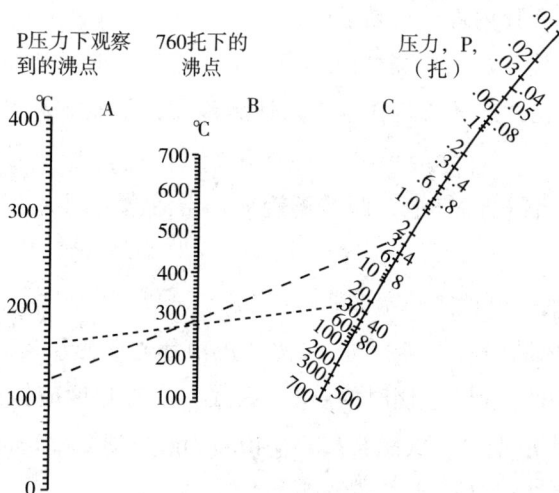

图 2 - 21　压力 - 温度关系图

4. 测量压力的装置叫压力计，压力计有许多种，在不同压力范围内精度不同。精度和压力范围能满足有机制备的经典压力计有两种：麦氏真空计（10^{-2} ~ 10mmHg）和封闭 U 型水银压力计（5 ~ 20mmHg），如图 2 - 22 所示。麦氏真空计操作如下：倾斜可动部分到垂直位置，直至较高管子里的两个水银柱与较低毛细管上沿平齐。如果压力计已校正，从毛细管水银柱高度及压力计上标尺，可直接读出压力。如使用开口或 U 型水银压力计必须用当时的大气压减去水银柱净高。近年来，电子压力计也在有机实验室中得到广泛应用。

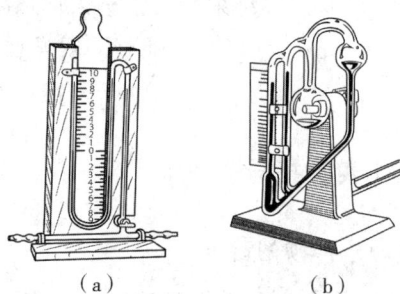

图 2 - 22　压力计
（a）封闭式；（b）开口式

5. 减压蒸馏时，压力计所测压力很重要，说明沸点时一定要有压力。例如苯甲醛在一个大气压下，180℃沸腾；35mmHg，87℃沸腾；因此其沸点表示为：bp 180℃/760mmHg 和

87℃/35 mmHg。

6. 减压蒸馏时，应维持油浴温度比馏出液温度高 25～30℃，以避免过热。

7. 待蒸馏的液体常含有少量低沸点溶剂。减压蒸馏时液体易起泡、爆沸，如果这样，调节解压阀，降低真空度，直至起泡减退。这一步骤可能要重复几次，直至溶剂完全除去。

8. 当水泵或油泵接到蒸馏装置上时，可以获得低压。水泵可达 25mmHg 左右，油泵可低于 1mmHg。油泵能获得的低压，与泵的性质、泵油质量及蒸馏装置接点密封有关。水泵的极限是水蒸气压，因而水泵压力与水管流出水的温度有关，天气较冷时，可获得 8～10mmHg 低压。

9. 蒸馏液用油泵、油浴减压蒸馏前，需先用水泵、水浴减压蒸馏，以除去蒸馏液中低沸点溶剂。

10. 减压蒸馏时要达到最高真空度，必须定期换油，蒸馏装置接点必须紧密。

11. 如毛细管上螺旋夹处在关闭状态，打开调节阀让空气进入装置，液体将会进入毛细管。

（四）思考题

1. 用图 2-21 估计下列各化合物在 1mmHg 时的沸点。

(1) 戊酸（bp 184℃）　　(2) 乙苯（bp 136℃）　　(3) 邻氯甲苯（bp 157℃）

2. 估计下列化合物在多大压力下，80℃时可以沸腾。

(1) 戊酸　　(2) 乙苯　　(3) 溴苯（bp 156℃）

3. 为什么减压蒸馏时的爆沸比普通蒸馏更麻烦？

4. 用水泵减压时，必须采用什么预防措施？

5. 在哪些方面减压蒸馏和水蒸气蒸馏有相似的优点？

6. 何种混合物用水蒸气蒸馏比用减压蒸馏分离效果更好？

Experiment 7　Vacuum Distillation

Experimental principle

The boiling point of a liquid is known to be the temperature at which the total vapor pressure is equal to the external pressure. It is most convenient to distill liquids under conditions such that the external pressure is the atmospheric pressure. In many instances, however, boiling temperature at this pressure are higher than desirable, because the compound being distilled may decompose, oxidize, or undergo molecular rearrangement at temperatures below its normal boiling point. Sometimes impurities present may catalyze such reactions at higher temperatures. These problems may often be alleviated by carrying out the distillation at pressures less than atmospheric, because under these conditions the boiling temperature is, of course, lower; the technique is commonly called vacuum distillation.

Two useful approximations of the effect of lowered pressure on boiling points are the following:

1. Reduction from atmospheric pressure to 25mm lowers the boiling point of a high-boiling compound (250～300℃) by about 100～125℃.

2. Below 25mm, each time the pressure is halved, the boiling point is lowered about 10℃. More accurate estimates of boiling points at various pressures may be made by the use of charts and nomographs found in the experiment method. Calculations may also be made using integrated forms of the Clausius-Clapeyron equation, as described in physical chemistry textbooks.

Apparatus and technique

The typical apparatus for vacuum distillation is pictured in Figure 2 – 20. The distilling flask, which should not be more than half-full, is heated by means of an oil bath or some other suitable means. The flask should be immersed to a depth above the level of the liquid in the flask as an aid in preventing bumping problems. The flask should never be heated directly with a flame because this causes localized hot spots and intensifies the problem of bumping. The oil bath may be heated with a burner or by means of electrical resistance coils immersed in the oil and connected to a variable transformer for temperature control.

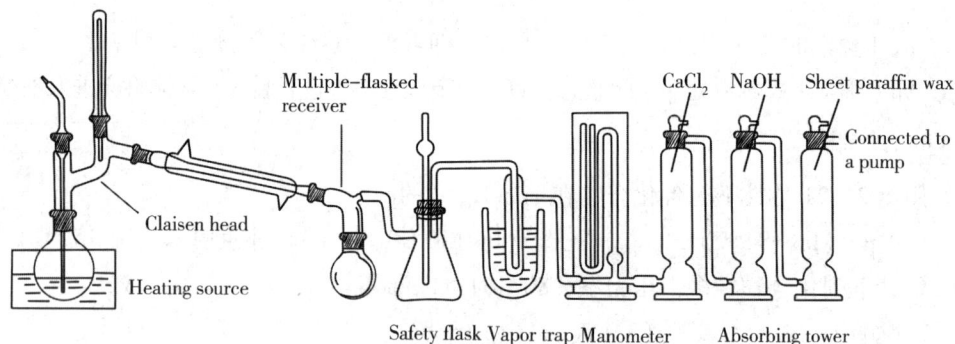

Figure 2 – 20   Typical apparatus for vacuum distillation

The capillary tube is used in conjunction with a Claisen head. The Claisen head prevents carry-over if bumping should occur. The capillary is adjusted so that it comes close to the bottom of the flask. A short section of heavy wall rubber tubing, with an open screw clamp, is attached to the capillary, as shown in Figure 2 – 20. This clamp is used to regulate the amount of air admitted to the system and the rate of production of bubbles.

Aside from the capillary, another common used method to avoid superheating is stirring. Magnetic stirrer can also be applied in this experiment.

The multiple-flasked receiver is connected to a safety flask which serves not only as a trap to prevent backup of water into the apparatus from the water pump in case of loss of water pressure, but also as a vacuum manifold, providing vacuum connections to the apparatus and manometer and bearing a vacuum release vale (stopcock). The manometer provides for measurement of the pressure at which the distillation is being effected.

In order to avoid contamination of the pump oil by any uncondensed materials from the distillation, it is important that the pump be protected by one vapor trap and several absorbing towers.

Ice-water, ice-salt and dry ice are common coolants used in vapor trap. The absorbing agent used in absorbing tower depends on the property of distilling liquid. Concentrated sulfuric acid, anhydrous calcium chloride, solid sodium hydroxide, granular active charcoal, sheet paraffin wax and molecular sieve are often used.

Experimental procedure

1. Materials and reagents

Methyl salicylate (wintergreen oil) 20ml

2. Procedure

(1) Examine the pump efficiency. The vacuum should be satisfactory.

(2) Assemble the apparatus as show in Figure 2 – 20. REMEMBER TO USE SAFETY GLASSES! Weigh each of the empty receiving flasks to be used in the collection of the various fractions to be obtained during the distillation. Lubricate and seal all glass joints during assembly as an aid against air leaks. Check the rubber fittings holding the thermometer and capillary in place to ensure that they are tight.

(3) Turn on the oil pump.

(4) Tighten the screw clamp until the tubing is nearly closed.

(5) Slowly close the stopcock on the safety flask.

(6) Record the pressure obtained after waiting a few minutes. If the pressure is not satisfactory, check all connection to see if they are tight. Do not proceed until a good vacuum is obtained.

(7) To release the vacuum in the distilling flask, open the stopcock and gradually allow the pressure to reach atmospheric pressure in the apparatus before shutting off the oil pump.

(8) Place the liquid to be distilled in the flask. Make sure the capillary tip extends nearly to the bottom of the flask and turn on the oil pump. The release valve on the safety flask should be *open*. Do not heat the flask until the system is fully evacuated. *Slowly* close the release valve, being ready to reopen it if necessary.

(9) Watch the bubbling action of the capillary to see that it is not too vigorous or too slow. Adjust the screw clamp until a fine steady stream of bubbles is formed with the stopcock closed.

(10) Begin to heat.

(11) Increase the temperature of the heat source. Eventually a reflux ring will contact the thermometer bulb and distillation will begin. Record the temperature range as well as the pressure range during the distillation. The distillate should be collected as the rate of about 1 drop per second.

(12) To change receiving flasks during distillation when a new component begins to distill (higher boiling point at the same pressure), these flasks are successively employed by rotating them into the receiving position.

Collect 101 ~ 103℃/12mmHg fraction

Literature: 126℃/40mmHg; 115℃/20mmHg; 105℃/14mmHg; 101℃/12mmHg; 95℃/10mmHg.

(13) At the end of the distillation, remove the heat source, allow the pot to cool somewhat, slowly open the screw clamp and release the vacuum. Then turn off the oil pump. Remove the receiving flask, and clean all glassware as soon as possible after disassembly to prevent the ground glass joints from sticking.

Experimental instruction

Notes

1. Never use glassware with cracks or thin-walled vessels, especially those with flat bottoms, such as Erlenmeyer flasks, in a system to be evacuated. Even with systems of only moderate size un-

der water-pump evacuation, pressures of many hundreds of pound may be exerted on the exterior surfaces of the assembly. Weak points may yield to implosion; the in-rushing air will shatter the glassware in a manner little different from an explosion.

2. Careful examination of the distilling flask to make sure that it does not have small cracks is recommended. If there is doubt about condition of the apparatus, the laboratory supervisor should be consulted.

3. SAFETY GLASSES MUST BE WORN AT ALL TIMES.

4. Do not begin heating the flask until the system is fully evacuated and the vacuum is stable.

Explanation

1. It is important that all of the rubber tubing (except for water connections to the condenser) be of the heavy wall type, so that the tubing will not collapse under the vacuum. If the rubber tubing shows evidence of cracks when it is bent or extended by pulling from both ends, it should be discarded and replaced with new tubing.

2. When distilling, a method is needed to form small bubbles to prevent superheating of the liquid, or to prevent "bumping." Conventional boiling stones will not work under a vacuum capillary (bubblers) are generally employed in most vacuum systems. A capillary is drawn from a piece of 6 – mm soft glass tubing and should be fine enough to allow only a slow stream of fine bubbles when air is blown through it into a test tube containing acetone. Alternatively, if the equipment is available, a magnetic stirring bar (a cylindrical bar magnet covered with Teflon or glass) in the flask may be employed with a magnetic stirrer.

3. Accurate estimates of the effect of pressure upon the boiling point of a liquid may be use of charts or a nomograph (Figure 2 – 21).

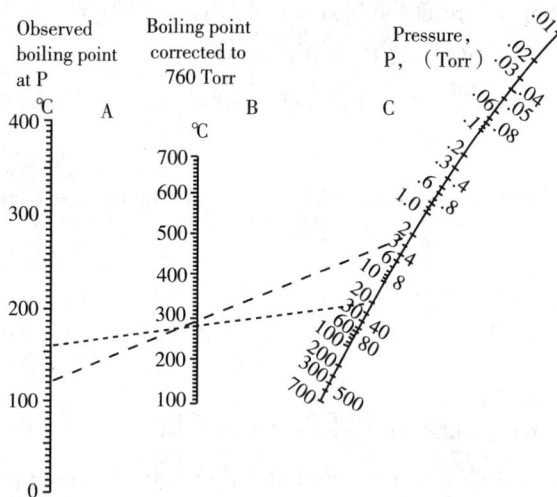

Figure 2 – 21 Pressure-temperature alignment nomograph
(dashed lines added for illustrative purposes).

Assume a reported boiling point of 120℃ at 2 mmHg. To determine the boiling point at 20 mmHg, connect 120℃ (column A) to 2 mmHg (column C) with a transparent plastic rule and observe where this line intersects column B (about 295℃). This value would correspond to the normal boiling point. Next, connect 295℃ (column B) with 20 mmHg (column C) and observe where this intersects column A (160℃). The approximate boiling point will be 160℃ at 20 mmHg.

4. The pressure is measured by a device called a manometer. There are many styles of manometers for measuring the pressure in the system, each designed for maximum precision over a small range of pressures. Two general-purposeclassic manometers that together cover a sufficient range with adequate precision of preparative work are the tilting Mcleod gauge ($10^{-2} \sim 10$mmHg) and closed-end U-tube mercury manometer ($5 \sim 200$mmHg), which are shown in Figure 2 – 22. The electronic manometers are also widely used in current organic chemistry laboratories.

The Mcleod gauge is operated by tilting the movable section of the gauge toward the upright position until the higher of the two mercury columns is level with the top of the bore of the lower capillary column. If the gauge has been calibrated properly, the pressure can be read directly from the height of the lower capillary column against the gauge markings.

With the open-tube manometer (Figure 2 – 22) it is necessary to subtract the net height of the mercury column in the manometer from the barometric pressure.

5. The manometer measures the pressure at which the distillation is being conducted; this value is important and is reported with the boiling point. For example, benzaldehyde boils at 180℃ at atmospheric pressure and at 87℃ at 35 mmHg, and these two boiling points are reported in the format: bp 180℃ (760 mmHg) and 87℃ (35 mmHg).

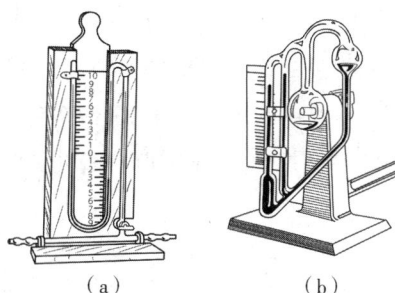

Figure 2 – 22　Manometer
(a)Closed – End U – tube Manometer;
(b)McLeod gauge

6. The difference between the actual and measured pressure can be minimized by distilling the liquid at a slow but steady rate. Superheating the vapor can be avoided by maintaining the oil bath at a temperature no more than $25 \sim 30$℃ higher than the head temperature.

7. If the distilling liquid contains small quantities of low-boiling solvents, as is often the case, foaming and bumping are likely to occur in the distillation flask. If this occurs, adjust the release valve until the foaming abates. This may have to be done several times until the solvent has been removed completely.

8. Reduced pressures may be obtained by connecting an aspirator ("water pump") or a mechanical oil pump to the distillation apparatus. An aspirator will commonly reduce the pressure to about 25mmHg and an oil pump to below 1mm. The exact pressure obtained in the lower range by an oil pump is highly dependent on the condition of the pump and its oil and on the tightness of the connections of the distillation apparatus. The vacuum produced by a water aspirator is limited by the vapor pressure, and hence by the temperature of the water issuing from the water lines; in cold climates, pressures as low as $8 \sim 10$mmHg may be obtained

9. The distilling liquid should be distilled on a water bath reduced the pressure by an aspirator before on an oil bath reduced the pressure by an oil pump.

10. It is important to clean the oil periodically and maintain tight connections in the distillation apparatus to achieve the lowest possible pressures for a particular pump.

11. If air is admitted into the apparatus at some other point while the screw clamp controlling the capillary remains closed, liquid may back up into the capillary tube.

Exercises

1. Estimate from the nomograph in Figure 2 – 21 the boiling point of each compound at 1 mm-Hg pressure.

(1) pentanoic acid (bp 184℃)

(2) ethylbenzene (bp 136℃)

(3) o-chlorotoluene (bp 157℃)

2. Estimate the pressure under which each compound could be vacuum distilled at 80℃.

(1) pentanoic acid

(2) ethylbenzene

(3) bromobenzene (bp 156℃)

3. Why is bumping more troublesome in vacuum distillation than in ordinary distillation?

4. What precautions must be observed in using an aspirator for vacuum distillation?

5. In what way are the advantages of steam distillation and vacuum distillation similar?

6. What kind of mixture may better be separated by seam distillation than by vacuum distillation?

实验八 分液漏斗萃取

【目的要求】

1. **掌握** 多步萃取的原理及操作方法。
2. **了解** 萃取和洗涤的原理、用途及操作方法。

【实验原理】

液 – 液萃取是从混合物中分离有机化合物的常用方法。事实上，合成或分离天然产物都需要这种技术以纯化产物。简单萃取涉及溶质在互不相溶的两种溶剂间的分配，这种分配可用分配系数 K 定量表示（式 2 – 7）。液体 S 和 S' 互不相溶，溶质 A 与 S 和 S' 混合物接触，溶质将在两相间分配，在一定温度下，分配达到平衡，溶质在两相中的浓度之比为常数。

$$K = \frac{S \text{中} A \text{浓度}}{S' \text{中} A \text{浓度}} \qquad (2-7)$$

理论上，A 的分配系数应等于 A 在纯溶剂 S 和 S' 中的溶解度之比，实际上仅是近似，因为没有两种液体完全不相溶。溶剂间相互溶解，将改变溶剂特性，从而略微影响 K 值。式 2 – 7 可写成 2 – 8 和 2 – 9。

$$K = \frac{S \text{中} A \text{克数}/S \text{毫升数}}{S' \text{中} A \text{克数}/S' \text{毫升数}} \qquad (2-8)$$

$$K = \frac{S \text{中} A \text{克数}}{S' \text{中} A \text{克数}} \times \frac{S' \text{毫升数}}{S \text{毫升数}} \qquad (2-9)$$

如 S 和 S' 体积相等，S 中 A 的克数与 S' 中 A 克数之比等于 K；如果 S 体积翻倍，S' 体积不变，则 S 中 A 的克数与 S' 中 A 克数之比将翻倍，因为 K 是常数。故在萃取时，将 A 提

取至溶剂 S 中，可通过增加溶剂 S 的体积提高 A 的回收量。

分配定律（式 2 - 7）的进一步推论在萃取操作的实践中非常重要。若用一定总体积的溶剂 S，从溶剂 S′ 中提取溶质，可证明将总体积分几次进行多步萃取要比总体积萃取一次更有效。分配系数越大，有效分离溶质所需的重复萃取的次数越少。

现假定溶剂 S′ 中只有两种溶质，为有效分离，萃取溶剂 S 应满足下列条件：一种溶质分配系数远大于 1，而另一种远小于 1。满足这些条件时，当分配达到平衡，一种溶质主要分配在溶剂 S，而另一个主要分配在溶剂 S′。两个液层的物理分离可使两种化合物（至少部分）被分离。

【仪器和技术】

分液漏斗有许多不同的形状，从近乎球形到拉长的梨形（图 2 - 23）。漏斗越长，两相在被振摇后分层所需时间越长。分液漏斗的活塞有玻璃和聚四氟乙烯两种，后者不需要润滑，萃取液不会受到活塞润滑脂的污染，因而更好。在化学反应结束后的后处理过程中，常要使用分液漏斗。例如，将所需产物从不相溶的一相萃取到另一相；或"洗涤"有机层，从所需有机化合物中除去不需要的物质，如酸、碱等。

使用分液漏斗，需遵守如下一些基本准则。

1. 装料　装液前，先关闭活塞，漏斗下置一干净烧杯，以防塞子未关紧而泄漏。分液漏斗不能填装超过 3/4 容积的液体，尤其在萃取时。然后用玻璃、塑料或橡皮塞塞住漏斗上口；绝大多数漏斗都配备玻璃或塑料塞子。

2. 抓握和使用　如需要振摇，用下法抓握漏斗：右撇子用左手食指顶住塞子，拇指、食指、中指抓住漏斗；右手母指、食指、中指卷曲在活塞周围［图 2 - 24（a）］。以此方式把握漏斗，可确保振摇时塞子和活塞固定紧密。左撇子左右对调。

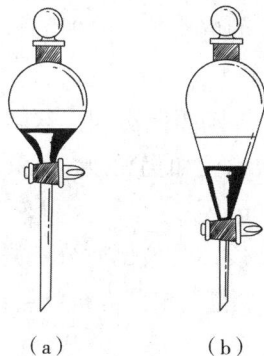

（a）

（b）

不要指向自己或他人

（c）

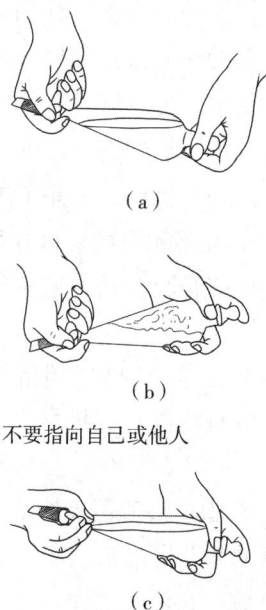

（a）　　　（b）

图 2 - 23　分液漏斗

（a）球形分液漏斗；（b）梨形分液漏斗

图 2 - 24　使用分液漏斗进行分离操作

（a）抓握分液漏斗的合适方法；

（b）振摇分液漏斗；（c）分液漏斗放气

3. 振摇 按图 2－24（b）振摇分液漏斗及内容物，让不相溶的液体充分混合。振摇将增加不相溶液体间的接触面积，加速建立溶质在两相间的分配平衡。但过于剧烈或长时间的振摇可能产生不希望出现的乳化现象（下面讨论）。

漏斗每隔几秒钟就必须放气一次，以避免漏斗内部压力积聚。放气是通过倒置漏斗来完成的，下部支管指向斜上方，朝向无人处缓慢打开，释放压力 ［图 2－24（c）］。如果漏斗没有小心地放气，液体可能会猛烈地冲出，溅到你或同伴身上。使用挥发性、低沸点溶剂（如乙醚、二氯甲烷）时，放气尤为重要；当用酸中和碳酸钠或碳酸氢钠时，因有 CO_2 产生，必须放气。如漏斗不经常放气，塞子可能会意外冲出；极端情况下，漏斗可能会炸裂。如前所述，只需握住漏斗，用卷曲在活塞周围的手指旋开活塞，即可放气，无需重新调整抓握漏斗的方式。

振摇完毕（如振摇剧烈，通常一两分钟即可），最后一次放气，置于铁圈上（图 2－25）静置分层。可事先将橡皮管从侧面剪开，覆盖在铁圈上，并用铜丝将其固定。待两层液体完全分开后，下层通过下口活塞小心放入锥形瓶。如有少量不溶物聚集在两相之间，使得界面不清，最好将其与不需要的液层一起除去，这样做会不可避免地损失少量所需液层；另一方法是在分层前进行重力或真空过滤，预先除去不溶物。

4. 液层鉴别 分液前，必须确定分液漏斗中的水层和有机层，通常密度大的液体在下层，因此被分离液体的密度是液层鉴别的重要线索。但这一通则并非万无一失，因为液层中溶质的高浓度可能会逆转两层液体的相

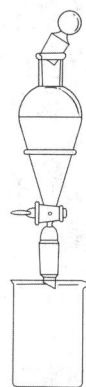

图 2－25 分液漏斗置于铁圈上，烧杯用来在漏斗泄漏时收集液体

对密度。不要因为错误的液层鉴别而丢弃所需的液层。在确认你需要哪一层之前，两层都要保留，以确保所需的产品被正确地分离。

因为有一层常是水，另一层是有机层，所以有一个简单、方便地鉴别两层液体的方法。用吸管吸几滴上层液体，加到含有 0.5ml 水的试管中，如果上层是水，液滴和试管中水混溶、消失，但如上层是有机层，液滴不溶，仍清晰可见。

5. 乳化 有时，互不相溶的液体在振摇后会生成胶体混合物而乳化，不能清晰地分层。如可能产生乳化，则应轻轻摇动，避免剧烈振摇。发生乳化的混合物经长时间放置，有时能重新分层。

（1）向漏斗中加几毫升饱和氯化钠溶液（盐水），轻轻摇动重新分层。这增加了水层的离子强度，迫使有机物进入有机层。这一过程可重复几次，但如仍无效，就必须采用其他方法。

（2）在布氏漏斗中加一薄层助滤剂，真空过滤，除去杂质，滤液倒回分液漏斗。如果不用助滤剂，滤纸的微孔可能会堵塞，过滤速度变慢。有时少量树胶状有机物会导致乳化，通常去除这些物质后，乳化可消失。

（3）加少量水溶性洗涤剂，重新分离混合物。这种方法不如前两种方法所期望的那样理想，尤其所需化合物在水层时，因为加入的洗涤剂成为一种杂质，随后必须除去。

（4）处理相转移催化反应的产物时，有时会遇到难处理的乳化，少量空气泡似乎能稳定这种乳状液。如果分液漏斗是厚壁的，可使用水泵温和减压，以加速分层。

（5）如果这些方法都无效，可能需要更换不同的萃取溶剂。

【实验步骤】

1. 样品

乙酸水溶液	15ml
乙醚	15ml
氢氧化钠溶液	
含硫酸铜和苏丹Ⅲ的乙醇－水溶液	20ml
石油醚（bp 60～90℃）	10ml×3

2. 步骤

（1）简单萃取　分配系数测定。

在小分液漏斗中，加入15ml乙酸水溶液和15ml乙醚，小心握住分液漏斗，一只手在旋塞处，另一只手在顶部塞子处。小心倒置漏斗，下部支管斜向上朝向无人处旋开活塞，放气。关闭活塞，用力振摇分液漏斗，再次放气。将分液漏斗置于铁圈上，打开上口活塞，静置。下层液体自下口活塞放出，将两层分开。量出水层体积。取10ml水层，用标准氢氧化钠溶液滴定，测定水相中乙酸的浓度。计算水相中乙酸的浓度及醚层中乙酸的量。利用这些结果，依据式2-7算出分配系数。

（2）多步萃取　在分液漏斗中，加入20ml硫酸铜和苏丹Ⅲ的乙醇－水溶液和10ml石油醚，振摇、放气，静置分层。将两层分开，收集石油醚层。水层再用10ml石油醚萃取，收集石油醚层。用10ml石油醚进行第三次萃取。将三次的石油醚层合并，加入无水氯化钙干燥20分钟以上。滤除干燥剂，随即用常压蒸馏法去除石油醚，得到较纯净的苏丹Ⅲ。

【实验指导】

（一）预习要求

1. 检索和记录苏丹Ⅲ、五水硫酸铜、石油醚（bp 60～90℃）、乙醇的化学结构（或组成）、理化常数、MSDS信息，了解其操作、储存和回收方法，个人防护要点。

2. 了解液－液萃取的原理，了解萃取溶剂的选择方法。

3. 知晓萃取的简单步骤。

（二）注意事项

1. 乙醚是挥发性易燃易爆溶剂。使用乙醚时，实验室不能有明火。

2. 使用分液漏斗时，记住要经常放气，以避免分液漏斗内压过高。解除压力时，漏斗支管不能指向任何人，支管内液体可能会喷出。

3. 如分液漏斗配备玻璃活塞，活塞上必须涂润滑脂，避免处理有机溶剂时粘连。如不涂，活塞如同"冻"在固定位置，分液漏斗无法使用。

4. 根据试剂标签，乙酸和苏丹Ⅲ是刺激性物质，实验过程中建议使用安全护目镜和耐化学品手套。

（三）实验说明

1. 根据相似相溶原理，低级醇溶于水，酯溶于醇或醚等。

2. 用稀氢氧化钠（碳酸钠或碳酸氢钠）可以提取有机溶液中的有机酸，或除去有机合成中存在的少量杂质酸。碱性水溶液将游离酸转化成相应的钠或钾盐而溶于水或稀碱溶液。

3. 稀盐酸可以相同方式提取混合物中碱性物质，或除去碱性杂质。稀酸将碱（胺、氨等）转化成水溶性盐（胺的盐酸盐、氯化铵等）。

4. 为减少两层液体相互污染，下层液体自活塞放出，上层液体从分液漏斗上口倒出。

5. 有机溶剂与水溶液混合、振摇后，有机溶剂是"湿的"，即使有机溶剂与水的混溶性不高，但有机溶剂中仍会溶解一些水。为除去有机层中的水，需使用干燥剂。最常用的干燥剂是无水无机盐，当它暴露在潮湿空气或湿溶液中，它会获得水合水。加干燥剂时，根据溶剂的体积在瓶底形成两三毫米厚的干燥剂层，至少放置 15 分钟，静置后，过滤除去干燥剂（表 2 – 4）。

表 2 – 4　可过滤除去的固体干燥剂

	酸度	水合物	容量[a]	完全度[b]	速度[c]	应用
硫酸镁	中性	$MgSO_4 \cdot 7H_2O$	高	中等	快	通用
硫酸钠	中性	$Na_2SO_4 \cdot 7H_2O$ $Na_2SO_4 \cdot 10H_2O$	高	低	中等	通用
氯化钙	中性	$CaCl_2 \cdot 2H_2O$ $CaCl_2 \cdot 6H_2O$	低	高	快	烃 卤化物
硫酸钙	中性	$CaSO_4 \cdot 1/2H_2O$ $CaSO_4 \cdot 2H_2O$	低	高	快	通用
碳酸钾	碱性	$K_2CO_3 \cdot 1/2H_2O$ $K_2CO_3 \cdot 2H_2O$	中等	中等	中等	胺，酯 碱，酮
氢氧化钾	碱性	—	—	—	快	仅胺
分子筛 （3Å 或 4Å）	中性	—	高	非常高	—	通用

[a] 单位重量干燥剂的除水量。
[b] 指干燥剂在溶液中吸水达到平衡时，溶液中残留的水量。
[c] 指作用（干燥）速度。

6. 为快速蒸馏除去大量的溶剂，大多数实验室配有旋转蒸发仪。

（四）思考题

1. 如果用有机溶剂提取水溶液，你不能确定分液漏斗中哪一层是有机层，如何迅速解决这个问题？

2. 用不相溶的溶剂从水中提取乙酸，你认为哪种方法最有效？

3. 什么是分配系数？

4. 好的萃取溶剂应具有哪些性质？

5. 解释下面事实：氢氧化钠水溶液可以提取乙醚中的乙酸。

6. 用下列溶剂提取稀水溶液中的有机物，有机层是上层还是下层？

（1）三氯甲烷　　（2）环己烷　　（3）正庚烷　　（4）二氯甲烷

7. 用甲苯（d 0.87）提取 2 – 溴乙醇（d 2.41）水溶液。

（1）你能确定有机溶液在上层吗？

（2）用什么方法能确定哪一层是非水层？

8. 采取乙醚为萃取剂，有什么缺点？

9. 为什么在萃取分液前，必须打开分液漏斗上口的塞子？

Experiment 8　Extractions Using Separatory Funnels

Experimental principle

A widely used method of separating organic compounds from mixtures is that of liquid-liquid extraction. In fact, virtually every organic synthesis or isolation of a natural product requires one or more extractions of this type at some stage for the purification of a product.

In its simplest form, extraction involves the distribution of a solute between two immiscible solvents. The distribution is expressed quantitatively in terms of the distribution (or partition) coefficient, K(Equation 2 – 7). This expression indicates that a solute, A, in contact with a mixture of two immiscible liquids, S and S', will be distributed (partitioned) between the liquids so that at equilibrium the ratio of concentrations of A in each phase will be constant, at constant temperature.

$$K = \frac{\text{concentration of A in S}}{\text{concentration of A in S}'} \qquad (2-7)$$

Ideally, the distribution coefficient of A is equal to the ratio of the individual solubilities of A in pure S and in pure S'. In practice, however, this correspondence is generally only approximate, since no two liquids are completely immiscible. The extent to which they dissolve in each other alters their solvent characteristics and thus slightly affects the value of K.

Equation 2 – 7 may be rewritten as shown in equations 2 – 8 and 2 – 9, given below:

$$K = \frac{\text{concentration of A in S/ml of S}}{\text{concentration of A in S}'/\text{ml of S}'} \qquad (2-8)$$

$$K = \frac{\text{grams of A in S}}{\text{grams of A in S}'} \times \frac{\text{ml of S}}{\text{ml of S}'} \qquad (2-9)$$

Note that when the volumes of S and S' are equal, the ratio of the grams of A in S and in S' will equal the value of K. If the volume of S is doubled and the volume of S' is kept the same, the ratio of the grams of A in S to the grams of A in S' will be increased by a factor of two. This follows because K is a constant. Therefore, if A is to be recovered by extraction into solvent S, the amount of A recovered will be increased by using larger quantities of solvent S.

A further consequence of the distribution law (Equation 2 – 7) is of practical importance in performing an extraction. If a given total volume of solvent S is to be used to separate a solute from its solution in S', it can be shown to be more efficient to effect several successive extractions with portion of that volume than one extraction with the full volume of solvent. The larger the distribution coefficient, the fewer the number of repetitive extractions that are necessary to separate the solute effectively.

Consider now a solution of two compounds in solvent S'. For effective separation of these two compounds by extraction with solvent S, the distribution coefficient of one should be significantly greater than 1.0, whereas the distribution coefficient of the other should be significantly smaller than 1.0. If these conditions are met, one compound will be mainly distributed insolvent S and the other in solvent S', at equilibrium. Physical separation of the two liquid layers would then result in at least a partial separation of the two compounds.

Apparatus and technique

Separatory funnels are available in many different shapes, ranging from almost spherical to an elongated pear shape (Figure 2 – 23); the more elongated the funnel, the longer the time required for the two liquid phase to separate after the funnel is shaken. Although separatory funnels may be equipped with either a glass or Teflon stopcock, the latter does not require lubrication and thus is the preferred type because the solutions being separated do not get contaminated with stopcock grease. Separatory funnels are most commonly used during work-up procedures after completion of a chemical reaction. For example, they are used for extracting the desired product from one immiscible liquid phases into another and for "washing" organic layers to remove undesired substances such as acids or bases from the desired organic compound.

There are a number of general guidelines for using separatory funnels that merit discussion:

1. Filling separatory funnels The stopcock should be closed and a clean beaker placed under the funnel before any liquid are added to the funnel in case the stopcock leaks or is not completely closed. A separatory funnel should never be more than three-quarters full, especially when doing an extraction. The upper opening of the funnel is then stoppered either with a ground-glass, plastic, or rubber stopper; most separatory funnels are now fitted with a ground-glass or plastic stopper.

2. Holding and using separatory funnels If the contents of the funnel are to be shaken, it is held in a specific manner. If the user is right-handed, the stopper should be placed against the base of the index finger of the left hand and the funnel grasped with the first two fingers and the thumb. The thumb and the first two fingers of the right hand can then be curled around the stopcock [Figure 2 – 24(a)]. Holding the funnel in this manner permits the stopper and the stopcock to be held tightly in place during the shaking process. A left-handed person might find it easier to use the opposite hand for each position.

3. Shaking separatory funnels A separatory funnel and its contents should be shaken as shown in Figure 2 – 24(b) to mix the immiscible liquids as intimately as possible. The shaking process increases the surface area of contact between the immiscible liquids so that the equilibrium distribution of the solute between the two layers will be attained quickly; however, overly vigorous or lengthy shaking may produce undesired emulsions (discussed below).

The funnel must be vented every few seconds to avoid the buildup of pressure within the funnel. Venting is accomplished by inverting the funnel with the stopcock pointing upward and away from you and your neighbors and slowly opening it to release any pressure [Figure 2 – 24(c)]. If the funnel is not carefully vented, liquid may be violently expelled, covering you and your laboratory partners with the contents. Venting is particularly important when using volatile, low-boiling solvents such as diethyl ether or methylene chloride; it is also necessary whenever an acid is neutralized with either sodium carbonate or sodium bicarbonate, since CO_2 is produced. If the funnel is not vented frequently, the stopper may be accidentally blown out; under extreme circumstances the funnel might blow up. The funnel may be vented simply by holding it as described previously and opening the stopcock by twisting the fingers curled around it without readjusting your grip on the funnel.

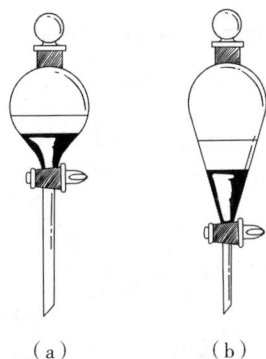

Figure 2 – 23 Separatory funnel

（a）pear-shaped；（b）conical

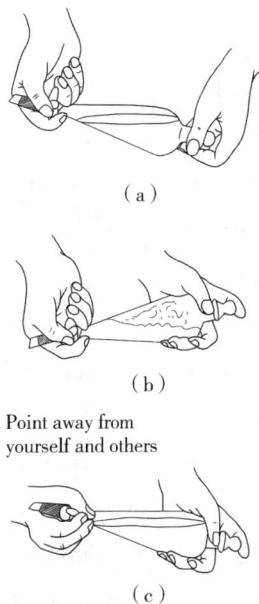

Point away from yourself and others

Figure 2 – 24 Extraction using a separetory funnel

（a）proper method for holding separatory；

（b）Shaking a separatory funnel；

（c）Venting a separatory funnel

At the end of the period of shaking of（1 ~ 2min are usually sufficient if the shaking is vigorous）, the funnel is vented a final time. It is then supported in an iron ring（Figure 2 – 25）, and the layers are allowed to separate. This may be accomplished by slicing the tubing along its side and slipping it over the ring. Copper wire may be used to fix the tubing permanently in place. The lower layer in the separatory funnel is then carefully dispensed into a flask through the stopcock while the interface between the two layers is watched. If small quantities of insoluble material collect at the boundary between the layers and make it difficult to see this interface, it is best to remove these solid with the undesired liquid layer; a small amount of the desired layer is inevitably lost by this procedure. An alternative procedure is to remove the solids by gravity or vacuum filtration before separating the layers.

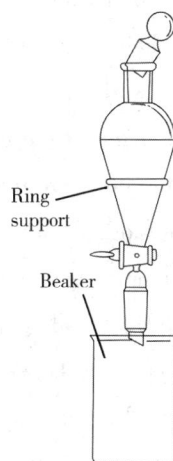

Ring support

Beaker

Figure 2 – 25 Separatory funnel positioned on iron ring with beaker located to catch liquid if funnel leaks

4. Layer identification It is important to ascertain which of the two layers in a separatory funnel is the aqueous layer and which is the organic; this may be easily accomplished with a little care and thought. Since the layers will usually separate so that the denser solvent is on the bottom, knowledge of the densities of the liquids being separated provides an important clue for this identification. This generalization is not foolproof, however, because a high concentration of a solute in one layer may reverse the relative densities of the two liquids. You must not confuse the identity of the two layers in the funnel and then discard the layer containing your product. Both layers should always be saved until there is no doubt about the identity of each and the desired product has been isolated.

Since one of the layers is usually aqueous and the other is organic, there is a simple and fool-proof method to identify the two layers. Withdraw a few drops of the upper layer with a pipet and add these drops to about 0.5ml of water in a test tube. If the upper layer is aqueous, these drops will be miscible with the water in the test tube and will dissolve, but if the upper layer is organic, the droplets will not dissolve and will remain visible

5. Emulsions   Occasionally the two immiscible liquids will not separate cleanly into two distinct layers after shaking because of an emulsion that results from a colloidal mixture of the two layers. If prior experience leads you to believe that an emulsion might form, you should avoid shaking the funnel too vigorously; instead, swirl it gently to mix the layers. Encountering an emulsion during an experiment can be extraordinarily frustrating, because there are no infallible convenient procedures for breaking up emulsions. An emulsion left unattended for an extended period of time sometimes separates. However, it is usually more expedient to attempt one or more of the following remedies:

(1) Add a few milliliters of a saturated solution of aqueous sodium chloride, commonly called brine, to the funnel and gently reshake the contents. This increases the ionic strength of the water layer, which helps force the organic material into the organic layer. This process can be repeated, but if it does not work the second time, other measures must be taken.

(2) Filter the heterogennneous mixture by vacuum filtration through a thin pad of a filter-aid, and return the filtrate to the separatory funnel; if a filter-aid is not used, the pores of the filter paper may become clogged and the filtration will be slow. Sometimes emulsions are caused by small amounts of gummy organic materials whose removal will often remedy the problem.

(3) Add a small quantity of water-soluble detergent to the mixture and reshake the mixture. This method is not as desirable as the first two techniques, particularly if the desired compounds are in the water layer, because the detergent adds an impurity that must be removed later.

(4) Sometimes intractable emulsions that appear to be stabilized by small trapped air bubbles are encountered during the work-up of phase-transfer reactions. If the separatory funnel is thick-walled, apply a gentle vacuum with a water aspirator to speed the separation of the phases.

(5) If all these procedures fail, it may be necessary to select a different extraction solvent.

Experimental procedure

1. Materials and reagents

acetic acid solution	15ml
diethyl ether	15ml
sodium hydroxide solution	
CuSO$_4$ and Sudan Ⅲ in aqueous ethanol solution	20ml
petroleum ether(bp 60 ~ 90℃)	10ml × 3

2. Procedure

（1）Simple extraction　Determination ofdistribution coefficients.

Place 15ml of the acetic acid solution and 15ml of diethyl ether in a small separatory funnel. Hold the separatory funnel carefully with one hand on the stopcock and the other on the stopper area. Invert the funnel carefully and swirl it. Tip the stopcock end up and vent the funnel by opening the stopcock. Close the stopcock and shake the funnel more vigorously. Vent again. Mount the separatory funnel on a ring stand and open the top. Separate the layers by draining the aqueous layer out the bottom stopcock. Measure the new volume of the aqueous phase. Determine the new concentration of the acetic acid in the aqueous phase by titrating a 10ml aliquot with standard sodium hydroxide solution. Calculate the concentration of acetic acid in the aqueous phase, the amount extracted into the ether phase, and use the results to determine the distribution coefficient as described in Equation 2 – 7.

（2）Multiple extractions

Place 20ml of the $CuSO_4$ and Sudan Ⅲ in aqueous ethanol solution and 10ml of petroleum ether into a separatory funnel and shake with venting. Separate the layers and collect the petroleum ether layer. Extract the aqueous phase with a second 10ml portion of petroleum ether and again collect the petroleum ether layer. Do a third extraction with 10ml of petroleum ether. The petroleum ether layer is then dried with $CaCl_2$ for at least 20 min. Filter out the desiccant and distill out petroleum ether with a simple distillation device. At last the Sudan Ⅲ product is obtained.

Experimental instruction

Notes

1. Diethyl ether is volatile and flammable solvents. No flames should be allowed in the laboratory during this experiment.

2. Remember to vent the separatory funnel frequently during its use to avoid buildup of pressure. Do not point the stem of the funnel at anyone when you release the pressure. Any liquid in the stem may be ejected forcefully

3. In the manipulation of organic solvents in a separatory funnel with a glass stopcock, it is important that the stopcock be kept properly greased to avoid sticking. If this is not done, the stopcock is likely to become "frozen" in a fixed position and the separatory funnel will be rendered useless.

4. Acetic acidand Sudan III are irritants according to the labels and thus, for this activity, the use of safety goggles and chemical-resistant gloves, is recommended.

Explanation

1. A substance is most soluble in that solvent to which it is structurally most closely related. Thus, simple alcohols are soluble in water; esters are soluble in alcohol and ether, and so on.

2. Dilute sodium hydroxide solution (also sodium carbonate or bicarbonate) can be used to extract an organic acid from its solution in an organic solvent, or to remove traces of acid that are present as an impurity in an organic preparation. The use of aqueous alkali depends upon the conversion of the free acid to the corresponding sodium or potassium salt, which is soluble in water or dilute al-

kali.

3. Dilute hydrochloric acid can be used in a similar way to extract basic substances from mixtures or to remove impurities. The use of dilute acids depends upon converting the base (amines, ammonia, etc.) into a water-soluble salt (amine hydrochloride, ammonium chloride, etc.).

4. To minimize contamination of the two layers, the lower layer should always be removed from the bottom of the separatory funnel and the upper layer from the top of the funnel.

5. After an organic solvent has been shaken with an aqueous solution, it will be "wet," that is, it will have dissolved some water even though its miscibility with water is not great. To remove water from the organic layer a drying agent is used. A drying agent is an anhydrous inorganic salt which acquires waters of hydration when exposed to moist air or a wet solution. The dry agent is added to make a 2 or 3 mm layer in the bottom of the flask, depending on the volume of the solution and allowed to stand for at least 15 minutes. After a period of standing, the crystals are removed by filtration (Table 2 - 4).

Table 2 - 4 Solid Drying Agents That Can Be Removed by Filtration

	Acidity	Hydrated	Capacity[a]	Completeness[b]	Rate[c]	Use
Magnesium sulfate	neutral	$MgSO_4 \cdot 7 H_2O$	high	medium	rapid	general
Sodium sulfate	neutral	$Na_2SO_4 \cdot 7 H_2O$ $Na_2SO_4 \cdot 10 H_2O$	high	low	medium	general
Calcium chloride	neutral	$CaCl_2 \cdot 2 H_2O$ $CaCl_2 \cdot 6 H_2O$	low	high	rapid	hydrocarbons halides
Calcium sulfate (Drierite ©)	neutral	$CaSO_4 \cdot 1/2 H_2O$ $CaSO_4 \cdot 2 H_2O$	low	high	rapid	general
Potassium carbonate	basic	$K_2CO_3 \cdot 1/2 H_2O$ $K_2CO_3 \cdot 2 H_2O$	medium	medium	medium	amines, esters bases, ketones
Potassium hydroxide	basic	–	–	–	rapid	amines only
Molecular sieves (3Å or 4 Å)	neutral	–	high	extremely high	–	general

[a] Amount of water removed per given weight of drying agent.

[b] Refers to the amount of H_2O still in solution at equilibrium with drying agent.

[c] Refers to rate of action (drying).

6. For rapid evaporation of larger volumes of solvent, rotary evaporators are standard equipment in most advanced laboratories.

Exercises

1. If, when extracting an aqueous solution with an organic solvent, you are uncertain of which layer in the separatory funnel is the organic layer, how could you quickly settle the issue?

2. What conclusion can you draw about the most efficient method of extracting acetic acid from an aqueous solution by means of an immiscible solvent?

3. What is meant by the term distribution coefficient?

4. What properties do you look for in a good solvent for extraction?

5. Explain the fact that acetic acid can be extracted quantitatively from an ether solution by di-

lute aqueous sodium hydroxide solution.

6. In the extraction of an organic compound from a dilute aqueous solution, will the organic solvent form the upper or lower layer when each of the following solvents is used?

(1) chloroform

(2) cyclohexane

(3) n-heptane

(4) methylene chloride

7. If toluene (density 0.87) is used to extract ethylene bromohydrin (density 2.41) from an aqueous solution,

(5) Could you be certain that the organic solution would form the upper layer?

(6) By what test could you determine whichthe nonaqueous layer is?

8. What are the disadvantages of using ether as extractant?

9. Why is it necessary to open thestopper at the top of the separatory funnel before separating the two layers?

实验九 薄层色谱和柱色谱

【目的要求】

1. **掌握** 薄层色谱和柱色谱分离的方法。
2. **了解** 薄层色谱和柱色谱的原理及应用。

【实验原理】

色谱法是利用混合物中各组分在两相（一相为固定相，一相为流动相）间的分配平衡不同，将各组分分开的方法。不同物质在流动相和固定相间的分配系数不同，化合物与固定相作用弱，主要在流动相，通过色谱快；化合物与固定相作用强，通过色谱慢。理想情况下，混合物中各组分有不同的分配系数，通过色谱速度不同，各组分可完全分开。

薄层色谱（TLC）是吸收色谱，吸附剂薄薄地铺在平板上，一滴溶液滴加于靠近薄层板一端，薄层板放在一容器中（展开槽），展开槽中放置足够展开剂，展开剂略低于样品点。展开剂沿薄层板上行，带动混合物中各组分以不同速度上行，产生几个点，排成一条线，与容器内溶剂液面正交（例如：图 2-26），并计算保留因子或比移值（R_f = 溶质移动的距离/溶液移动的距离）。TLC 可用于鉴别化合物，如薄层板性能一定，相对于标样或溶剂前沿（溶剂沿薄层板上行位置），化合物展开速度一定。

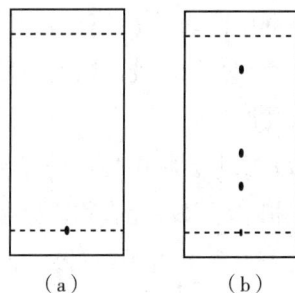

图 2-26 薄层色谱
(a) 原板；(b) 展开板

柱色谱则将固定相填充在一根特制的下端带活塞的长玻璃管中。填充固定相吸附剂时，通常可以采取干法与湿法两种不同的装柱方式。前者直接将干燥的吸附剂粉末缓缓倒入柱内，同时不断使用橡胶塞、洗耳球等弹性材料轻敲柱体，帮助粉末夯实并排出吸附剂颗粒间的空气，而后小心沿柱内壁倾入流动相溶剂，使溶剂充满柱体且略超出固定相上沿。而湿法装柱，则事先将吸附剂粉末与流动相溶剂充分搅拌混合，而后全部倾入柱中。

装柱完成后，在柱顶固定相上表面小心地加入一层待分离的混合物，混合物需水平、均匀地铺满固定相上表面。随即自柱上端投入流动相溶剂，打开色谱柱下方活塞，通过重力作用或额外加压使溶剂沿固定相向下流动进行洗脱。由于待分离混合物中各组分与固定相之间作用力不同，因而其洗脱速度也有差异。收集不同阶段的洗脱溶液即可完成不同组分的分离。

【仪器和技术】

色谱最常用的吸附剂是硅胶和氧化铝，柱色谱中使用的吸附剂颗粒较大，而薄层色谱用的则是细粉，有更大的表面积和分离能力。

根据吸附剂及待分离化合物类型，选择展开剂。不同溶剂的展开能力，即它们推动一特定物质沿固定相行进的能力，通常有下列次序。

①石油醚（bp30~60℃） ②己烷 ③四氯化碳 ④甲苯 ⑤二氯甲烷 ⑥三氯甲烷
⑦乙醚 ⑧乙酸乙酯 ⑨丙酮 ⑩1-丙醇 ⑪乙醇 ⑫甲醇 ⑬水

展开能力增强

薄层色谱通常用于检验或分离少量混合物。用量少是薄层的显著优势，有时可达10^{-9}g极限。点样时要小心，样点不能过大。样品量较大，如0.5mg样品可用吸附剂较厚的大薄层板。根据混合物中分子类型，在可见色谱图上确定各组分的位置。如果混合物中所有组分都有色，薄层板展开后，目测确定各化合物斑点。如化合物无色，有两种常用显色方法：使用含荧光染料的吸附剂或用碘蒸气显色。如使用含荧光染料的吸附剂，展开后的薄层板在低强度紫外灯下照射时，因荧光被板上化合物猝灭，在明亮荧光背景下产生暗斑。这种技术要求混合物中各组分都能猝灭荧光。有些化合物不能猝灭荧光，尤其是碳氢化合物及其他相对无极性化合物。碘蒸气显色是利用混合物中各组分化合物与碘能形成电荷转移络合物，不含π电子或路易斯碱基团的化合物与碘不形成电荷转移络合物，因而不能用碘蒸气显色。

柱色谱则可用于相对多量的混合物分离。洗脱过程中，若各组分具有明显颜色，则通过肉眼直接观察色带的下行情况即可完成组分的分离。反之若各组分无色，则可使用一系列试管连续接收不同阶段的洗脱液，而后取少量洗脱溶液进行薄层色谱展开，即可判断不同试管中的组分情况。

【实验步骤】

1. 用TLC分离顺、反偶氮苯　从指导教师处领取长10cm的硅胶薄层板（无荧光指示板）和0.5ml市售偶氮苯10%甲苯溶液。用毛细管吸取样品，在TLC板上点样，点样斑点距底边约2cm，竖边约1cm，点样斑点直径1~2mm。将硅胶薄层板晾干后放在阳光下1~2

小时，也可以将薄层板放在太阳灯下照约 20 分钟。随后再用原溶液点样，点样斑点距底边距离与第一个点样点相同，距第一个点样斑点约 1cm，将硅胶薄层板晾干。

用带盖广口瓶或小烧杯盖一表面皿作展开槽，配制正己烷∶三氯甲烷 = 9∶1（体积）溶液，将配好的溶液倒入展开槽，液面高约 1cm。沿展开槽壁放一滤纸，如图 2 - 27 所示。振摇展开槽，让溶剂蒸气饱和展开槽。薄层板展开时，溶剂饱和蒸气可以抑制薄层板上溶剂蒸发，而滤纸有助于溶剂蒸气饱和。将薄层板放入展开槽（小心！不能让溶剂溅到板上），样品点必须高于展开剂液面，展开剂将沿薄层板上行，当展开剂前沿距薄层板顶边不到 1.5cm 时，取出薄层板。将薄层板晾干，记下两个样品原点上方斑点数，比较哪个斑点更接近原点，该斑点即为顺式偶氮苯。

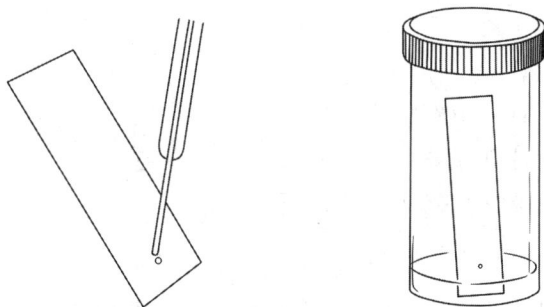

图 2 - 27　点样和展开

2. 用 TLC 分离叶绿素　在研钵里，放几片新鲜菠菜叶与几毫升 2∶1（体积比）的石油醚（bp 30 ~ 60℃）和乙醚（体积）溶液，仔细研磨。用吸管将液体转入小分液漏斗，加等体积水，旋摇，注意若剧烈振摇液体可能导致乳化。静置分层，分出、弃去下面的水层。有机层再用水洗涤两次，水相弃掉。水洗可除去乙醇及从叶子里提取的水溶性物质。将有机层倒入小锥形瓶，加 2g 无水硫酸钠干燥。放置几分钟后倾出溶液，如颜色不深，将溶液浓缩。然后从指导教师处领取 10cm×2cm 硅胶板，用毛细管将带色溶液点在硅胶板上，样品点距末端约 1.5cm。点样时，应避免样品点直径扩散超过 2mm。将硅胶板晾干，用三氯甲烷作展开剂，按前法展开。

展开后的硅胶板上有时可能会有 8 个有色斑点，按 R_f 逆减，这些斑点已被确证：胡萝卜素（两个点，橙色）、叶绿素 a（蓝绿）、叶黄素（四个点，黄色）和叶绿素 b（绿色）。

计算展开板上所有斑点的 R_f 值，同时，为了保留板上信息，将展开板上溶剂前沿、点样点和各斑点按比例画在记录本上。

3. 使用柱色谱分离二茂铁与乙酰二茂铁　如图 2 - 28 所示，取小型色谱柱一根，使用干法向其中填充氧化铝吸附剂至柱高的 2/3 左右。向柱中沿内壁缓慢加入正己烷至覆盖氧化铝上表面。取 0.090g 二茂铁与乙酰二茂铁的混合物（事先按 1∶1 比例混合均匀），使用 1.5ml 正己烷将其溶解并转移至柱中。溶解容器及柱内壁残留的样品可使

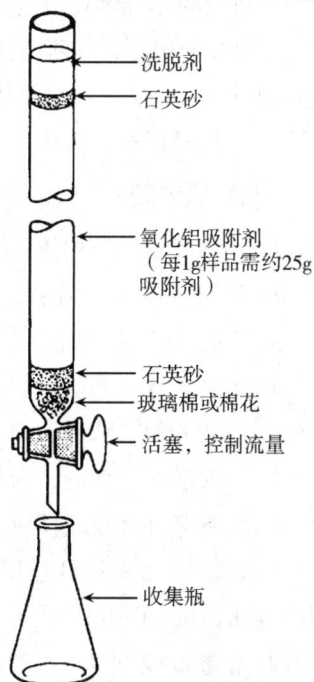

图 2 - 28　柱色谱

用少量环己烷洗涤且一并转入柱内。柱下可放置一 25ml 锥形瓶准备接收洗脱液。

从柱顶加入正己烷，利用重力进行洗脱。洗脱过程中根据情况不断投入洗脱液，防止洗脱液液面低于固定相上表面。洗脱过程中，柱内出现明显的黄色（二茂铁）、橙色（乙酰二茂铁）分离的色带。收集黄色色带对应的洗脱液至一干燥的锥形瓶中。待黄色色带完全洗脱后，改用 1∶1 的正己烷-乙醚混合溶液进行洗脱，随即橙色色带逐渐下移。使用另一个干燥锥形瓶收集橙色色带对应的洗脱液。

分别将两组洗脱液在旋转蒸发仪上蒸干溶剂，得到固体称重，计算二茂铁与乙酰二茂铁的回收率。

【实验指导】

（一）预习要求

1. 明确应用乙醚时的注意事项。

2. 了解 R_f 的意义和计算方法。

3. 了解薄层色谱的操作步骤。

（二）注意事项

1. 使用石油醚萃取叶绿素时，附近不能有明火，因其非常易燃。

2. 柱色谱装柱时必须保证固定相紧密均匀，无裂缝无气泡。

（三）实验说明

1. TLC 简单、快速，可用于混合物组成的常规分析，也可用于确定柱色谱的最佳洗脱剂。然而，必须牢记挥发性化合物（bp ＜100℃）不能用 TLC 分析。

2. 如用于鉴定，可将已知物和未知物在相同条件下进行比较，选用一系列不同展开剂（如有可能，还可选用不同吸附剂）。作最终鉴定时，文献 R_f 只能作为参考，应尽可能用未知物与可能的化合物直接比较。

3. TLC 的优点在于所需样品少（1 毫克以下）、所用时间短（一般不到 10 分钟）。TLC 在监测反应、确定反应中间体方面非常有用。

4. 一块薄层板只能用一种溶剂或混合溶剂展开，而柱色谱可以梯度洗脱。

（四）思考题

1. 两种偶氮苯异构体，哪一个热力学稳定性较高，为什么？

2. 从偶氮苯 TLC 结果，描述阳光作用。

3. 进行 TLC 实验时，为什么样品点不能浸入展开槽的溶剂里？

4. 解释为什么薄层板展开时不能让薄层板上溶剂蒸发？

5. 在实验第二部分，石油醚萃取液为什么要加无水硫酸钠？

6. 在实验第一部分，为什么要将原混合物点样？

7. 解释为什么反式偶氮苯 R_f 值比顺式大？

8. 两个组分 A 和 B 已用 TLC 分开，当溶剂前沿从样品原点算起，移动了 6.5cm 时，A 距原点 0.5cm，而 B 距原点 3.6cm。计算 A 和 B 的 R_f 值。

9. 在进行柱色谱分离时，为何样品需水平均匀地铺洒在固定相上方？若不水平，会出现什么样的情况？

Experiment 9 Thin-Layer and Column Chromatography

Experimental principle

Chromatography can be defined as the separation of a mixture into various fractions by distribution between two phases, one phase being stationary and essentially two-dimensional (a surface), and the remaining phase being mobile. The underlining principle of chromatography is that different substances have different partition coefficients between the stationary and mobile phases. A compound that interacts weakly with the stationary phase will spend most of its time in the mobile phase and move rapidly through the chromatographic system. Compounds that interact strongly with the stationary phase will move very slowly. In the ideal case, each component of a mixture will have a different partition coefficient between the mobile and stationary phases, and consequently each will move through the system at a different rate, resulting in complete separations.

Thin-layer chromatography (TLC) is a special application of adsorption chromatography in which a thin layer of the adsorbent supported on a flat surface is utilized instead of a column of the adsorbent.

A drop of the solution to be separated is placed near one edge of the plate, and the plate is placed in a container, called a developing chamber, with enough of the eluting solvent to come to a level just below the "spot" (Figure 2 – 26). The solvent migrates up the plate, carrying with it the components of the mixture at different rates. The result may then be a series of spots on the plate, falling on a line perpendicular to the solvent level in the container (see, for example, Figure 2 – 26). The retention factor (R_f) of a component can then be measures as: R_f = distance of solute movement/distance of solution movement.

TLC can be used as a tentative means of identification of a compound. If plate conditions are kept constant, a compound will progress up the plate at the same rate relative to an added standard or with respect to the solvent front (the position on the plate to which the solvent has migrated).

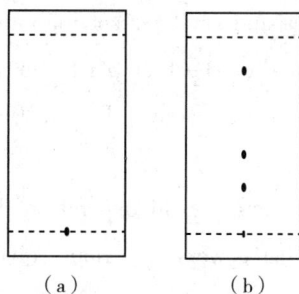

Figure 2 – 26 **The application of a solution to a TLC plate (left)**
and development of the plate in a screw-capped bottle (right)

In column chromatography, the stationary phase, a solid adsorbent, is packed in a vertical glass column with dry or slurry approach. In the dry pack technique, the adsorbent is carefully and slowly poured into the column directly. The column is gently but firmly tapped with a rubber stopper on the end of a pencil or stir rod. This tapping helps air trapped in the adsorbent powder to escape. Afterward, the solvent is carefully poured by the edge of the column to cover the adsorbent. The slurry pack technique is fundamentally the same, except, the adsorbent is mixed with, or suspended in, a small amount of solvent, and this slurry is poured into the column.

The mixture to be analyzed by column chromatography is placed inside the top of the column. The liquid solvent (the eluent) is passed through the column by gravity or by the application of air pressure. Equilibrium is established between the solute adsorbed on the adsorbent and the eluting solvent flowing down through the column. Because the different components in the mixture have different interactions with the stationary and mobile phases, they will be carried along with the mobile phase to varying degrees and a separation will be achieved. The individual components, or elutants, are collected as the solvent drips from the bottom of the column.

Column chromatographyusually uses gravity to move the mobile phase through the glass column. The sample to be separated should be dissolved with the minimum amount of solvent. When the column is drained until the solvent is right at the top of the stationary phase layer. The solution is then added dropwise to the top of the column. As the solution layer increases, the column is again drained until the mobile phase layer (solvent) is again at the top of the stationary phase layer. This is repeated until all the sample is added to the top of the column. Solvent is then added dropwise to the top of the column, trying to add the solvent down the sides of the column walls so as not to disturb the top of the column. As the solvent layer builds to 1 ~ 2 cm, the column is drained until the solvent layer is again at the top of the column. This is repeated 5 ~ 10 times, or until it is clear the sample has moved a few mm down the column. The sample is now loaded. Add solvent carefully, dropwise at first, and then by careful pouring until the column is full. From now on, never let the solvent layer drain below the top of the stationary phase layer. As the solvent drains, add more to keep the column full.

Apparatus and technique

The most commonly used adsorbents in chromatography are silica gel and alumina. The adsorbents used in TLC are of much smaller particle size than those used in column chromatography, providing for a much greater surface area and greater resolving capability. Ready-to-use TLC plates on which the adsorbent is layered on a thin sheet of plastic or aluminum are commercially available. These plates generally come in 5cm × 20cm and 20cm × 20cm sizes and are easily cut to the desired dimensions with scissors.

The choice of eluent for chromatography will depend on the adsorbent used and the types of compounds to be separated. The eluting powers of various solvents, that is, their ability to move a given substance through the stationary phase, are generally found to occur in the order shown (increasing eluting power):

Petroleum ether (bp 30 ~ 60℃), Hexane, Carbon tetrachloride, Toluene, Dichloromethane, Chloromethane, Diethyl ether, Ethyl acetate, Acetone, 1-Propanol, Ethanol, Methanol, Water.

The TLC is generally used as a detection technique but also as apurification method to separate a small amount of mixtures. A distinct advantage of TLC is the very small quantity of sample required.

A lower limit of detection of 10^{-9} g is possible in some cases. The spot of sample must be applied to the TLC plate with care; it should not be large. However, larger samples such as 0.5mg may be used on larger TLC plates, which have thicker coats of adsorbent.

Visualization of the chromatogram to locate the position of each of the components of a mixture depends on the type of molecules present in the mixture. If all the components of the mixture are colored, then visual inspection of the developed pate is sufficient to locate the spots. If this is not the case, the two most commonly used methods for visualizing compounds are the use of an adsorbent that contains a fluorescent dye and the use of iodine vapor. With the former technique, the developed plate is irradiated with a "black" light (a low-intensity ultraviolet lamp), the fluorescence of the dye being quenched by the compounds on the plate producing a dark spot against a light blue background of the fluorescing dye. This method requires that the components of a mixture all are capable of quenching the fluorescence of the dye. This is not always the case particularly with hydrocarbons and other relatively nonpolar compounds. The use of iodine vapor for visualization depends on the ability of the components of the mixture to form charge-transfer complex with iodine. Compounds that do not contain π or Lewis basic functions do not form charge-transfer complexes with iodine.

The column chromatography is generally used as a purification technique to separate a rather large amount of mixtures. If the compounds separated in a column chromatography procedure are colored, the progress of the separation can simply be monitored visually. More commonly, the compounds to be isolated from column chromatography are colorless. In this case, small fractions of the eluent are collected sequentially in labeled tubes and the composition of each fraction is analyzed by TLC.

Experimental procedure

1. Separation of *syn*-and *anti*-Azobenzenes by TLC

Obtain from your instructor a 10cm strip of silica gel chromatogram sheet (without fluorescent indicator) and about 0.5ml of a 10% toluene solution of commercial azobenzene. Place a spot of this solution on the TLC plate about 1 cm from one edge and about 2cm from the bottom, using a capillary tube to apply the spot. The spot should be 1 or 2mm in diameter. Allow the spot to dry and then expose the plate to sunlight for one or two hours. Alternatively, the plate may be placed beneath a sunlamp for about 20 min. After this time, apply another spot of the original solution on the plate at the same distance from the bottom as the first and leave about 1 cm between the spots. Again, allow the plate to dry.

A wide-mouth bottle with a tightly fitting screw-top cap may be used as a developing chamber (Figure 2 – 27). Alternatively, a beaker covered with a watch glass may be used. Prepare a 9 : 1 (by volume) mixture of hexane: chloroform and place a 1cm layer of this mixture in the bottom of the developing chamber. Fold a piece of filter paper, and place it into the developing chamber, as shown in Figure 2 – 27. Saturate the chamber with the vapors of the solvent by shaking. This inhibits the evaporation of solvent from the plate during the development of the chromatogram. The piece of filter paper helps maintain this saturated state.

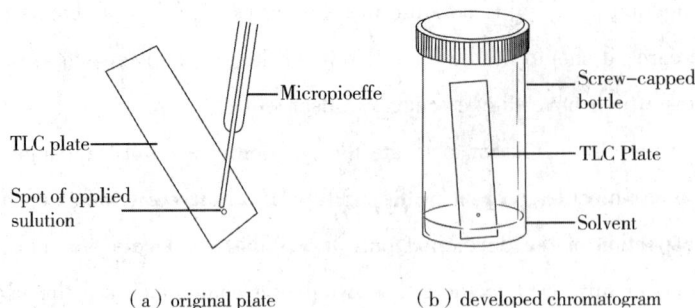

(a) original plate   (b) developed chromatogram

Figure 2 – 27　Thin-layer chromatogram

Place the chromatogram plate in the chamber, being careful not to splash the solvent onto the plate. The spots must be above the solvent level. Allow solvent to climb to within about 1. 5cm of the top of the plate and then remove the plate and allow it to air-dry. Note the number of spots arising from each of the two original spots and compare the intensities of the two spots nearest the starting point, which correspond to syn-azobenzene.

2. Separation of Green Leaf Pigments by TLC

Place in a mortar several fresh spinach leaves and a few milliliters of a 2 : 1 mixture of petroleum ether (bp 30 ~ 60℃) and ethanol, and grind the leaves well with a pestle. By means of a pipet, transfer the liquid extract to a small separatory funnel and swirl with an equal volume of water; shaking may cause formation of an emulsion. Separate and discard the lower aqueous phase. Repeat the water washing twice, discarding the aqueous phase each time. The water washing serves to remove the ethanol as well as other water-soluble materials that have been extracted from the leaves. Transfer the petroleum ether layer to a small Erlenmeyer flask and add 2g of anhydrous sodium sulfate. After a few minutes decant the solution from the sodium sulfate, and if the solution is not deeply and darkly colored, concentrate it by evaporating part of the petroleum ether, using a gentle stream of air.

Obtain from your instructor a 10cm × 2cm strip of silica gel chromatogram sheet. Place a spot of the pigment solution on the sheet about 1. 5cm from one end, using a capillary tube to apply the spot. Avoid allowing the spot to diffuse to a diameter of no more than 2mm during application of the sample. Allow the spot to dry, and develop the chromatogram according to the general directions given in the second paragraph of part 1, but use chloroform as the developing solvent.

It is sometimes possible to observe as many as eight colored spots. In order of decreasing R_f values, these spots have been identified as the carotenes (two spots, orange), chlorophyll a (blue-green), the xanthophylls (four spots, yellow), and chlorophyll b (green).

Calculate the R_f values of any spots observed on your developed plate. Also, as an aid in maintenance of a permanent record of the plate, draw to scale a picture of the developed plate in your notebook.

3. Separation of Ferrocene and Acetylferrocene by Column Chromatography

As shown in Figure 2 – 28, use the dry pack technique to build a small column with two-thirds full of alumina. Add hexane into the column to cover the alumina layer. Obtain 0. 090 g of the 1 : 1 mixture of ferrocene and acetylferrocene and dissolve them in 1. 5ml of hexane. Pour the solution on the surface of the alumina. Using a Pasteur pipet, wash down any mixture that adheres to the wall of the column with a few drops of hexane. Place a 25ml Erlenmeyer flask under the valve of the column.

Open the valve on the column and elute the column with hexane. Continue adding hexane to the column as necessary so that it does not run dry. As the column is eluted, ferrocene will travel down as a yellow band. Collect this yellow solution in the Erlenmeyer flask. When the yellow has been completely eluted, place a beaker under the column, and let the level of hexane lower until it is about 1 cm above the top of the alumina. Fill the column to the top of the glass with a 1 : 1 mixture of hexane and diethyl ether. Open the stopcock and continue to collect the colorless solution that elutes off the column in the beaker. During this time, an orange band will travel down the alumina. When this orange band (acetylferrocene) reaches the bottom of the column, replace the beaker with a new Erlenmeyer flask and collect the orange solution. Once a-

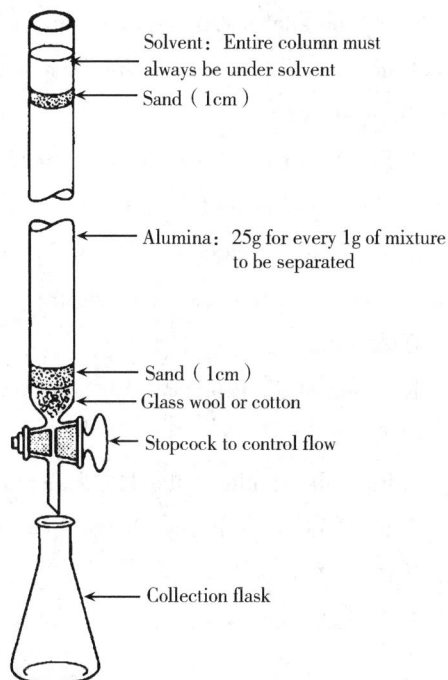

Figure 2 – 28　Column chromatography

gain, it is very important throughout the elution that the column never be allowed to run dry! When elution of both yellow and orange bands is completed, shake out the contents of the column into a beaker. Rinse out the glass column with water, adding the rinses to the beaker. The mixture of alumina and liquid (including the solvents that eluted in between the bands) must be disposed of in the appropriate Laboratory Byproducts jar.

Evaporatethe collected solutions of ferrocene and acetylferrocene on the rotary evaporator. Weight those two products separately and calculate the recovering yield.

Experimental instruction

Notes

Have no flames in the vicinity of petroleum ether when you use it to extract the green pigments, as it is extremely flammable.

Explanation

1. This chromatographic technique is very easy and rapid to perform. It lends itself well to the routine analysis of mixture composition and may also be used to advantage in determining the best eluting solvent for subsequent column chromatography. However, it should be borne in mind that volatile compounds (bp < ~100℃) cannot be analyzed by TLC.

2. For identification purposes, a comparison of a known and unknown should be carried out under identical condition with a number of different solvent systems and, if possible, different adsorbents. R_f values from the literature are not reliable enough for use in final identification; they should be used only as general guides. Whenever possible, a direct comparison between an unknown and a

possible known compound should be made.

3. The value of the use of TLC lies in the relatively small amount of time and material required to carry out an analysis, generally on the order of 10 minutes or less and less-than-milligram quantities of material. TLC is very useful for monitoring the progress of reactions, in the detection of reaction intermediates.

4. Elution, more properly refers to as the development of the chromatogram, is accomplished by the capillary movement of the solvent up the layer of the adsorbent. Unfortunately, generally only one solvent, or solvent mixture, can be used to develop a single plate instead of the use of gradient solvent systems as in column chromatography.

Exercises

1. Which of the two isomers of azobenzene would you expect to be the more thermodynamically stable? Why?

2. From the results of the TLC experiment with the azobenzenes, describe the role of sunlight.

3. In a TLC experiment whythe spot must not be immersed in the solvent in the developing chamber?

4. Explain why the solvent must not be allowed to evaporate from the plate during the development.

5. Why is anhydrous sodium sulfate added to the petroleum ether extract in part 2?

6. Why is a spot of the original mixture put on the plate in part 1?

7. Explain why the R_f of *anti*-azobenzene is greater than the R_f of *syn*-azobenzene.

8. Two components, A and B, were separated by TLC. When the solvent front had moved 6.5 cm above the level of the original sample spot, the spot of A was 0.5 cm and that of B was 3.6 cm above the original spot. Calculate the R_f for A and for B.

9. Why is it important to keep the sample band level and even when performing a column chromatographic separation? Describe what can happen if the sample band is very uneven.

第三部分　基础性有机合成实验

Part III　Basic Organic Synthetic Experiments

实验十　溴乙烷制备

【目的要求】

1. **掌握**　分馏的方法。
2. **熟悉**　普通蒸馏、萃取等基础实验操作。
3. **了解**　液体的干燥原理及方法；溴乙烷制备的原理与方法。

【实验原理】

最简便的制备溴乙烷的方法之一是将乙醇与溴化钠或溴化钾和硫酸混合物一起加热。溴化物与硫酸混合，生成溴化氢，溴化氢与乙醇反应生成溴乙烷。

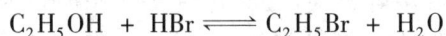

$$NaBr + H_2SO_4 \longrightarrow HBr + NaHSO_4$$
$$C_2H_5OH + HBr \rightleftharpoons C_2H_5Br + H_2O$$

溴化氢与乙醇的反应为可逆反应，为获得较高产率，必须促使平衡向生成产物的方向移动。在本反应中采用将溴乙烷从反应混合物中蒸出的办法，使平衡向产物方向移动。

因为反应中需要加入硫酸，故会引起以下副反应。

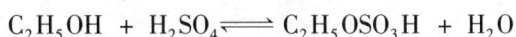

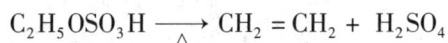

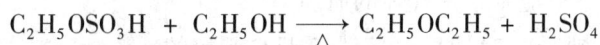

$$C_2H_5OH + H_2SO_4 \rightleftharpoons C_2H_5OSO_3H + H_2O$$
$$C_2H_5OSO_3H \xrightarrow{\triangle} CH_2=CH_2 + H_2SO_4$$
$$C_2H_5OSO_3H + C_2H_5OH \xrightarrow{\triangle} C_2H_5OC_2H_5 + H_2SO_4$$
$$2HBr + H_2SO_4 \longrightarrow Br_2 + SO_2 + 2H_2O$$

伯醇发生亲核取代反应时的温度一般不高，因此该反应的副反应不是很严重。

【实验步骤】

1. 原料与试剂

溴化钠（无水）	15g（0.15mol）
浓硫酸	19ml（35g，0.35mol）
95%乙醇	10ml（7.9g，0.163mol）

2. 步骤　在100ml圆底烧瓶中放入10ml 95%乙醇和9ml水，在冷却和旋摇下，慢慢加入19ml浓硫酸。将混合物冷却至室温，并在摇动下加入15g已在研钵中研细的溴化钠，再投入2或3粒沸石，按图3-1安装分馏装置。冷凝管下接牛角管，牛角管的末端应浸入50ml锥形瓶内的冰水，锥形瓶则浸入250ml烧杯内的冰水。

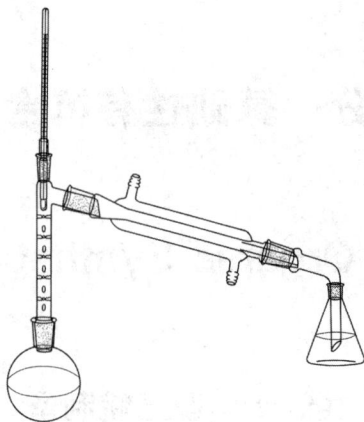

图 3-1　制备溴乙烷装置

　　油浴小心加热，开始加热温度不能太高，慢慢升高温度，然后进行分馏，直至牛角管末端看不见油珠，大约需要 40 分钟。反应开始时，混合物明显起沫，反应结束时，液体静静沸腾，不再有挥发物形成。反应结束后，为了防止馏出液到吸，应先移去接收瓶，然后停止加热。

　　将溴乙烷粗品和冰水倒入分液漏斗，静置分层，溴乙烷层（下层）放入一个 50ml 干燥的浸在冰水浴的锥形瓶中，冰水冷却下慢慢加入浓硫酸，直至溴乙烷层澄清（约 4ml）。将混合物倒入一干燥小分液漏斗中，静置几分钟后仔细分去硫酸 - 乙醚混合物（下层）。

　　将浓硫酸处理过的粗溴乙烷倒入一干燥的蒸馏瓶，加 2 或 3 粒沸石。装上温度计和冷凝管，装置如图 2 - 12 所示。加热蒸馏，用已称重的锥形品收集产品，锥形瓶外用冰水浴冷却，蒸馏收集 36 ~ 40℃ 的馏分。产量约 10 ~ 11g。

　　文献值：溴乙烷 bp38.5℃。

【实验指导】

（一）预习要求

1. 复习醇和氢卤酸反应制备卤代烃的原理。

2. 了解本实验在制备溴乙烷时是如何打破反应平衡的。

3. 复习简单蒸馏操作以及分液漏斗的使用和保养等基础操作。

4. 查阅本实验的主要试剂、原料及产物的主要物理常数。

（二）注意事项

1. 如牛角管插入水面很深，水可能倒吸进冷凝管、进入反应瓶，导致不良后果。

2. 加入浓硫酸是为了除去副产物乙醚。

3. 为分清界面，应该从不同方向仔细观察分液漏斗。

4. 由于溴乙烷易挥发，称重后要迅速回收。

（三）思考题

　　1. 在制备溴乙烷的起始反应混合物中，要加一些水，如部分学生没有加水，对溴乙烷产率有何影响？加两倍量水，对产率有何影响？

　　2. 纯化时，用浓硫酸洗涤溴乙烷粗品，除去什么杂质，为什么？

3. 下列反应中，各产物已分离得到。

$$(CH_3)_2CCH_2CH_3 \xrightarrow{HBr} (CH_3)_2CHCHCH_3 + (CH_3)_2CCH_2CH_3$$

$$\underset{OH}{|} \qquad\qquad \underset{Br}{|} \qquad\qquad \underset{Br}{|}$$

$$\qquad\qquad\qquad\qquad\qquad 10\% \qquad\qquad 90\%$$

写出合理的反应机理并指出是 S_N1 反应还是 S_N2 反应。

4. 反应中有时会产生桔黄色蒸气，为什么？

Experiment 10 Preparation of Ethyl Bromide

Experimental principle

One of the most convenient way to prepare ethyl bromide is to heat ethanol with a mixture of sodium or potassium bromide and sulfuric acid. The bromide-sulfuric acid combination liberates the hydrogen bromide for the reaction.

$$NaBr + H_2SO_4 \longrightarrow HBr + NaHSO_4$$
$$C_2H_5OH + HBr \rightleftharpoons C_2H_5Br + H_2O$$

The reaction of hydrogen bromide with ethanol is reversible. In order to obtain high yield, it is necessary to shift the equilibrium toward the product. ,This can be accomplished by removing ethyl bromide from the reaction mixture.

Although the added sulfuric acid is desirable, it may also give rise to side reactions:

$$C_2H_5OH + H_2SO_4 \rightleftharpoons C_2H_5OSO_3H + H_2O$$
$$C_2H_5OSO_3H \xrightarrow{\triangle} CH_2=CH_2 + H_2SO_4$$
$$C_2H_5OSO_3H + C_2H_5OH \xrightarrow{\triangle} C_2H_5OC_2H_5 + H_2SO_4$$
$$2HBr + H_2SO_4 \longrightarrow Br_2 + SO_2 + 2H_2O$$

For primary alcohols the temperatures used for the substitution reaction are generally not high enough to cause these side reactions to be of great importance.

Experimental procedures

1. Materials and reagents

anhydrous sodium bromide	15g (0.15mol)
concentrated sulfuric acid	19ml (35g,0.35mol)
95% ethanol	10ml (7.9g,0.163mol)

2. Procedures

With swirling and cooling, 19ml of concentrated sulfuric acid is slowly added to the mixture of 10ml of 95% ethanol and 9ml of water in a 100ml round-bottomed flask. After cooling the mixture to room temperature, with agitation, 15g anhydrous sodium bromide which has been previously ground to fine powder in a mortar is added and then 2 or 3 boiling chips are added. Fit this flask for fractionation with a condenser carrying an adapter, the mouth of which is just below the surface of some ice and water in a 50ml Erlenmeyer flask immersed in a 250ml beaker full of the mixture of ice and water, according to Figure 3-1.

Heat carefully by the oil bath. The temperature should not be too high at the beginning. Slowly increase the temperature until the oil drops can't be seen at the end of the adapter. It'll cost about 40 minutes. During the process of the reaction, the mixture foams considerably and at last it settles to a quietly simmering liquid as the reaction comes to an end and no more volatile material is formed.

Pour the crude ethyl bromide and ice water into a separatory funnel, properly mounted on a ring stand and tap off the ethyl bromide layer (bottom layer) into a 50ml dry Erlenmeyer flask immersed in an ice-water bath. Slowly add some concentrated sulfuric acid until disappearance of turbidity (about 4ml). Transfer the mixture to a small, dry separatory funnel, and let it stand a few minutes, then separate the layers carefully, and tap off the sulfuric acid-ethyl ether mixture (bottom layer).

Pour the ethyl bromide, which has been treated with concentrated sulfuric acid, into a dry distilling flask, equipped with a thermometer and a dry condenser. Add 2 or 3 boiling chips, then distill. Collect the portion distilling at $36 \sim 40°C$ in a preweighed small Erlenmeyer flask packed in the ice in a beaker. The yield is about $10 \sim 11$g.

Literature: bp of ethyl bromide 38.5°C。

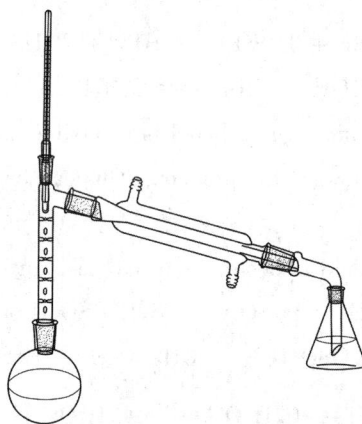

Figure 3 – 1   Apparatus for preparation of ethyl bromide

Experimental instruction

Notes

1. If the adapter dips too far below the surface of the water, it may be possible for water to ride into the condenser tube and into the reaction flask with disastrous results.

2. This treatment is designed to remove the diethyl ether, which is formed as a by-product in the reaction.

3. In order to distinguish the interface, you may find it necessary to view the funnel from several different angles.

4. Since bromoethane is volatile, it should be weighed and handed to the instructor immediately.

Exercises

1. Observe that some water is added to the initial reaction mixture in the preparation of ethyl bromide. How might the yield of ethyl bromide be affected by the failure on the part of the student to add the water? What products would be obtained? How might the yield of ethyl bromide be affected by adding twice as much water as is called for?

2. In the purification process the impure ethyl bromide is "washed" with concentrated sulfuric

acid. What impurities would a wash of this sort remove? Why?

3. The following reaction was carried out and the indicated products were isolated.

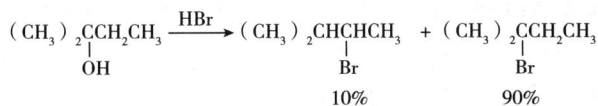

$$(CH_3)_2CCH_2CH_3 \xrightarrow{\text{HBr}} (CH_3)_2CHCHCH_3 + (CH_3)_2CCH_2CH_3$$

$$\underset{OH}{} \qquad\qquad \underset{Br}{} \qquad\qquad \underset{Br}{}$$

$$10\% \qquad\qquad 90\%$$

Suggest reasonable mechanisms for this reaction, and indicate whether each is S_N1 or S_N2.

实验十一　环己烯的制备

【目的要求】

1. **掌握**　以硫酸为催化剂在实验室制备环己烯的原理及方法。
2. **熟悉**　分馏、蒸馏、分液等基础操作。
3. **了解**　有机化学实验中液体的干燥原理及方法。

【实验原理】

醇在酸性条件下加热可以发生分子内脱水生成烯烃，可用于烯烃的制备，反应中常用的催化剂有浓硫酸、磷酸、对甲苯磺酸、硫酸氢钾或三氧化二铝、分子筛等。

本实验用浓硫酸为催化剂，通过环己醇的脱水制备环己烯。此反应可逆，反应生成的环己烯在反应条件下能与水作用又生成醇，必须把生成的环己烯从反应混合物中及时移去。

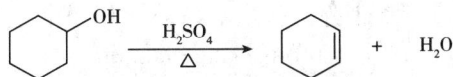

在平衡混合物中，环己烯（bp 83℃）沸点最低，可以一边生成一边蒸出，使平衡向右移动，从而获得较高产率的环己烯。

【实验步骤】

1. 原料和试剂

环己醇	20.0g（21.2ml, 0.20mol）
浓硫酸	2ml
5%碳酸钠溶液	4ml
无水硫酸钠	2~4g

2. 步骤　在100ml圆底烧瓶中，放置20g（0.20mol）环己醇，然后加2ml浓硫酸。充分振摇使之混合均匀，再加2粒沸石，按图2-14安装分馏装置，接收瓶应浸入冰水浴。油浴加热反应瓶，控制分馏柱顶部馏出温度不超过90℃，收集馏出液。在蒸馏的大部分时间内，顶部馏出温度不会超过70℃。当反应瓶中剩少量残液并出现白雾时，停止加热。

将馏出液中加入少量精盐饱和，然后加3~4ml 5%碳酸钠溶液中和微量的酸。然后转入小分液漏斗，静置分层，除去水层后有机层转入干燥的50ml锥形瓶中，加1~2g无水硫酸钠，不时摇动5~10分钟，将干燥的有机混合物倾入另一个干燥的50ml锥形瓶中，加

1~2g 无水硫酸钠，不时摇动，5 分钟后滤入干燥的 50ml 蒸馏瓶中。为获得纯品环己烯，粗品必须彻底干燥。加几粒沸石，用事先干燥的简单蒸馏装置蒸馏，用事先称重的干燥的 25ml 锥形瓶为接收瓶，接收瓶用冰水浴冷却，真空接液管上要接一氯化钙干燥管。收集 80~85℃馏分，产量约 8~10g。

文献值：环己烯 bp 82.98℃。

【实验指导】

（一）预习要求

1. 复习烯烃的一般制法和醇在酸性条件下脱水成烯的反应原理。

2. 了解盐析法的基本原理及应用。

（二）注意事项

1. 可用 85% 磷酸催化，但效果不好，反应速度慢且产率低。

2. 反应中，环己烯和水形成最低共沸物（bp 70.8℃，含水 10%）；环己醇与环己烯形成共沸物（bp 64.9℃，含环己醇 30.5%）；环己醇与水形成共沸物（bp 97.8℃，含水 80%）。

3. 水和环己烯形成共沸物。

4. 如果低沸点馏分较多，可重新干燥然后再蒸馏一次。

（三）思考题

1. 蒸馏烯和干燥剂混合物会有什么结果？换句话说，最后蒸馏前，为什么要过滤分开有机层和干燥剂？

2. 下列伯醇哪个更易进行 E1 消除，哪个更易进行 E2 消除？解释原因。

$$CH_3CH_2OH \quad (CH_3)_3CCH_2OH$$

3. 写出下列各醇脱水产物的结构，并指出主产物。

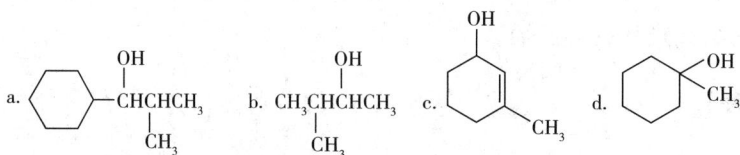

4. 在环己醇反应脱水时，采用回流而不用蒸馏装置，将会有什么结果？假定其他操作不变。

5. 写出酸催化环己醇脱水生成环己烯的机制。

6. 什么是最低共沸物？

7. 画出环己烯加溴产物的结构（包括立体结构）。理论上，这个二溴化合物能拆分吗？

Experiment 11　Preparation of Cyclohexene

Experimental principle

An alcohol can be heated under acidic conditions to generate olefin, which can be used in the preparation of olefin. The catalysts commonly used in the reaction are concentrated sulfuric acid, phosphoric acid, p-toluenesulfonic acid, potassium hydrogen sulfate or aluminum oxide, molecular sieve, etc.

Cyclohexene was prepared by dehydration of cyclohexanol using concentrated sulfuric acid as catalyst. This reaction is reversible. The cyclohexene formed by the reaction can interact with water to form alcohol under reaction conditions, so the cyclohexene formed must be removed from the reaction mixture in time.

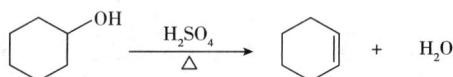

$$\text{cyclohexanol} \xrightarrow[\Delta]{H_2SO_4} \text{cyclohexene} + H_2O$$

Cyclohexene is the lowest boiling component of the equilibrium mixture and can be distilled from the reaction as it is formed. Thus, cyclohexene can be formed in good yield.

Experimental procedures

1. Materials and reagents

cyclohexanol	20g(0.20mol)
concentrate sulfuric acid	2ml
5% sodium hydroxide solution	4ml
Anhydrous sodium sulfate	2~4g

2. Procedures

Place 20g (0.20mol) of cyclohexanol in a 100ml round-bottom flask and add 2ml of concentrated sulfuric acid to this flask. Thoroughly mix the contents of the flask by swirling it. Add two boiling chips, and assemble the flask for fractional distillation according to Figure 2 – 13. The receiving flask should be immersed in an ice-water bath. Heat the reaction flask with an oil bath, collecting all distillates, but keeping the head temperature below 90℃. If the reaction mixture is not heated too strongly, the head temperature will remain below about 70℃ for most of the period of reaction. When a small amount of residual liquid is left in the reaction bottle and white mist appears, discontinue heating.

Saturate the distillate with a small amount of refined salt, then add 3~4 ml 5% sodium carbonate solution to neutralize the trace acid, and then transfer the mixture to a small separatory funnel, allow the layers to separate and remove the aqueous layer.

Transfer the organic layer to a dry 50ml Erlenmeyer flask and add 1~2g of anhydrous sodium sulfate. Occasionally swirl the mixture during a period of 5~10 min; then decant the dried organic mixture into another dry 50ml Erlenmeyer flask, and add a fresh 1~2 g portion of anhydrous sodium sulfate. Swirl the flask occasionally during the next 5 min or so and then filter the liquid into a dry 50ml distilling flask. The product must be dry at this stage in order to obtain pure cyclohexene. Add boiling chips and distil the mixture through a pre-dried simple distillation apparatus. Collect the fraction boiling between 80 and 85℃ in a preweighed ice-cooled dry 25ml Erlenmeyer flask. A calcium chloride drying tube should be attached to the nipple of the vacuum adapter. The yield is about 8~10g.

Literature: bp of cyclohexene 82.98℃.

Experimental instruction

Notes

1. 85% Phosphoric acid can also be used as the catalyst but is somewhat less satisfactory. The

reaction is slower and the yields are lower. Use 5ml of this acid if you are instructed to use it.

2. During the reaction,cyclohexene and water form a minimum-boiling azeotrop (bp 70. 8℃ , 10% water) ,cyclohexanol and cyclohexene form a minimum-boiling azeotrope (bp 64. 9℃ ,30. 5% cyclohexanol) ,cyclohexanol and water form a azeotrope (bp 97. 8℃ ,80% water) .

3. Water and cyclohexene form a minimum-boiling azeotrope.

4. If there is an appreciable low-boiling fraction, dry this again, and redistill it.

Exercises

1. What would be the consequence of distilling the slurry of alkenes and the drying agent? In other words,why is the organic solution separated from the drying agent by filtration prior to the final distillation?

2. Which of the following primary alcohols would be most likely to dehydrate by the E1 mechanism? By the E2 mechanism? Explain.

$$CH_3CH_2OH \qquad (CH_3)_3CCH_2OH$$

3. Give structures for the products of dehydration of each of the following alcohols. For each,order the products with respect to preference of formation.

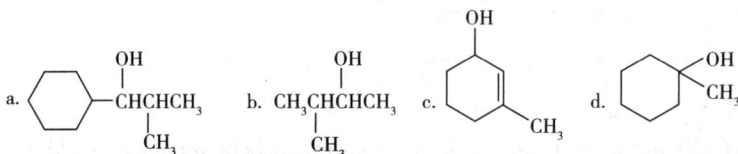

4. What consequences would be expected if the dehydration step of this procedure were conducted under reflux rather than with distillation? Assume that the work-up of the reaction would be unchanged.

5. Give a detailed mechanism for the acid-catalyzed dehydration of cyclohexanol to cyclohexene.

6. Define a "minimum-boiling azeotrope."

7. Give the structure,including stereochemistry,of the product of addition of bromine to cyclohexene. Is this dibromide,at least in principle,separable into enantiomers? Explain.

实验十二　乙酰苯胺制备

【目的要求】

1. 掌握　苯胺乙酰化的原理及操作方法。
2. 熟悉　分馏柱的使用及重结晶操作。

【实验原理】

乙酰化常用来保护伯胺和仲胺。游离胺能参与许多反应,乙酰胺的碱性比胺弱,参与这些典型反应的倾向较小;乙酰胺难以氧化;芳胺酰化后,芳环上亲电取代反应的活性比胺小。氨基很容易通过酰胺在酸或碱催化下水解重新生成。

芳香胺和脂肪胺可用酸酐、酰氯或与冰醋酸加热来进行酰化,用乙酸时,需将反应中生成的水除去。冰乙酸价格便宜,但是反应活性较低,需要更高的反应温度和较长的反应时间。

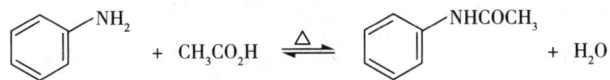

$$\underset{}{\text{NH}_2} + CH_3CO_2H \rightleftharpoons \underset{}{\text{NHCOCH}_3} + H_2O$$

【实验步骤】

1. 原料和试剂

苯胺	5ml（5.1g，0.055mol）
冰乙酸	7.4ml（7.4g，0.13mol）
锌粉	0.1g

2. 步骤 在 50ml 圆底烧瓶中，放置 5ml（5.1g，0.055mol）苯胺、7.4ml（7.4g，0.13mol）冰乙酸和约 0.1g 锌粉。加两粒沸石，装上短分馏柱和温度计，接上冷凝管，安装成蒸馏装置（图 3-2）。

油浴加热，保持微沸而蒸气不进入分馏柱。15 分钟后，逐渐升高温度，将反应中生成的水和少量乙酸缓慢、恒速地蒸出（馏出温度 100~110℃），约一小时后，反应生成的水和大部分乙酸已蒸出，温度计读数下降，表示反应已基本完成，停止加热。

剧烈搅拌下，将反应混合物趁热倒入盛有 100ml 冰水的烧杯中，冷却后抽滤收集析出的固体，用少量冷水洗涤，得到乙酰苯胺粗产物。粗产物用水重结晶，干燥称重，产量约 4~5g，mp 113~114℃。

图 3-2 制备乙酰苯胺装置

乙酰苯胺纯品为白色片状晶体，文献值：mp 114.3℃。

【实验指导】

（一）预习要求

1. 复习羧酸形成羧酸衍生物以及羧酸衍生物发生取代反应的原理。
2. 分析比较本实验和实验十在原理和仪器装置上的异同。
3. 复习基本操作中固体有机化合物重结晶部分。
4. 说明本实验粗产物中可能存在的杂质以及去除的方法。

（二）注意事项

1. 久置的苯胺颜色变深，使用前最好减压蒸馏，因为有色杂质影响乙酰苯胺质量。
2. 加锌粉防止苯胺氧化。
3. 蒸出液约 4ml。
4. 防止化合物结块。
5. 每克干粗品大约需要 20ml 水。
6. 如颜色较深，再重结晶一次。

（三）思考题

1. 苯胺是碱而乙酰苯胺不是，解释这种差异。
2. 如果 10g 苯胺与过量乙酐作用，计算乙酰苯胺理论产量。

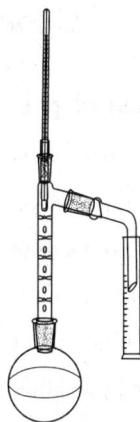

3. 当胺与乙酸作用乙酰化时，为什么用过量酸？为什么要将反应生成的水蒸出？

4. 制备对硝基苯胺时，硝化前为什么要将苯胺转化为乙酰苯胺？

5. 苯胺和下列化合物反应，将得到什么产物？

（1）琥珀酸酐，加热　　　　　（2）二甲基乙烯酮

6. 写出下列制备的反应式

（1）从苯胺合成邻硝基苯胺　　（2）从苯合成间硝基苯胺

7. 由苯胺制备乙酰苯胺，有哪几种酰化剂？各有何优点？

Experiment 12　Preparation of Acetanilide

Experimental principle

Acetylation is often used to "protect" a primary or secondary amine functional group. Acetylated amines are less susceptible to oxidation, less reactive in aromatic substitution reactions, and less prone to participate in many of the typical reactions of free amines, since they are less basic. The amino group can be regenerated readily by hydrolysis in acid or base.

Arylamines (and aliphatic amines) may be acetylated by means of acetic anhydride or acetyl chloride or by heating the amine with glacial acetic acid under conditions that permit removal of the water formed in the reaction. Glacial acetic acid is cheaper but has lower reactivity, which requires higher reaction temperature and longer reaction time.

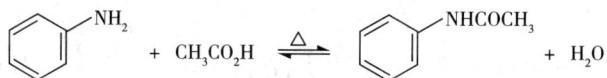

Experimental procedures

1. Materials and reagents

aniline 5ml	(5.1g, 0.055mol)
glacial acetic acid	7.4ml (7.4g, 0.13mol)
zinc powder	0.1g

2. Procedures

In a 50ml round-bottom flask, place 5ml (5.1g, 0.055mol) aniline, 7.4ml (7.4g, 0.13mol) glacial acetic acid and 0.1g zinc powder. Provide the flask with a short fractionating column fitted with a thermometer and arranged for distillation (Figure 3 − 2). Add two boiling chips and heat the flask gently by oil bath, so that the solution boils quietly and the vapor does not rise into the column.

After 15min increase the heating slightly so that the water formed in the reaction, together with a little acetic acid, distills over very slowly at a uniform rate (vapor temperature 100~110℃). After about an hour, when the water formed in

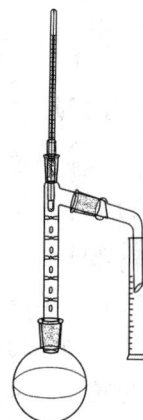

Figure 3 − 2　Apparatus for preparation of acetanilide

reaction and most of acetic acid has been distilled, head temperature will drop.

Discontinue the heating and pour the reaction mixture out at once into about 100ml of ice and water in a large beaker with vigorously stirring. After cooling, the solid was collected by suction filtration and washed with a small amount of cold water. The crude products were recrystallized with water, dry and weigh the solid. The yield is about 4 ~ 5g, mp 113 ~ 114℃. Literature: mp 114. 3℃.

Experimental instruction

Notes

1. The aniline stored for a long time is dark colored. It had better be distilled by vacuum distillation before use because the colored impurity may affect the quality of acetanilide.

2. Add zinc powder to prevent aniline from oxidating.

3. The total volume of distillate is about 4ml.

4. Prevent the compound from clumping.

5. About 20ml of water per gram of dry crude product.

6. If the color is darker, recrystallize again.

Exercises

1. Aniline is basic while acetanilide is not basic. Explain this difference.

2. Calculate the theoretical yield of acetanilide which would be expected if 10g of aniline were allowed to react with an excess of acetic anhydride.

3. When acetic acid is used for acetylation of an amine, why is it desirable to use an excess of the acid and to distill off the water formed in the reaction?

4. In the preparation of *p*-nitroaniline, why is aniline converted to acetanilide before nitration?

5. What products are obtained from aniline and each of the following reagents?

(1) Succinic anhydride, followed by heating

(2) Imethylketene

6. Outline a series of reactions for each preparation.

(1) *o*-nitroaniline from aniline

(2) *m*-nitroaniline from benzene

实验十三 乙酰乙酸乙酯的制备

【目的要求】

1. **掌握** 乙酰乙酸乙酯的制备原理及操作方法；简单的无水操作方法。
2. **熟悉** 蒸馏、萃取、减压蒸馏等基础操作。
3. **了解** 金属钠的使用方法；机械搅拌装置的拆装顺序和应用。

【实验原理】

含有 α - H 的酯在强碱催化下，发生 Claisen 酯缩合反应，生成 β - 酮酸酯。乙酸乙酯在乙醇钠催化下，发生酯缩合反应生成乙酰乙酸乙酯。在含有痕量乙醇的绝对干燥的乙酸

扫码"学一学"

乙酯中，加金属钠，乙醇与金属钠反应生成的乙醇钠用于催化此反应，生成乙酰乙酸乙酯。

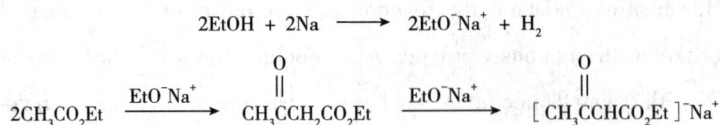

$$2EtOH + 2Na \longrightarrow 2EtO^-Na^+ + H_2$$

$$2CH_3CO_2Et \xrightarrow{EtO^-Na^+} CH_3\overset{\overset{O}{\|}}{C}CH_2CO_2Et \xrightarrow{EtO^-Na^+} [CH_3\overset{\overset{O}{\|}}{C}CHCO_2Et]^-Na^+$$

乙酰乙酸乙酯亚甲基氢更活泼（$pK_a = 10.65$），在此反应条件下生成乙酰乙酸乙酯的钠化合物，因此反应最后一步是不可逆的。

乙酰乙酸乙酯钠化合物酸化后即最终生成乙酰乙酸乙酯。

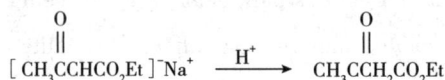

$$[CH_3\overset{\overset{O}{\|}}{C}CHCO_2Et]^-Na^+ \xrightarrow{H^+} CH_3\overset{\overset{O}{\|}}{C}CH_2CO_2Et$$

【实验步骤】

1. 原料和试剂

乙酸乙酯   28ml（25.3g，0.283mol）

钠   2.0g（0.087mol）

50%乙酸   12ml

饱和氯化钠水溶液

无水硫酸镁

2. 步骤

在100ml三颈瓶上装机械搅拌器和回流冷凝管，冷凝管上口接一氯化钙干燥管（图3-3）。将28ml（0.283mol）乙酸乙酯加入三颈瓶中，快速加入干净并切成薄片的2.0g（0.087mol）金属钠。反应立即开始，开动搅拌，保持瓶内溶液呈微沸状态。开始反应较剧烈，待反应缓和后，在油浴上加热反应，使反应始终保持微沸状态，直至金属钠全部溶解，反应约需1小时。此时反应混合物应为红色带有绿色荧光（有时有少量沉淀）。

反应液稍冷后，缓慢加入50%乙酸酸化（约需12ml），直至反应液呈弱酸性，若有固体析出，可加少量水使其溶解。将反应液倒入分液漏斗，加入等体积的氯化钠饱和溶液，用力振摇后放置分层。分出酯层，用无水硫酸镁干燥，然后滤入蒸馏瓶。为减少乙酰乙酸乙酯沾在瓶壁和干燥剂上的损失，用2ml乙酸乙酯洗涤瓶子和干燥剂，洗涤液通过漏斗滤入蒸馏瓶。用沸水浴加热蒸馏除去未反应的乙酸乙酯。将蒸馏残余液用油浴加热减压蒸馏，收集76～80℃/18mmHg馏分，乙酰乙酸乙酯产量约5～5.5g。

图3-3　制备乙酰乙酸乙酯装置

乙酰乙酸乙酯为无色液体，文献值 bp：181℃/760mmHg，92℃/40mmHg，82℃/20mmHg，78℃/18mmHg，74℃/14mmHg，71℃/12mmHg。

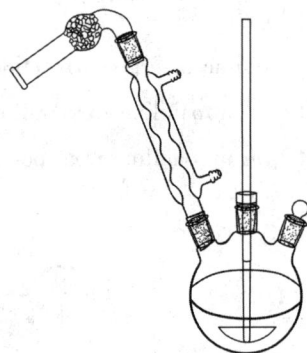

【实验指导】

（一）预习要求

1. 复习克莱森酯缩合反应的基本原理。

2. 了解本实验对试剂、原料、仪器及操作过程的要求。

3. 复习普通蒸馏、萃取、减压蒸馏操作。

4. 复习金属钠的使用方法及注意事项。

（二）注意事项

1. 乙酸乙酯品质非常重要，必须绝对无水且应含有 1~2% 乙醇。普通乙酸乙酯提纯方法如下：用等体积的饱和氯化钙溶液洗涤，无水硫酸镁干燥，过滤，蒸馏，收集 76~78℃ 馏分。

2. 本反应使用切成薄片的金属钠和钠丝的效果一样好。避免金属钠曝露在空气中，在空气中，部分金属钠会转变成氢氧化钠。

3. 为避免乙酸乙酯逸出，油浴温度不能太高。

4. 一般要求金属钠全部消失，但极少量未反应的金属钠并不妨碍进一步操作。

5. 这是乙酰乙酸乙酯钠盐。

6. 所用 50% 乙酸按体积比配制。用 pH 试纸检验，pH 约为 6，要避免加入过量乙酸，因为乙酸会增加酯在水中的溶解度。

7. 如采用常压蒸馏，乙酰乙酸乙酯很容易分解。

8. 产率可按金属钠用量计算。本实验最好连续进行，间隔时间太长，会由于副产物生成而降低产率。

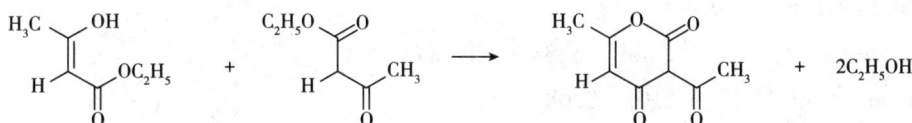

9. 分析显示，乙酰乙酸乙酯存在互变异构体。

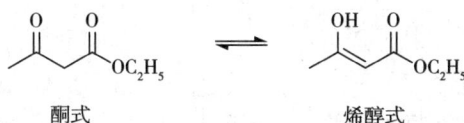

酮式　　　　　　　　　　　　烯醇式

（三）思考题

1. 写出下列反应的产物和机理。

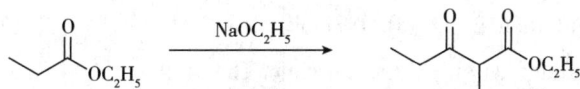

2. 为什么与羰基相连碳上的氢有酸性？

3. 制备乙酰乙酸乙酯时，为什么试剂必须绝对无水，仪器为什么要清洁干燥？

4. 当金属钠消失后，溶液为什么是红色？

5. 使用 50% 乙酸和饱和氯化钠溶液的目的是什么？

6. 使用氯化钙干燥管时，应注意什么？

Experimental 13　Preparation of Ethyl Acetoacetate

Experimental principle

The ester containing α-H undergoes a Claisen ester condensation reaction under strong base catalysis to form a β-ketoester. Ethyl acetate undergoes an ester condensation reaction under the catalysis of sodium ethoxide to form ethyl acetoacetate. In absolute dry ethyl acetate containing traces of ethanol, sodium is added, and sodium ethoxide formed by the reaction of ethanol with sodium is used to catalyze the reaction to form ethyl acetoacetate.

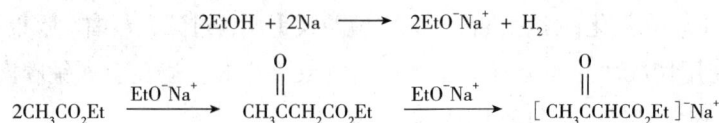

$$2EtOH + 2Na \longrightarrow 2EtO^-Na^+ + H_2$$

$$2CH_3CO_2Et \xrightarrow{EtO^-Na^+} CH_3\overset{\overset{O}{\|}}{C}CH_2CO_2Et \xrightarrow{EtO^-Na^+} [CH_3\overset{\overset{O}{\|}}{C}CHCO_2Et]^-Na^+$$

The methylene hydrogen of ethyl acetoacetate is more reactive ($pK_a = 10.65$), so the sodium compound of ethyl acetoacetate is formed under reaction conditions. The last step of this reaction is irreversible.

Ethyl acetoacetate is formed after sodium acetoacetate is acidified finally.

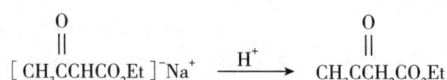

$$[CH_3\overset{\overset{O}{\|}}{C}CHCO_2Et]^-Na^+ \xrightarrow{H^+} CH_3\overset{\overset{O}{\|}}{C}CH_2CO_2Et$$

Experiment procedures

1. Materials and reagents

ethyl acetate	28ml (25.3g, 0.283mol)
sodium	2.0g (0.087mol)
50% acetic acid	12ml
saturated aqueous sodium chloride	
anhydrous magnesium sulfate	

2. Procedures

Equip a 100ml three-necked round-bottom flask with a mechanical stirrer, and with a reflux condenser. Attach a calcium chloride drying tube to the top of the condenser (Figure 3 – 3). Add 28ml (0.283mol) ethyl acetate to the flask, and then 2.0g (0.087mol) clean finely sliced sodium is added as quickly as possible. The reaction starts immediately. Start the stirring, and keep the reaction mixture in the flask slightly boiling. If it gets too violent, immerse the flask in a cold water bath. When the rapid reaction slows down, the reaction mixture is heated on an oil bath. Keep the reaction mixture slightly

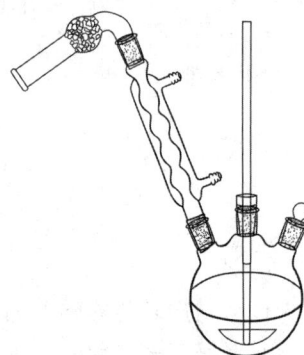

Figure 3 – 3 Apparatus for preparation of ethyl acetoacetate

boiling until the sodium has completely dissolved. This usually requires about one hour. At this stage the reaction mixture should be a clear red liquid with a green fluorescence (A solid may appear).

This solution is then cooled and made slightly acid by slowly adding 50% acetic acid (about 12ml) until the solution is just slightly acid to blue litmus paper. If a solid appears, add a little of water to dissolve it. Pour the contents (not the boiling chip) into a separatory funnel, add an equal volume of saturated aqueous sodium chloride. Shake the mixture vigorously, and stand to separate into layer. The ester layer is separated and dried with anhydrous magnesium sulfate.

Filter through a funnel into a dry distilling flask. In order to minimize losses from ethyl acetoacetate clinging to the walls of the Erlenmeyer flask and the drying agent, rinse the flask with 2ml of ethyl acetate and pass the rinse through the funnel into the distilling flask. Remove unreacted ethyl acetate from the ethyl acetoacetatae by distilling the filtrate on a boiling water bath. The residue is distilled under reduced pressure and the yield of ethyl acetoacetate boiling at 76 ~ 80℃/18mmHg is about 5 ~ 5.5g.

Ethyl acetoacetate is colorless. Literature bp: 181℃/760mmHg, 92℃/40mmHg, 82℃/20mmHg, 78℃/18mmHg, 74℃/14mmHg, 71℃/12mmHg.

Experimental instruction

Notes

1. The grade of ethyl acetate used is very important. It must be entirely free from water and should contain about 1% ~ 2% of alcohol. Ordinary ethyl acetate may be purified in the following manner: wash it with an equal volume of saturated aqueous calcium chloride and dry over anhydrous magnesium sulfate. Then it is filtered, distilled and collected the fraction boiling at 76 ~ 78℃.

2. Sodium wire and finely sliced sodium are equally good to use in this reaction. It is important to avoid exposure of the sodium to the air which converts part of it into sodium hydroxide.

3. In order to avoid ethyl acetate escaping the oil bath temperature should not be too high.

4. It is usually asked that all the sodium metal disappear, but only thin unreacted slivers will not affect the following operation.

5. It is sodium salt of ethyl acetoacetate.

6. The solution of 50% acetic acid was prepared by volume ratio. Use a pH test paper, and the pH is about 6. It is advisable to avoid a large excess of acetic acid since it increases the solubility of the ester in water.

7. During distillation, ethyl acetoacetate is easy to decompose at its atmospheric boiling point.

8. The yield may be based on sodium. The experiment had better be performed successively. If an interval of time is too long, by-products are formed and the yield will decrease.

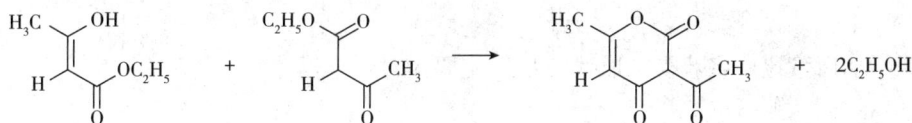

9. Include an analysis of the peaks indicating that ethyl acetoacetate exhibits tautomerism.

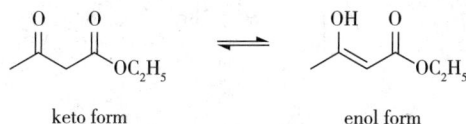

keto form   enol form

Exercises

1. Give the product and mechanism for the following reaction.

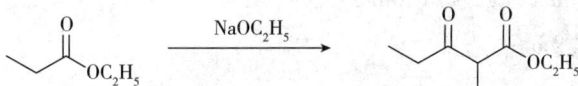

2. Why is the hydrogen on the carbon adjacent to the carbonyl carbon acidic?

3. In the preparation of ethyl acetoacetatae, why is it essential that the reagents be free from water, and the apparatus perfectly clean and dry?

4. Why is the solution red in color? When the sodium has completely dissolved.

5. What are the purposes of the 50% acetic acid and saturated aqueous sodium chloride?

6. What should be paid attention to when an anhydrous calcium chloride drying tube is used?

实验十四　溴苯制备

【目的要求】

掌握　制备溴苯的原理及操作方法；学习有毒及有刺激性物质的取用及处理方法。

【实验原理】

如不加热，苯和氯及溴常温下不发生反应，但在催化剂如铝汞齐、吡啶或铁存在下，苯和氯及溴常温下立即发生反应，首先产生单卤代产物。催化剂的作用是增加卤素的亲电性。吡啶催化的苯溴化反应机理如下：

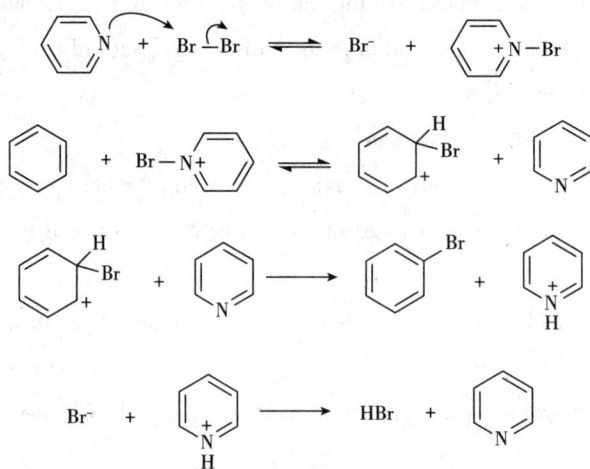

如果增加卤素比例将获得二取代产物（主要为对位异构体）。

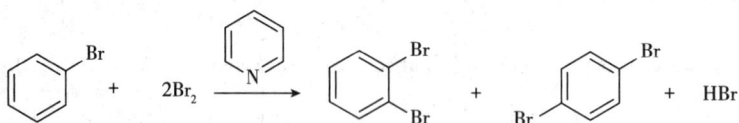

【实验步骤】

1. 原料和试剂

干燥苯	16ml（14g，0.180mol）
溴	8ml（25g，0.156mol）
干燥吡啶	0.2ml
10%氢氧化钠溶液	

2. 步骤 在250ml二颈瓶中，放置16ml（14g，0.180mol）苯（小心）和0.2ml干燥吡啶，装上滴液漏斗和冷凝管，在冷凝管上端装一个溴化氢吸收装置（图3-4）。烧瓶部分浸入冷水浴，冷水浴用三脚架和石棉网支撑，用滴液漏斗小心加入8ml（25g，0.156mol）溴。立即发生剧烈反应，反应生成的溴化氢气体逸出，被烧杯中的水吸收，待反应变缓后，加热水浴，维持水浴温度25~30℃一小时，然后水浴温度升至65~70℃，反应45分钟或直至溴消失（无红色蒸气）并且几乎没有溴化氢逸出为止。将深色反应混合物转入分液漏斗，先用水洗涤，然后用10%氢氧化钠洗涤，直至洗涤液对石蕊试纸显碱性，最后再用水洗涤。反应混合物洗涤后，用无水硫酸镁或无水氯化钙干燥，再用折叠滤纸滤入一小蒸馏瓶，缓慢蒸馏，收集150~170℃馏分。剩余物趁热倒入一小瓷缸。将bp150~170℃馏出液再蒸馏一次，收集154~157℃馏分，溴苯产量约12g。

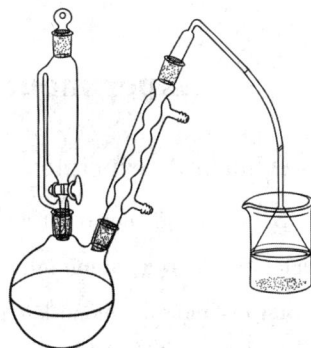

图3-4 制备溴苯装置

文献值：溴苯 bp 156.4℃。

【实验指导】

（一）预习要求

1. 复习苯环上进行亲电取代反应的原理。

2. 预习溴的性质及其取用注意事项。

3. 了解刺激性气体（如HBr）的吸收方法及其注意点。

4. 说明在本实验中提高产品的产量和质量所需采用的措施。

（二）注意事项

1. 用片状氢氧化钾干燥。

2. 仪器必须完全清洁干燥。

3. 溴具有强腐蚀性和强刺激性，取用时必须在通风橱中进行，必须佩戴橡胶手套和防毒面具，小心操作。如不慎触及皮肤，立即用稀乙醇洗，然后涂抹硼酸凡士林。

4. 将150ml水和20ml 10%氢氧化钠在250ml烧杯中混合，漏斗必须接近水面但没有浸入水。

5. 对二溴苯 bp 219℃，邻二溴苯 bp 224℃。

6. 瓷缸中的剩余物，可以用乙醇重结晶，分离得到纯的对二溴苯。每克用4ml乙醇（工业乙醇）溶解，0.5g活性炭脱色，趁热过滤，冰水浴冷却，真空过滤收集结晶，产量约2g，文献 mp 89℃。

7. 二次蒸馏可除去痕量苯。

（三）思考题

1. 什么是 Lewis 酸？

2. 芳环上的溴化反应为什么要有 Lewis 酸存在？

3. 为什么溴是邻、对位定位基？

4. 在溴苯与溴的反应中，为什么对二溴苯是主产物？为什么只有少量邻或间二溴苯形成？

Experiment 14　Preparation of Bromobenzene

Experimental principle

Benzene does not react appreciably with chlorine and bromine in the cold, but in the presence of catalysts, such as aluminium amalgam, pyridine or iron, reaction takes place readily, affording in the first instance the mono-halogenated derivative as the main product. The function of the catalyst is to increase the electrophilic activity of the halogen and the mechanism of the bromination of benzene with pyridine as the catalyst can be represented by the following scheme.

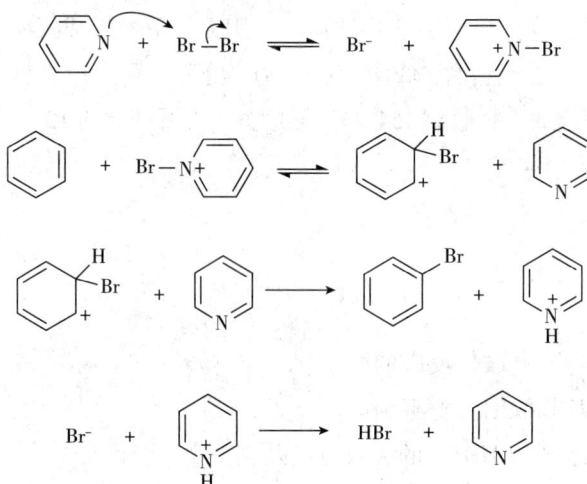

Di-substituted products (largely the para isomer) are obtained if the proportion of the halogen is increased.

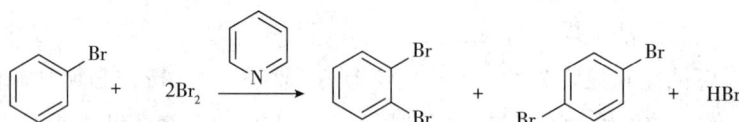

Experimental procedures

1. Materials and reagents

dry benzene　　　16ml

bromine　　　　　8ml

dry pyridine　　　0.2ml

10% sodium hydroxide

anhydrous magnesium sulphate or anhydrous calcium chloride

2. Procedures

Place 16ml (14g, 0.180mol) of dry benzene (CAUTION) and 0.2ml dry pyridine in a 250ml two-necked, round-bottom flask. Attach a reflux condenser and an addition funnel to the flask and fit a device on the top of the condenser for absorbing the hydrogen bromide gas subsequently evolved (Figure 3 − 4). Partially immerse the flask in a bath of cold water, supported upon a tripod and gauze. Carefully add 8ml (25g, 0.156mol) of bromine from the funnel to the flask.

A vigorous reaction soon occurs and hydrogen bromide is evolved which is absorbed by the water in the beaker; when the reaction slackens, warm the bath to 25 ~ 30℃ for 1 hour. Finally raise the temperature of the bath to 65 ~ 70℃ for a further 45min or until all the bromine has disappeared (no red vapours visible) and the evolution of hydrogen bromide has almost ceased. Transfer the dark-coloured reaction product to a separatory funnel and shake successively with water, with sufficient 5% ~ 10% sodium hydroxide solution to ensure that the washings are alkaline to litmus, and finally with

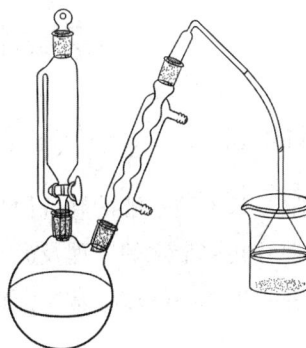

Figure 3 – 4　Apparatus for Preparation of Bromobenzene

water. Dry with magnesium sulphate or anhydrous calcium chloride. Filter through a fluted filter paper into a small distilling flask and distil slowly. Collect the crude bromobenzene at 150 ~ 170℃; Pour the residue while still hot into a small porcelain basin. Redistill the liquid of bp 150 ~ 170℃ and collect the bromobenzene at 154 ~ 157℃; the yield is about 12g.

Literature: bp 156.4℃.

Experimental instruction

Notes

1. It is dried over potassium hydroxide pellets.

2. It is essential that the apparatus be perfectly clean and dry.

3. A mixture of 150ml of water and 20ml of 10% sodium hydroxide is placed in a 250ml beaker. The funnel should be closed to the surface of the water and not immersed in the water.

4. Bromine is highly corrosive and irritating. It must be used in a fume hood. Rubber gloves and gas masks must be worn. In case of skin contact, wash immediately with dilute ethanol and apply boric acid petroleum jelly.

5. Boiling point of *p*-dibromobenzene is 219℃ and *o*-dibromobenzene is 224℃.

6. Isolate the pure *p*-dibromobenzene from the residue in the basin by recrystallization from hot ethanol with the addition of 0.5g of decolourising charcoal; use about 4ml of ethanol (industrial spirit) for each gram of material. Filter the hot solution through a fluted filter paper, cool in ice and filter crystals at the crystals at the pump. The yield of *p*-dibromobenzene, mp 89℃, is about 2g.

7. The trace of benzene is removed by redistillation.

Exercises

1. What is a Lewis acid?

2. Why is the presence of a Lewis acid required during the bromination of the aromatic ring?

3. Why is bromine an ortho-para director?

4. In the reaction between bromine and bromobenzene, why is para-dibromobenzene the dominant product, and why is very little ortho-or meta-dibromobenzene formed?

实验十五　苯甲酸乙酯的制备

【目的要求】

1. 学习苯甲酸乙酯的制备原理及操作方法。
2. 学习共沸带水的原理及分水器的使用方法。
3. 进一步熟练萃取、常压蒸馏、减压蒸馏等操作。

【实验原理】

羧酸和醇在酸催化下生成酯的反应称为酯化反应，常用的催化剂有硫酸、卤化氢和苯磺酸等，这是常用的制备酯的方法之一。本实验以硫酸为催化剂，通过苯甲酸和乙醇的反应制备苯甲酸乙酯。

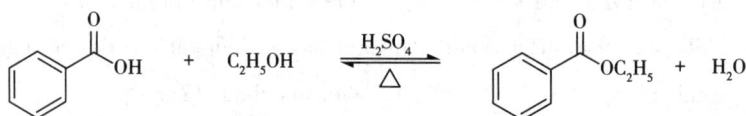

$$\text{C}_6\text{H}_5\text{COOH} + \text{C}_2\text{H}_5\text{OH} \underset{\triangle}{\overset{\text{H}_2\text{SO}_4}{\rightleftharpoons}} \text{C}_6\text{H}_5\text{COOC}_2\text{H}_5 + \text{H}_2\text{O}$$

此反应为可逆反应，为使平衡向生成酯的方向移动，提高酯的收率，一般使用过量的酸或醇，或者除去反应中生成的酯或水，或者两者同时使用。本反应使用过量乙醇，将反应生成的水从反应混合物中除去，使平衡向生成酯的方向移动。另外，使用大大过量的强酸催化剂，水转化为其共轭酸 H_3O^+，不具有亲核性，可以抑制逆反应的进行。

【实验步骤】

1. 原料和试剂

苯甲酸	6.1g（0.05mol）
无水乙醇	15ml（11.8g，0.257mol）
环己烷	35ml（23.7g，0.325mol）
浓硫酸	2ml
乙酸乙酯	30ml
饱和氯化钠	
无水氯化钙	

2. 步骤

在100ml圆底烧瓶中，放置6.1g（0.05mol）苯甲酸和15ml无水乙醇，沿瓶壁小心加入2ml浓硫酸，摇动圆底烧瓶使混合均匀。加入搅拌子，装上回流冷凝管，开动搅拌，用油浴加热回流半小时，反应物稍冷，加入35ml环己烷，在回流冷凝管和圆底烧瓶之间装一分水器（图3-5）。

继续搅拌，油浴加热回流，三元共沸，环己烷-乙醇-水被蒸出，蒸气冷凝后冷凝液滴入分水器，冷凝液在分水器中分为二层。回流反应时，允许上层液体回到反应瓶，防止下层液体回到反应瓶。当下层液体液面接近分水器支管时，放出部分下层液体。继续回流，直至上层澄清，看不

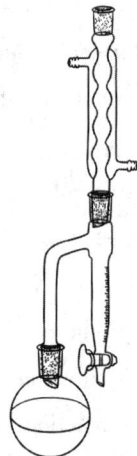

图3-5　制备苯甲酸乙酯装置

到水珠通过上层进入下层。放出分水器中的馏出液并回收，提高加热温度，蒸馏反应混合物，将反应瓶中的环己烷和乙醇蒸入分水器，并不时放出分水器中的液体并回收，以防止冷凝液返回反应瓶。直至大部分乙醇、环己烷都已蒸出，回收蒸出液。

反应瓶中的剩余物冷却后倒入盛有 50ml 水的烧杯，反应瓶用少量乙醇荡洗，荡洗液倒入烧杯。在搅拌下分批加入少量固体碳酸钠，直至没有二氧化碳逸出，反应混合物溶液呈中性。将反应混合物转入分液漏斗静置分层，分出有机层，水层用乙酸乙酯提取（15ml × 2），合并有机层和提取液，用 20ml 饱和氯化钠溶液洗涤，仔细分层，有机层放入一干燥锥形瓶，加无水氯化钙充分干燥。

液体滤入干燥蒸馏瓶，蒸除乙酸乙酯。将剩余物减压蒸馏，收集 bp 101 ~ 103℃/20mmHg 馏分。产量约 8 ~ 10g。

文献值：bp 212℃/760mmHg，108℃/30mmHg，101.5℃/20mmHg，86.5℃/10mmHg，70 ~ 71℃/4mmHg。

【实验指导】

（一）预习要求

1. 复习酸和醇发生酯化反应的原理。
2. 了解共沸蒸馏的原理。
3. 了解分水器分水的原理。
3. 复习萃取、普通蒸馏、减压蒸馏等基本操作。

（二）注意事项

1. 瓶内温度必须降到 80℃以下，以防止混合物起泡冲料。
2. 水和许多物质可形成共沸物（见表 3 - 1）。
3. 水含量上层比下层少。
4. 上层和下层都只含少量的水，大部分都是乙醇和环己烷，上层和下层都易燃，操作时要特别小心，以避免火灾。
5. 回流时间约 2.5 ~ 3 小时。

表 3 - 1　水共沸物

组分 A		组分 B		共沸物			
物质	沸点，℃	物质	沸点，℃	A 百分含量（重量）	水百分含量（重量）	B 百分含量（重量）	沸点，℃
硝酸	86.0			68	32		120.5
甲酸	100.7			77.5	22.5		107.3
正丙醇	97.2			71.7	28.3		87.7
特丁醇	82.5			88.2	11.8		79.9
乙醇	78.3			95.6	4.4		78.1
苯	80.1			91.1	8.9		69.4
苯	80.1	乙醇	78.3	74.1	7.4	18.5	64.9
环己烷	81	乙醇	78.3	75.5	4.8	19.7	62.6
2 - 丙醇	82.4			87.8	12.2		80.4
苯酚	181.8			9.2	90.8		99.5

（三）思考题

1. 本实验中采用了哪些措施提高反应收率？

2. 设计一个用苯甲酸和叔丁醇制备苯甲酸叔丁酯的方法。

3. 酯的碱性水解为什么称为皂化反应？为什么优于酸催化水解？

4. 什么情况下，用过量醇，促进平衡向产物移动，没有实用性？

Experiment 15 Preparation of Ethyl Benzoate

Experimental principle

The reaction of carboxylic acid and alcohol under the catalysis of acid to produce ester is called esterification reaction, which is one of the common methods to prepare ester. Common catalysts include sulfuric acid, hydrogen halide and benzene sulfonic acid. In this experiment, ethyl benzoate is prepared by reaction of benzoic acid and ethanol with sulfuric acid as catalyst.

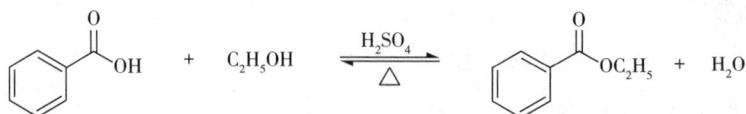

Since the reaction is reversible, the equilibrium must be shifted toward to obtain good conversion to the ester. This can be accomplished by using excessive alcohol or carboxylic acid and removing the water or ester from the reaction mixture as it is formed. In addition, a large excess of the strong acid catalyst is used; water is converted to its conjugate acid, H_3O^+, which is non-nucleophililc and cannot promote the reversion of the desired ester to reactants.

Experimental procedure

1. Materials and reagents

benzoic acid	6. 1g（0. 05mol）
ethanol	15ml（11. 8g,0. 257mol）
cyclohexane	35ml（23. 7g,0. 325mol）
concentrated sulfuric acid	2ml
Ethyl acetate	30ml
saturated aqueous sodium chloride	
anhydrous calcium chloride	

2. Procedures

In a 100ml round-bottom flask, place 6. 1g（0. 05mol）of benzoic acid and 15ml of ethanol. Carefully pour 2ml of concentrated sulfuric acid down the wall of the flask and swirl the flask to obtain good mixing. Add stirring bar, and attach a refux condenser, Start the stirring and reflux the mixture for 30min in an oil bath. Cool the contents of the flask slightly, remove the condenser, add 35ml of cyclohexane, and fit a Dean-Stark trap between the flask and the reflux condenser. (Figure 3 −5).

Continuing stirring and gently heat the mixture at reflux. A ternary azeotrope mixture, cyclohexane-ethanol-water, is distilled out. As the azeotrope condenses and falls into the water separator, distillate appears two layers. Allow the top layer to return to the flask and prevent the bottom layer from returning to the reaction mixture during the reflux period. When the bottom layer comes close to the sidearm of the Dean-Stark trap the portion of it is removed. Continue to reflux until the top layer is clear and water droplets no longer appear in it. Remove the condensate in the Dean-Stark trap, increase the heating so that the vapor from the flask is condensed in the Dean-Stark trap, and prevent the condensate from returning to the flask by removing it. Distill the reaction mixture until the excess of ethanol and cyclohexane has been distilled out. Cool the residue in the flask, pour it into about 50ml of water in a beaker, rinse the reaction flask with a little of ethanol, and

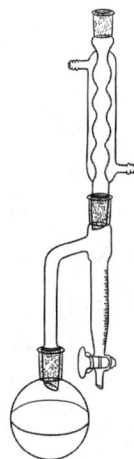

Figure 3 – 5　Apparatus for Preparation of Ethyl Benzoate

pour this into the beaker. Add successive small portions of sodium carbonate, while stirring the mixture, until no carbon dioxide escapes and the aqueous solution is neutral.

Transfer the mixture to a separatory funnel, allow the layers to separate, and separate the organic liquid from the aqueous layer. Extract the aqueous layer with ethyl acetate (15ml × 2), combine the organic liquid and the extract liquor, wash it with 20ml of saturated aqueous sodium chloride, and separate the layers carefully. Place the organic layer in a dry Erlenmeyer flask, add a small amount of anhydrous calcium chloride, cork the flask firmly.

Filter the liquid into a dry flask and distill off the ethyl acetate. The residue is distilled under reduced pressure and collect the 101 ~ 103℃/20mmHg fraction. The yield is about 8 ~ 10g.

Literature: bp 212℃/760mmHg, 108℃/30mmHg, 101. 5℃/20mmHg, 86. 5℃/10mmHg, 70 ~ 71℃/4mmHg.

Experimental instruction

Notes

1. The contents of the flask must be cooled to a temperature below 80℃, in order to prevent the mixture from foaming and bumping.

2. Water forms azeotrope with many substances.

3. The water content of top layer is lower than that of bottom layer.

4. The top and bottom layers are both flammable. Avoid fire hazards.

5. Reflux for 2. 5 ~ 3h.

Table 3 – 1　Azeotropic Mixtures of Water

Component A		Component B		Azeotropic mixture			Boiling Point,℃
Substance	Boiling Point,℃	Substance	Boiling Point,℃	Percent of A (weight)	Percent of Water(weight)	Percent of B (weight)	
Nitric acid	86. 0			68	32		120. 5 (max.)
Formic acid	100. 7			77. 5	22. 5		107. 3 (max.)
n-Propyl alcohol	97. 2			71. 7	28. 3		87. 7 (min.)

continued

Component A		Component B		Azeotropic mixture			Boiling Point, ℃
Substance	Boiling Point, ℃	Substance	Boiling Point, ℃	Percent of A (weight)	Percent of Water(weight)	Percent of B (weight)	
t-Butyl alcohol	82. 5			88. 2	11. 8		79. 9（min.）
Ethanol	78. 3			95. 6	4. 4		78. 1（min.）
Benzene	80. 1			91. 1	8. 9		69. 4（min.）
Benzene	80. 1	Ethanol	78. 3	74. 1	7. 4	18. 5	64. 9（min.）
Cyclohexane	81	Ethanol	78. 3	75. 5	4. 8	19. 7	62. 6（min.）
2-propanol	82. 4			87. 8	12. 2		80. 4（min.）
Phenol	181. 8			9. 2	90. 8		99. 5（min.）

Exercises

1. What measures have been taken in this experiment to improve the reaction yield?

2. Suggest a method for preparing t-butyl benzoate from benzoic acid and t-butyl alcohol.

3. Why is the hydrolysis of an ester by an alkali called saponification? Why is this preferable to the use of an acid catalyst such as sulfuric acid?

4. Under what circumstances would it is impractical to use an excess of ROH to drive the equilibrium toward products? What alternatives for the synthesis of esters are available?

实验十六　三苯甲醇的制备

【目的要求】

1. **掌握**　用格氏反应制备三苯甲醇的原理及操作方法；无水操作技术。
2. **熟悉**　萃取、普通蒸馏、水蒸气蒸馏和重结晶等操作。
3. **了解**　简单化合物合成的实验设计方法；无水乙醚的制备方法。

【实验原理】

醇是一类非常重要的有机物，低级醇常用作溶剂或药物辅料，醇也可转化为烯、卤代烃、醛酮、羧酸等其他的各种有机化合物，是重要的有机合成和药物合成中间体或原料，无论工业上还是实验室经常需要制备醇。醇的制备方法很多，格氏试剂和醛酮或酯的反应，经常用于制备一些结构比较复杂的醇。

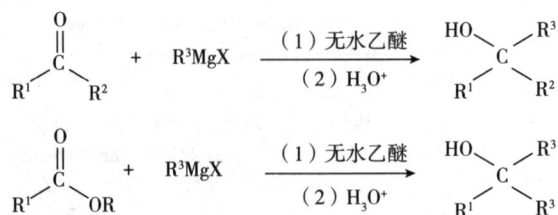

当 R^1、R^2、R^3 为苯基时，即可制备三苯甲醇。本实验以苯基溴化镁和苯甲酸乙酯为原料合成三苯甲醇。

卤代烃和溴苯在无水乙醚（或四氢呋喃）中反应，得到烃基卤化镁，称作格氏试剂。

$$R^3{-}X + Mg \xrightarrow{\text{无水乙醚}} R^3{-}MgX$$

由于格氏试剂可以和水、二氧化碳和氧气反应，因此涉及格氏试剂的反应必须在无水条件下进行，所用试剂和溶剂必须无水，所用仪器必需充分干燥，反应有时需要惰性气体保护下进行。

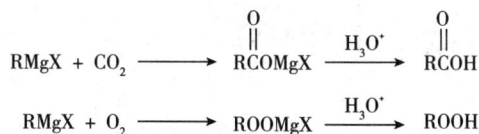

$$RMgX + CO_2 \longrightarrow RCOMgX \xrightarrow{H_3O^+} RCOH$$

$$RMgX + O_2 \longrightarrow ROOMgX \xrightarrow{H_3O^+} ROOH$$

当用乙醚为溶剂时，乙醚蒸气可以排出大部分的空气，一般可以不用惰性气体保护。制备格氏试剂时通常可加入少量碘引发反应。

本实验以无水乙醚为溶剂，利用溴苯和金属镁的反应制备苯基溴化镁（无水乙醚的制备参考本书第一部分之五：常用有机溶剂及纯化；溴苯的制备参考本书实验十四）。

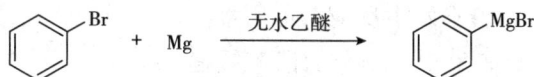

苯基溴化镁和溴苯经芳基偶联反应（Wurtz-Fittig 反应），生成少量联苯，这是反应的副产物之一。

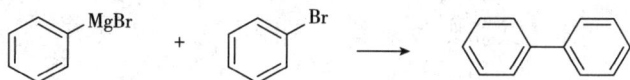

苯基溴化镁和苯甲酸乙酯经过下列反应制得三苯甲醇（苯甲酸乙酯的制备参考本书实验十五：苯甲酸乙酯的制备）。

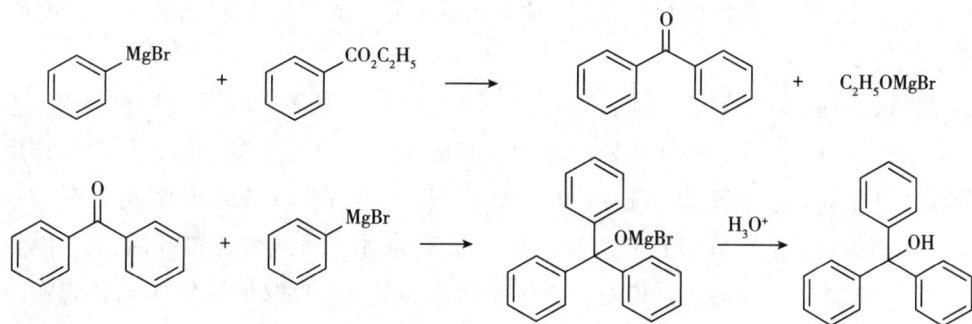

反应混合物酸化后，有机层（醚溶液）含有三苯甲醇、苯甲酸乙酯、溴苯、联苯、二苯甲酮和苯等，格氏试剂水解产生苯。

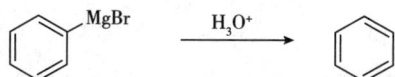

乙醚和苯可通过蒸馏除去，粗产物中含有需要的三苯甲醇和副产物联苯等，可通过水蒸气蒸馏的方法蒸出副产物联苯和未反应的溴苯，三苯甲醇粗产物可通过重结晶纯化。

（三）实验步骤

1. 原料和试剂

镁　　　　　　1.25 g（0.05 mol）

溴苯　　　　　　5.7ml（8.52g，0.054mol）

苯甲酸乙酯　　　2.4ml（2.51g，0.0167mol）

绝对乙醚　　　　33ml

10%硫酸　　　　50ml

乙醚

晶状碘

5%碳酸钠溶液

环己烷

2. 步骤　在250ml 三颈瓶上，分别装置机械搅拌、回流冷凝管和滴液漏斗，在冷凝管的上口装置氯化钙干燥管。在瓶内放置 1.25g（0.05mol）镁屑，25ml 绝对乙醚和一小粒碘。在滴液漏斗中，放置 5.7ml（8.52g，0.054mol）溴苯，开动搅拌，自滴液漏斗中滴下 1～2ml 溴苯，若不发生反应，可用水浴加热。反应开始后，将滴液漏斗中剩余的溴苯缓慢滴加到反应混合物里，控制滴加速度，保持溶液不加热时呈微沸状态（约15 分钟滴完）。溴苯加完后，在水浴上回流约 30 分钟。当金属镁溶解后反应结束，此时可能仍有一些暗色杂质颗粒未溶。停止加热，立即进行下步反应。

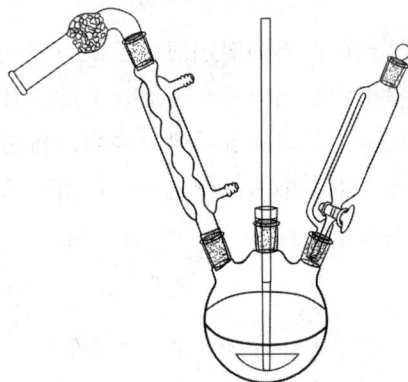

图3-6　制备三苯甲醇装置

将格氏试剂冷却至15～20℃，在滴液漏斗中加2.4ml（2.51g，0.0167mol）苯甲酸乙酯与8ml 绝对乙醚的溶液。在搅拌下，将该溶液缓慢滴入格氏试剂中（约20 分钟滴完），滴加过程中可冷却反应瓶以控制反应。苯甲酸乙酯加完后继续回流 30 分钟。停止搅拌，将反应混合物冷却。

在250ml 烧杯中，放置25g 冰，50ml 10%硫酸，在搅拌下，将反应混合物倒入烧杯，使加成物分解。分出醚层，水层用乙醚萃取（15ml×2）。合并乙醚溶液，依次分别用5%碳酸钠溶液和饱和食盐水各7ml 洗涤一次。然后把乙醚溶液转入250ml 圆底烧瓶，安装蒸馏装置，水浴加热，蒸馏除去乙醚。残余物中加20ml 水，将残留物捣碎后进行水蒸气蒸馏，直至馏出液无油状物为止。将残余物冷却抽滤，用滴管吸取少量95% 乙醇洗涤滤渣2次，干燥得黄色粗品。粗品用环己烷重结晶（10ml/g 粗产品），趁热过滤后，将滤液浓缩至约原体积的 1/2，冷却，抽滤得白色晶体。产量 2～3g，mp 160～162℃。

文献值：mp 162～164℃。

【实验指导】

（一）预习要求

1. 复习格氏试剂的性质及其在有机合成中的应用。

2. 了解制备格氏试剂的方法及进行格氏反应的条件。

3. 复习醇的制备方法及原理。

4. 复习萃取、普通蒸馏、水蒸气蒸馏和重结晶等操作。

5. 说明本实验中为了使反应在无水条件下进行所采取的有关措施。

（二）注意事项

1. 进行格氏反应时，反应试剂必须无水、无醇，仪器必须绝对清洁、干燥。

2. 必须使用干净，无氧化层的镁。

3. 乙醚必须绝对无水。

4. 碘颜色消失、出现混浊和自发沸腾表明反应开始。

5. 为保证实验成功，必须待反应开始后，再加入大部分乙醚和溴苯。

6. 加热不能太剧烈以免乙醚从冷凝管逸出。

7. 蒸出的乙醚及时回收。

（三）思考题

1. 写出苯基溴化镁与下列化合物的反应，包括反应混合物弱酸水解。

（1）二氧化碳　　（2）乙醇　　（3）氧

（4）对甲苯基氰　　（5）甲酸乙酯

2. 从苯基溴化镁如何合成下列化合物。

（1）1,2 - 二苯基乙醇

（2）苯甲醛

（3）苄醇

3. 工业乙醚常含有乙醇，如果用这种乙醚而不是无水乙醚，乙醇对格氏试剂形成有什么影响？解释原因。

4. 如果使用溴代环己烷作为添加剂，帮助引发反应，制备苯基溴化镁和正丁基溴化镁，将遇到什么问题？

5. 即便用干燥管，隔绝潮气，不必要的将格氏试剂溶液暴露在空气中仍不合理，为什么？

6. 为什么将格氏试剂溶液冷至室温后，再滴加苯甲酸乙酯溶液？

7. 酯滴入格氏试剂，反应生成的固体是什么？

Experiment 16　Preparation of Triphenylmethanol

Experimental principle

Alcohols are a very important class of organic compounds. Low-grade alcohols are often used as solvents or pharmaceutical excipients. Alcohols can also be converted to other organic compounds such as olefins, halogenated hydrocarbons, aldehydes, ketones, carboxylic acids, etc. Alcohols are important intermediates or raw materials for organic synthesis and drug synthesis, and often prepared in industry and laboratory. There are many methods for preparing alcohols. The reaction of Grignard reagent with aldehydes, ketones or esters is often used to prepare alcohols with complex structures.

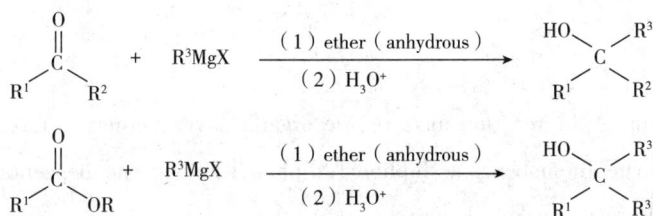

Triphenylmethanol can be prepared when R^1, R^2 and R^3 are phenyl. Triphenylmethanol was synthesized from phenylmagnesium bromide and ethyl benzoate in this experiment.

Halogenated hydrocarbons react with bromobenzene in anhydrous ether (or THF) to produce alkyl magnesium halide, which is called Grignard reagent.

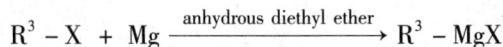

$$R^3 - X + Mg \xrightarrow{\text{anhydrous diethyl ether}} R^3 - MgX$$

Because Grignard reagent can react with water, carbon dioxide and oxygen, the reaction involving Grignard reagent must be carried out under anhydrous conditions, the reagent and solvent used must be anhydrous, the instrument used must be fully dried, and the reaction sometimes needs to be carried out under the protection of inert gas.

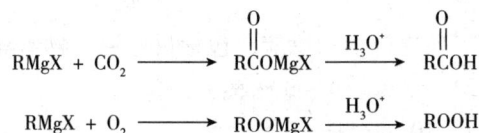

$$RMgX + CO_2 \longrightarrow RCOMgX \xrightarrow{H_3O^+} RCOH$$
$$RMgX + O_2 \longrightarrow ROOMgX \xrightarrow{H_3O^+} ROOH$$

When ether is used as the solvent, ether vapor disgels most of the air, usually without inert gas protection. A small amount of iodine is usually added to initiate the reaction in the preparation of Grignard reagent.

In this experiment, anhydrous ether was used as solvent to prepare phenylmagnesium bromide by the reaction of bromobenzene and magnesium.

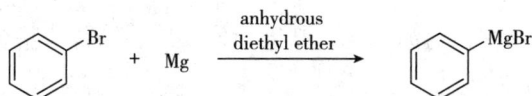

Magnesium phenyl bromide and bromobenzene react with aryl group (Wurtz-Fittig reaction) to produce a small amount of biphenyl, which is one of the by-products of the reaction.

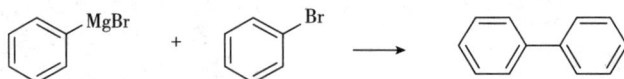

Triphenyl methanol is prepared by the following reaction of phenyl magnesium bromide and ethyl benzoate. (Reference experiment 15 of this book for preparation of ethyl benzoate).

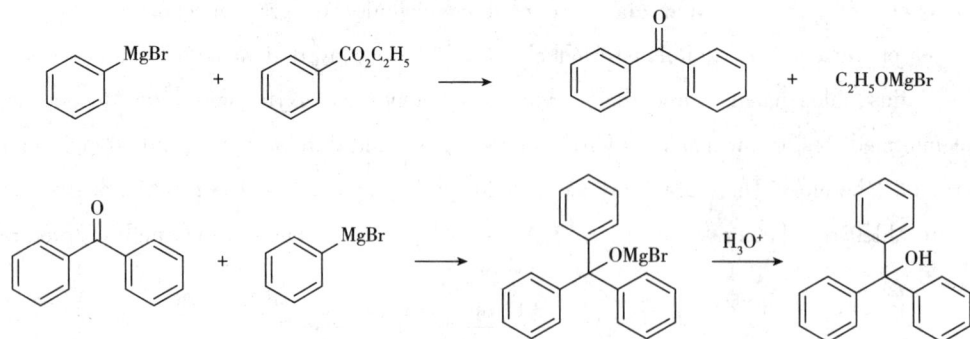

After acidification of the reaction mixture, the organic layer (ether solution) contains triphenyl methanol, ethyl benzoate, bromobenzene, biphenyl, diphenyl ketone and benzene etc. Phenyl magnesium bromide hydrolyzes to produce benzene.

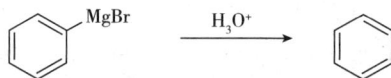

Ether and benzene can be distilled. The crude products contain the required Triphenylmethanol and by-product biphenyl. The by-product biphenyl and bromobenzene can be distilled by steam distillation. The crude products of Triphenylmethanol can be purified by recrystallization.

Experimental procedures

1. Materials and reagents

magnesium	1.25g (0.05mol)
bromobenzene	5.7ml (8.52 g,0.054mol)
ethyl benzoate	2.4ml (2.51g,0.0167mol)
anhydrous diethyl ether	33ml
10% sulfuric acid	50ml
crystal of iodine	
5% sodium carbonate solution	
cyclohexane	

2. Procedures

Equip a 250ml dry three-necked round-bottom flask with a mechanical stirrer, a reflux condenser and a dropping funnel. Attach calcium chloride drying tube to the top of the condenser (Figure 3 −6).

Introduce directly into the flask 1.25g (0.05mol) of magnesium turning, 25ml of anhydrous diethyl ether and a small crystal of iodine. Place 5.7ml (8.52g,0.054mol) bromobenzene in the dropping funnel. Start stirring, drop 1~2ml bromobenzene into the flask. If the reaction does not start at once, warm the flask gently in a bath of warm water. After

Figure 3 −6　Apparatus for Preparation of Triphenylmethanol

the reaction has started, continue adding the remaining bromobenzene dropwise into the reaction mixture at such a rate that the ether refluxes without external heating(about 15min).

After all of the halide has been added, reflux the mixture gently for 30min on a water bath. The reaction is complete when the solution normally has a tan to brown, and most of the magnesium will have disappeared. Remove the heating bath and proceed without delay to the next step.

Cool the reaction flask containing the Grignard reagent to 15~20℃ and place in the dropping funnel a solution of 8ml (8g,0.05mol) of pure ethyl benzoate in about 25ml of anhydrous ether. Drop the ethyl benzoate solution into the Grignard reagent slowly with continuous stirring. This reaction is exothermic, so you should control the rate of reaction by adjusting the rate of addition and by occasionally cooling the reaction flask as needed with the ice-water bath. The bromomagnesium derivative of the alcohol separates as a white precipitate. After all of the ethyl benzoate has been added, reflux another 30 min.

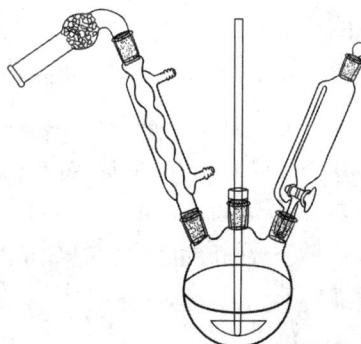

With stirring, pour the reaction mixture into a 250ml beaker containing 50ml of 10% sulfuric acid and about 25g of ice. Transfer the mixture to a separatory funnel, and separate the organic liquid from the aqueous layer. Extract the aqueous layer with diethyl ether (15ml×2), combine the ether extracts, wash the organic layer sequentially with 7ml 5% aqueous sodium carbonate and 7ml saturated sodium chloride solution. Transfer the organic layer into a 250ml round-bottom flask, remove the diethyl ether by simple distillation. Add 20ml water into the flask, the residue is mashed and steam distilled until the outflow is oil-free. The solid was collected by vacuum filtration and washed with little 95% ethanol twice, then dry the solid to obtain yellow crude product. Recrystallize the crude procuct with cyclohexane (ca. 10ml/g product). Isolate the product by vacuum filtration, dry and weigh it. The yield is about 2~3g, mp 160~162℃. Literature: mp 162~164℃.

Experimental instruction

Notes

1. In Grignard reactions it is essential that the reagents be free from ethanol and water, and the apparatus perfectly clean and dry.

2. The clean, unoxidized surfaces of magnesium must be used.

3. It is essential that the ether be of the anhydrous grade.

4. It is evidenced by disappearance of the iodine color, appearance of turbidity, and spontaneous boiling.

5. For the success of the experiment it is essential that the reaction begin before the main portions of the ether and bromobenzene are added

6. Do not heat the material so vigorously that ether vapors traverse the condenser.

7. Ether is a volatile, flammable and explosive substance with a low boiling point, so it is necessary to prevent open flame during distillation, maintain ventilation in the laboratory, receive cooling by ice water bath outside the bottle, and immediately recycle after steaming.

Exercises

1. Write equation for the action of phenylmagnesium bromide on the following compounds, including hydrolysis of the reaction mixture with dilute acid.

(1) Carbon dioxide

(2) Ethanol

(3) Oxygen

(4) *p*-tolunitrile

(5) Ethyl formate

2. How may the following compounds be prepared from phenylmagnesium bromide?

(1) 1,2-diphenylethanol

(2) Benzaldehyde

(3) Benzyl alcohol

3. Ethanol is often present in the technical grade of diethyl ether. If this grade rather than anhydrous were used, what effect, if any, would the ethanol have on the formation of the Grignard reagent? Explain?

4. Which problems might be encountered if bromocyclohexane were used as an additive to help

initiate the formation of phenylmagnesium bromide and *n*-butylmagnesium bromide? How does the use of 1,2-dibromoethane avoid such experimental difficulties?

5. Why is it unwise to allow the solution of the Grignard reagent to remain exposed to air for an unnecessary period of time even if it is protected from moisture by drying tubes?

6. Why is it unwise to begin addition of the solution of ethyl benzoate to the Grignard reagent before the latter has cooled to room temperature?

What is the solid that forms during the addition of the ester to the Grignard reagent?

实验十七 2-硝基雷琐酚的制备

【目的要求】

1. 学习在苯环上进行亲电取代反应的定位规律及磺化反应的应用。
2. 学习 2-硝基-1,3-苯二酚的合成方法。

【实验原理】

有机合成时，常引入其他基团，阻止或保护分子中某些潜在反应部位，免受反应试剂进攻。这种基团必须容易导入，一些关键合成反应步骤完成后，又易于除去。

由雷琐酚（1,3-二羟基苯）合成 2-硝基雷琐酚，雷琐酚先磺化生成 4,6-二磺酸基雷琐酚，两个最易硝化部位被保护。将 4,6-二磺酸基雷琐酚硝化，然后水蒸气蒸馏二磺酸雷琐酚硝化物酸性溶液，水解除去磺酸基，生成纯的 2-硝基雷琐酚。

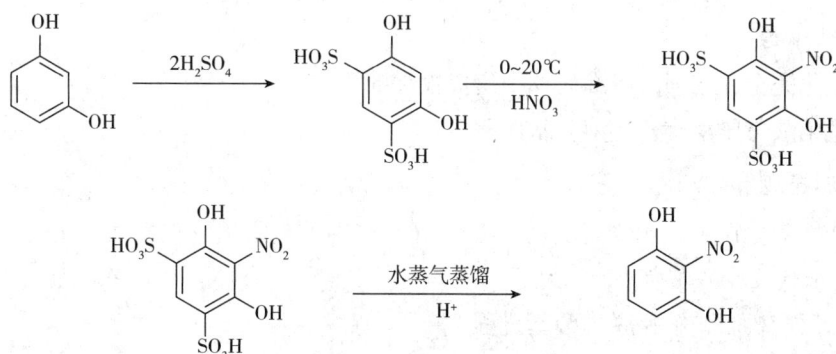

【实验步骤】

1. 原料和试剂

粉状雷琐酚	7.7g（0.07mol）
浓硫酸（98%，$d = 1.84$g/ml）	28ml（50.4g，0.515mol）
混酸 { 硝酸（70% ~72%，$d = 1.42$g/ml）	4.4ml（4.38g，0.0693mol）
浓硫酸（98%，$d = 1.84$g/ml）	6.2ml（11.9g，0.116mol）
95%乙醇	

2. 步骤

150ml 烧杯中，放置 7.7g（0.07mol）粉状雷琐酚，加 28ml（50.4g，0.515mol）浓硫酸（98%，$d = 1.84$）。几分钟后，如无黏稠的 4,6-二磺酸浆状物生成，混合物加热到 60~65℃。浆状物放置 15 分钟。

将 4.4ml（4.38g，0.0693mol）硝酸（70% ~ 72%，$d = 1.42$）和 6.2ml（11.9g，0.116mol）浓硫酸混合，混合酸用冰水浴冷却。浆状物用冰 - 盐浴冷至 5 ~ 10℃，烧杯上方悬一滴液漏斗，搅拌浆状物，用滴液漏斗缓慢滴加已冷却好的混酸。控制滴加速度，使反应混合物温度不超过 20℃。黄色混合物室温放置 15 分钟，然后保持混合物温度 50℃ 以下，小心加入 20g 碎冰。将混合物转入 500ml 圆底烧瓶，加 0.1g 尿素，进行水蒸气蒸馏。至冷凝管上无桔红色的 2 - 硝基雷琐酚，或冷凝管上有不要的黄色针状 4,6 - 二硝基雷琐酚（mp 215℃）时，停止蒸馏。

水蒸气蒸馏 5 分钟左右，通常有产物出现。如蒸馏瓶中冷凝蒸气太多，产品难以蒸出。如果这样，停止通水蒸气，加热蒸馏瓶（煤气灯或加热套）。除去水，增加蒸馏瓶中的酸浓度，当瓶中酸的浓度足以催化脱磺酸基的反应时，停止加热，重新水蒸气蒸馏。

如冷凝管中充满固化产品，停止通冷凝水几分钟，直至产品熔化进入接收瓶。

馏出液用冰水浴冷却，布氏漏斗过滤，稀乙醇重结晶。产品先溶于 95% 乙醇(3ml/g)，趁热过滤，然后缓慢加水至溶液混蚀（少量沉淀），放置缓慢冷却。产量 2.5 ~ 3.5g。纯 2 - 硝基雷锁酚 mp 84 ~ 85℃。

【实验指导】

（一）预习要求

1. 复习苯环上进行亲电取代反应的定位规律，熟记第一类定位基和第二类定位基及其致活和致钝强度的顺序。

2. 复习磺化反应的可逆性及其在合成中的应用。

3. 巩固机械搅拌、水蒸气蒸馏等基本操作。

（二）注意事项

1. 为磺化完全，雷琐酚应在研钵中研成很细的粉末。

2. 过量硝酸与尿素成盐，溶于水而除去。

（三）思考题

1. 为什么磺化在 4 和 6 位而不是 2 位？4,6 - 二磺酸基雷琐酚与雷琐酚比较，二磺化后活性（亲电取代反应）如何？

2. 写出反应机制，解释脱磺酸基过程。

3. 设计一个机制，解释 4,6 - 二雷琐酚的形成。

4. 与间苯二酚比较，2 - 硝基 - 1,3 - 苯二酚有什么特征红外吸收？

5. 如何利用氢核磁共振谱区别 2 - 硝基雷琐酚和 4,6 - 二硝基雷琐酚？

Experiment 17　Preparation of 2-Nitroresorcinol

Experimental principle

In the course of certain organic synthesis, it is often advantageous to introduce a group that will effectively block or protect certain potentially reactive sites on a molecule from attack by some specific reagent. Important features of such a group are that it should be easily introduced and easily removed after some crucial step in the synthesis has been performed.

In the process of converting resorcinol（1,3-dihydroxybenzene）to 2-nitroresorcinol,the starting compound is first sulfonated to give resorcinol-4,6-disulfonic acid in which two of the three positions most susceptible to nitration are now blocked. Nitration followed by steam distillation of an acidic solution of the nitrated disulfonic acid to remove the sulfonic acid groups results in pure 2-nitoresorcinol.

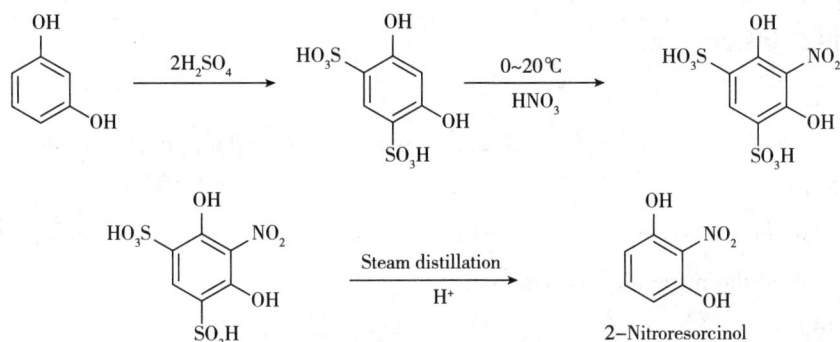

Experimental procedures

1. Material and reagents

powdered resorcinol	7.7g（0.07mol）
concentrated sulfuric acid（98%,$d = 1.84$g/ml）	28ml（50.4g,0.515mol）
mixed acid { nieric acid（70% ~72%,$d = 1.42$g/ml）	4.4ml（4.38g,0.0693mol）
concentrated sulfuric acid（98%,$d = 1.84$g/ml）	6.2ml（11.9g,0.116mol）
95% ethanol	
ice	

2. Procedures

Place 7.7g（0.07mol）of powered resorcinol in a 150ml beaker and add 28ml（50.4g,0.515mol）of concentrated sulfuric acid（98%,$d = 1.84$）. If a thick slurry of the 4,6-disulfonic acid does not form in a few minutes,warm the mixture to 60~65℃. Allow the slurry to stand for 15min.

Prepare a mixture of 4.4ml（4.38g,0.0693mol）of nitric acid（70% ~72%,$d = 1.42$）and 6.2ml（11.9g,0.116mol）of concentrated sulfuric acid,and cool it in an ice bath. Cool the slurry in an ice-salt bath to a temperature of 5~10℃,stir it,and slowly（dropwise）add the cold acid solution from an addition funnel suspended over the beaker. The temperature of the reaction mixture should not exceed 20℃. After the yellowish mixture has stood for 15min,it should be cautiously diluted with 20g of crushed ice so that the temperature never exceeds 50℃.

Transfer the mixture to a 500ml round-bottomed flask,add 0.1g of urea,and carry out an indirect steam distillation until no more of the orange-red,solid 2-nitroresorcinol appears in the condenser or until yellow needles of the undesired 4,6-dinitroresorcinol（mp 215℃）appear in thecondenser. The product will usually appear after about 5 min of steam distillation. The product may not steam-distill if too much steam has condensed in the distillation flask. In this event shut off the steam and heat the flask（a Bunsen burner or a heating mantle will be required）until sufficient water is removed to increase the sulfuric acid concentration in the flask to the point at which desulfonation will occur and product will again distill. If the condenser becomes filled with solidified product,turn off the cooling water for a few minutes until the product has melted and flowed into the receiver.

Cool the distillate in an ice bath and filter it with suction. Recrystallize the product from dilute aqueous ethanol by first dissolving it in 95% ethanol (ca. 3ml per gram of product) ,filtering it hot, adding water slowly until cloudiness (or small amounts of precipitate) persists ,and allowing the solution to cool slowly. The yield of 2-nitroresorcinol ,is 2. 5 ~ 3. 5g. The melting point of pure 2-nitroresorcinol is 84 ~ 85℃.

Experimental instruction

Notes

1. In order to be sulphated completely ,the resorcinol should have been previously ground to fine power in a mortar.

2. When urea is added ,the salt of the urea and the nitric acid is formed. As the salt dissolves in water ,the excess of the nitric acid is removed.

Exercises

1. Why might sulfonation be expected to occur most readily in the 4-and 6-positions rather than the 2-position? How does the overall reactivity (toward electrophilic attack) of the disulfonic acid compare with that of resorcinol?

2. Write out a step-by-step mechanism to explain the desulfonation process.

3. Devise a mechanism to account for formation of the 4 ,6-dinitroresorcinol.

4. What characteristic infrared absorptions would you expect to find in 2-nitroresorcinol that would not be present in resorcinol?

How could you use ^{1}HNMR to tell the difference between 2-nitroresorcinol and 4 ,6-dinitroresorcinol?

实验十八　芳香醛的康尼查罗反应

【目的要求】

学习通过芳香醛的康尼查罗反应来制备芳基甲醇和芳基甲酸的原理及操作方法。

【实验原理】

无 α - 氢的芳香醛，如苯甲醛、糠醛（呋喃 – 2 – 甲醛），不能进行羟醛缩合反应，但与浓碱溶液作用时，发生 Cannizzaro 反应，生成等摩尔的芳基甲醇和芳基甲酸。

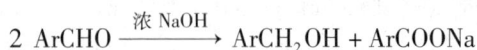

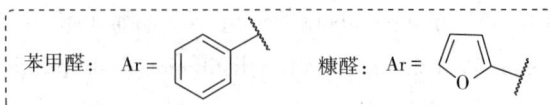

$$2\ ArCHO \xrightarrow{\text{浓 NaOH}} ArCH_2OH + ArCOONa$$

因芳基甲醇，如苯甲醇、呋喃 – 2 – 甲醇易溶于乙酸乙酯而芳基甲酸钠易溶于水，因而芳基甲醇容易用乙酸乙酯提取分离；水层加无机酸，水溶性芳基甲酸钠转化成芳基甲酸，芳基甲酸如苯甲酸、呋喃 – 2 – 甲酸不溶于冰水而析出。

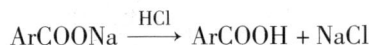

$$\text{ArCOONa} \xrightarrow{\text{HCl}} \text{ArCOOH} + \text{NaCl}$$

【实验步骤】

（一）苯甲醇和苯甲酸的制备

1. 原料和试剂

苯甲醛	10.5g（10ml，0.1mol）
氢氧化钠	7.5g
乙酸乙酯	60ml
饱和亚硫酸氢钠溶液	5ml
10%碳酸钠溶液	10ml
浓盐酸	40ml

无水硫酸镁

2. 步骤　在 100ml 三颈瓶上安装机械搅拌及回流冷凝管，加入 30ml 水和 7.5g 氢氧化钠，打开搅拌使固体溶解，稍冷后加入 10ml 新蒸苯甲醛，加热回流 1 小时，期间反应混合物由乳浊液变为透明液体。反应完毕，反应混合物冷却至室温，加入 35ml 冷水，搅拌下溶解析出的固体。混合物转入分液漏斗，用乙酸乙酯（30ml×2）萃取，同时保留有机相和水相。有机相依次用 5ml 饱和亚硫酸氢钠溶液、10ml 10%碳酸钠溶液、10ml 冷水洗涤，将有机层转移至锥形瓶，用无水硫酸镁干燥。滤去干燥剂，用少量乙酸乙酯洗涤瓶子和干燥剂，洗涤液一并滤入蒸馏瓶，沸水浴蒸馏除去乙酸乙酯。剩余物进行减压蒸馏，收集 75～77℃／12mmHg 馏分，苯甲醇产量 3.1g。文献：bp 205.4℃／762mmHg。

将 40ml 浓盐酸、40ml 水和 25g 碎冰放入烧杯，一边摇动烧杯一边将水相缓慢倒入其中，有白色固体析出，抽滤，滤饼用少量冷水洗涤，晾干，得苯甲酸粗品。为进一步纯化，可用水重结晶，得白色片状晶体。产量 3.7g，mp 120～122℃，文献：mp 122.4℃。

（二）呋喃－2－甲醇和呋喃－2－甲酸的制备

1. 原料和试剂

糠醛	19g（0.2mol）
33%氢氧化钠溶液	16ml
乙醚	45ml

25%盐酸

无水硫酸镁或无水碳酸钾

2. 步骤　在 100ml 三颈瓶中，加入 19g（16.4ml，0.2mol）糠醛，装上机械搅拌器，开动搅拌。冰水浴冷却至 10℃左右，搅拌下分批加入 16ml 33%氢氧化钠溶液。控制滴加速度，维持反应温度在 10～14℃之间。氢氧化钠滴加完后，室温搅拌 30 分钟，得黄色浆状物，加适量水（约 20ml），溶解沉淀。

暗褐色溶液转入分液漏斗，用乙醚萃取（15ml×3），合并醚层，用无水硫酸镁干燥（水层保留备用）。滤去干燥剂，滤液转移至圆底烧瓶中，先在水浴上蒸去乙醚，剩余物用油浴加热蒸馏。少量水和乙醚先蒸出，然后温度迅速升到呋喃－2－甲醇的沸点，收集 169～172℃馏分，产量 7～8g，文献 bp 171℃／750mmHg。

溶有呋喃－2－甲酸钠的水溶液用 25%盐酸酸化，至刚果红试纸变兰。冰水浴冷却，使

2 - 呋喃甲酸析出完全，抽滤，滤饼用少量冷水洗涤，晾干。

为进一步纯化，可用水重结晶，得白色针状晶体。产量约 8g，mp 129 ~ 130℃，文献：mp 133 ~ 134℃。

【实验指导】

（一）预习要求

1. 复习无 α - H 的醛自身氧化还原反应的原理、反应条件及应用。

2. 了解从反应产物中提取、分离有机醇和酸的一般操作过程。

3. 复习水溶剂重结晶、乙醚蒸馏等基本操作。

（二）注意事项

苯甲酸在 100℃ 开始升华。使用毛细管测熔点时，可在填充样品后通过密封毛细管的顶端来防止升华。使用比正常操作更多的样品，在略低于预期熔点的温度下将样品放入熔点仪。

（三）思考题

1. 苯甲醛与甲醛在浓氢氧化钾存在下反应，接着酸化。写出反应方程式和所有有机产物。

2. Cannizzaro 反应在稀氢氧化钾溶液中比在浓氢氧化钾溶液中慢很多，为什么？

3. 乙醛在碱催化下，与过量甲醛反应，生成季戊四醇。（交叉羟醛 + 交叉 Cannizzaro 反应）。分步写出方程式。

4. 为什么产率不能高于 50%？

Experiment 18   Cannizzaro Reaction of Aryl Aldehydes

Experimental principle

Aldehydes such as benzaldehyde and furfural, which do not contain an alpha (α) hydrogen, cannot undergo aldolization but rather in alkaline solutions undergo a Cannizzaro reaction to form equal numbers of molecules of alcohol and acid.

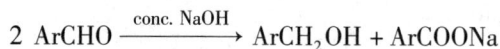

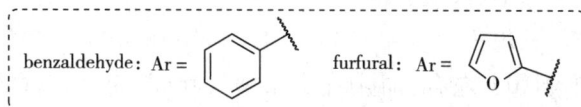

$$2 \ ArCHO \xrightarrow{\text{conc. NaOH}} ArCH_2OH + ArCOONa$$

benzaldehyde: Ar =   furfural: Ar =

Because aryl methanols, such as benzyl alcohol and furan-2-methanol, are soluble in ethyl acetate and sodium aryl formates are soluble in water, aryl methanols are easy to be extracted and separated by ethyl acetate, and water-soluble sodium aryl formates can be converted into aryl formic acids by adding inorganic acid into water layer. Aryl formic acids, such as benzoic acid and furan-2-carboxylic acid, will precipitate from the aqueous solution due to their insolubility in ice water.

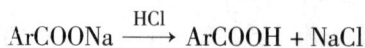

$$ArCOONa \xrightarrow{\text{HCl}} ArCOOH + NaCl$$

Experimental procedures

1. Preparation of benzyl alcohol and benzoic acid

（1）Materials and reagents

benzaldehyde	10. 5g（10ml,0. 1mol）
sodium hydroxide	7. 5g
ethyl acetate	60ml
saturated sodium bisulfite solution	5ml
10% sodium carbonate solution	10ml
hydrochloric acid	40ml
anhydrous magnesium sulfate	

（2）Procedures

30ml of water and 7. 5g of sodium hydroxide are placed in a 100ml three-necked round bottom flask provided with a mechanical stirrer and a reflux condenser. Stir the resulting mixture to dissolve the solid. Cool the solution slightly, and add 10ml of freshly distilled benzaldehyde. Reflux the mixture for 1h, during which the reaction mixture changes from emulsion to transparent liquid. After the mixture is cooled to room temperature, 35ml of cold water is added, and the precipitate is dissolved by stirring. The mixture is transferred into a separatory funnel and extracted with ethyl acetate （30ml×2）. Remember to keep organic phase and water phase respectively. The organic phase is washed sequentially with 5ml of saturated sodium bisulfite solution, 10ml of 10% sodium carbonate solution and 10ml of cold water. The separated organic layer is poured into an Erlenmeyer flask and dried with anhydrous magnesium sulfate. Then, filter out the desiccant and wash the bottle as well as desiccant with a small amount of ethyl acetate. Distill the filtrate on a water bath to remove the ethyl acetate. Then the residue is distilled under reduced pressure to collect 75 ~ 77 ℃/12mmHg fraction. The yield of benzyl alcohol was 3. 1g. Literature:bp 205. 4 ℃/762mmHg.

Put 40 ml of concentrated hydrochloric acid, 40 ml of water and 25g of crushed ice into a beaker. Shake the beaker while slowly pouring the water phase into it, and white solid will precipitate. Filter the solid by suction, wash the filter cake with a small amount of cold water, and dry it to get the crude benzoic acid. For further purification, water can be used for recrystallization to obtain white feathery crystals. The yield was 3. 7g,mp 120 ~ 122 ℃（Note 1）. Literature:mp 122. 4 ℃.

2. Preparation of furan－2－ylmethanol and furan－2－carboxylic acid

（1）Materials and reagents

furfural	19g（16. 4ml, 0. 2mol）
33% sodium hydroxide solution	16ml
diethyl ether	45ml
25% hydrochloric acid	
anhydrous magnesium sulfate or anhydrous potassium carbonate	

（2）Procedures

19g（16. 4ml, 0. 2mol）of furfural are placed in a 100ml three－necked, round－bottom flask provided with a mechanical stirrer and surrounded by an ice water bath. The stirrer is started and the furfural is cooled to about 10℃, and 16ml of 33% sodium hydroxide solution is added in portions at such a rate that the temperature of the reaction mixture is maintained between 10 ~ 14℃. The stirring is continued for 30min at room temperature after the addition of the sodium hydroxide solution. A yellow thick slurry is obtained, and then just enough water (about 20ml) is added to dissolve the precipitate.

Dark brown solution is transferred to a separatory funnel and extracted with diethyl ether (15ml × 3). After dried over anhydrous magnesium sulfate, the diethyl ether extraction is filtered into a round – bottom flask and distilled on a water bath. Then the residue is distilled on an oil bath. Some diethyl ether and water come over first and the temperature then rises rapidly to the boiling point of furyl – 2 – carbinol. The yield of furyl – 2 – carbinol boiling at 169 ~ 172℃ is 7 ~ 8g. Literature bp 171℃/750mmHg.

The water solution contained the sodium furan – 2 – carboxylate is made acid to Congo red paper with 25% hyfrochloric acid. On cooling, the furan – 2 – carboxylic acidcrystallizes and is filtered with suction. The filter cake is washed with cold water and air – dried.

For purification it may be recrystallized from hot water and white needle crystal is obtained. The yield is about 8g. mp129 ~ 130℃. Literature mp133 ~ 134℃.

Experimental instruction

Notes

Benzoic acid sublimates at 100 ℃. When using capillary to measure melting point, sublimation can be prevented by sealing the top of capillary tube after filling the sample. Use more samples than normal. Put the sample into the melting point instrument at a temperature slightly lower than the expected melting point.

Exercises

1. Write an equation for the reaction of a mixture of benzaldehyde or furfural and formaldehyde with concentrated potassium hydroxide solution, followed by acidification of the reaction mixture. Show all organic products.

2. The Cannizzaro reaction occurs much more slowly in dilute than in concentrated potassium hydroxide solution. Why is this?

3. Acetaldehyde, when treated with an excess of formaldehyde in the presence of a basic catalyst, furnishes pentaerythritol, $C(CH_2OH)_4$ (mixed aldol + crossed Cannizzaro reaction). Write equations, stepwise, for the reactions involved.

4. Why can't the yield exceed 50%?

实验十九　喹啉的制备

【目的要求】

学习用斯克劳普合成法制备喹啉的原理及操作方法。

【实验原理】

反应式

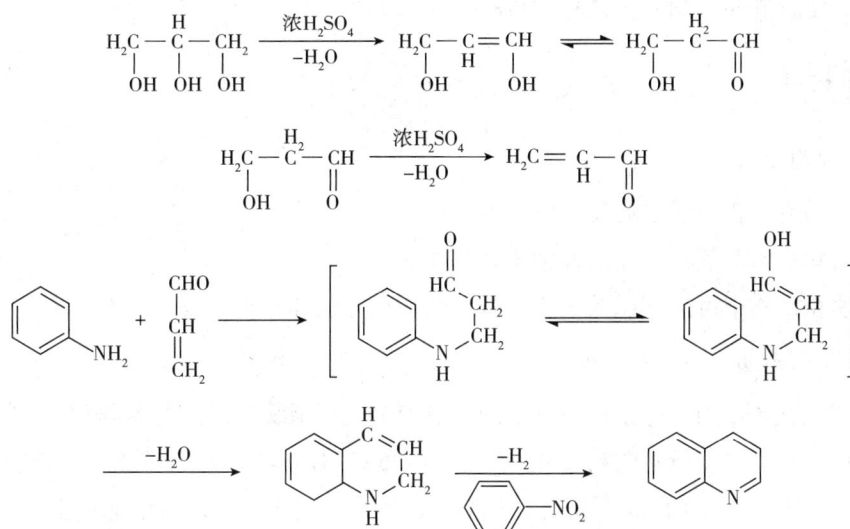

喹啉可以通过苯胺、无水甘油、浓硫酸和弱氧化剂硝基苯等一起加热而制得，称斯克劳普（Skraup）合成法。为避免反应过于剧烈，常加入少量硫酸亚铁。

【实验步骤】

1. 原料与试剂

无水甘油　　29.9ml（0.41mol）

苯胺　　　　9.3ml（0.1mol）

硝基苯　　　6.7ml（0.65mol）

浓硫酸　　　18ml（0.33mol）

30%氢氧化钠

硫酸亚铁　　4g

亚硝酸钠　　3g

乙醚

固体氢氧化钠

淀粉–碘化钾试纸

2. 步骤　在500ml圆底烧瓶中依次加入研磨成粉状的4g结晶硫酸亚铁、29.9ml无水甘油、9.3ml苯胺及6.7ml硝基苯，充分混合后，在振摇下缓缓加入18ml浓硫酸。装上回流冷凝管，微微加热。当有小气泡产生并开始沸腾时，立即移去热源。待反应趋于缓和时，再微微加热，保持反应物和缓地沸腾2.5小时。

待反应液稍冷后，进行水蒸气蒸馏，除去未反应的硝基苯，直至馏出液不显浑浊为止。瓶中残留物稍冷后，加入30%氢氧化钠溶液，中和反应混合物中的硫酸，使溶液呈碱性，再进行水蒸气蒸馏，蒸出喹啉及未反应的苯胺，直至馏出液变清为止。馏出液以浓硫酸酸化，待油状物全部溶解后，冰水浴中冷却至5℃左右。然后慢慢加入由3g亚硝酸钠和10ml水配成的溶液，直至取1滴反应液使淀粉–碘化钾试纸立即变蓝为止。将混合物在沸水浴加热 15 分钟，至无气体放出。反应液冷却后，用 30% 氢氧化钠液碱化，再进行水蒸气蒸馏。从馏出液中分出油层后，水层用乙醚萃取 2 次，每次用 25ml 乙醚。合并油层及乙醚萃取液，用氢氧化钠干燥过夜。蒸馏回收乙醚后直接加热蒸馏收集 bp 234～238℃ 的馏分，产量 8～10g。文献值 bp 238℃，114℃/17mmHg。

【实验指导】

（一）预习要求

1. 复习斯克劳普合成法的反应机制及应用。

2. 了解每次水蒸气蒸馏馏出液中所含物质名称。

3. 说明粗产物中可能存在的杂质、分离纯化的方法和原理。

（二）注意事项

1. 硫酸亚铁的作用是防止反应物之间的迅速氧化，减缓反应的剧烈程度。

2. 所用甘油的含水量不应超过 0.5%（d 1.26），若甘油中含水量较大，则喹啉的产率不高。为除去甘油中的水分，可将普通甘油在通风橱内置于瓷蒸发皿中加热至 180℃，冷至 100℃ 左右，放入盛有硫酸的干燥器中备用。

3. 试剂必须按所述次序加入，如果先加浓硫酸后加硫酸亚铁，则反应往往很剧烈，不易控制。

4. 此反应系放热反应，反应液呈微沸，表示反应已经开始，此时应停止加热。如果继续加热，则反应过于激烈，会使溶液冲出容器。因此当反应太剧烈时，可用湿布敷于烧瓶上冷却。

5. 每次碱化或酸化时，都必须将溶液稍加冷却，并充分搅拌后，再用试纸检验至呈明显的强碱或强酸性。

6. 由于重氮化反应在接近完成时，反应进行很慢，故应在加入亚硝酸钠溶液 2～3 分钟后再检验是否有亚硝酸存在。

7. 本实验系利用重氮化反应及重氮盐的特性，来除去喹啉中所夹杂的苯胺，其变化过程如下式。

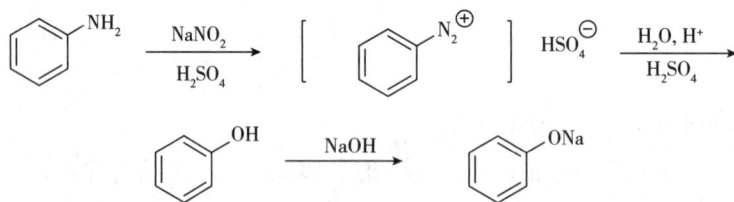

此外，也可用对甲基苯磺酰氯去除粗制喹啉中的苯胺，或用氯化锌分离喹啉与未作用的苯胺。后一方法的原理是：在盐酸溶液中氯化锌虽与它们可形成复盐，但两者溶解度不同：

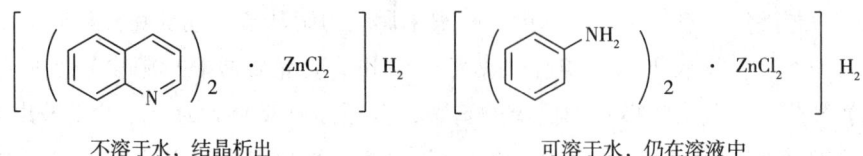

不溶于水，结晶析出　　　　　　　　　　　可溶于水，仍在溶液中

过滤收集析出的盐酸喹啉与氯化锌形成的复盐，加碱，至最初形成的氢氧化锌沉淀复

溶后，由醚提取喹啉即得。

8. 最好在减压下蒸馏，收集 110～114℃/14mmHg，118～120℃/20mmHg 或 130～132℃/40mmHg 的馏分，得到无色透明的产品。

9. 产率以苯胺计算，可不考虑硝基苯部分转化成苯胺而参与反应的量。

（三）思考题

1. 本实验中共使用 3 次水蒸气蒸馏操作，请回答下列问题。

（1）第一次水蒸气蒸馏的馏出液中，是否有苯胺和喹啉，为什么？

（2）第二次和第三次水蒸气蒸馏前为什么都要用碱中和反应液中的酸使溶液呈碱性？

（3）用什么简便的方法检验第二次水蒸气蒸馏的馏出液中是否含有苯胺？

2. 在 Skraup 合成中，用对甲苯胺或邻甲苯胺代替苯胺作原料，各应得到什么产物？硝基化合物应如何选择？

3. 试说明本实验中影响产率和产品质量的主要因素。

Experiment 19　Preparation of Quinoline

Experimental principle

Quinoline can be prepared by heating a mixture of aniline, glycerol and sulfuric acid with a weakly oxidizing agent like nitrobenzene. This strategy was called Skraup synthesis. In the Skraup synthesis of quinoline the principal difficulty has always been the violence with which the reaction takes place; it often gets beyond control in the majority of cases. By the addition of ferrous sulfate, the reaction generally proceeds relatively smoothly.

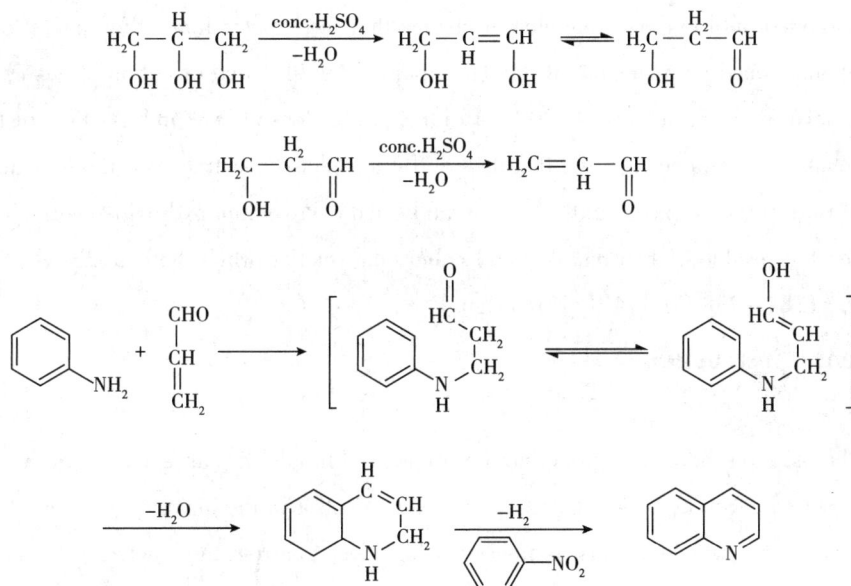

Experimental procedures

1. Materials and reagents

glycerol	29.9ml (0.41mol)
aniline	9.3ml (0.1mol)

nitrobenzene   6. 7ml（0. 65mol）

con. sulfuric acid   18ml（0. 33mol）

30% sodium hydroxide

ferrous sulfate   4g

sodium nitrite   3g

ether

solid sodium hydroxide

starch-potassium iodide paper

2. Procedures

To a 500ml round-bottomed flask, fitted with an efficient reflux condenser, are placed, 4g of powdered crystalline ferrous sulfate, 29. 9ml of glycerol, 9. 3ml of aniline and 6. 7ml of nitrobenzene in order. After mixing well, 18ml concentrated sulfuric acid is added slowly with shaking-up. The mixture was heated gently. As soon as the liquid begins to boil, heating is removed, since the heat evolved by the reaction is sufficient to keep the mixture boiling for one-half to one hour. When the boiling has ceased the heat is again applied and the mixture boiled for two and one-half hours.

It is then allowed to cool to about $100℃$ and the flask is connected with the steam-distillation apparatus. Steam is passed in until no further droplets of oil can be seen. This removes all the unchanged nitrobenzene. The current of steam is then interrupted, the receiver is changed and 30% sodium hydroxide solution is added cautiously to neutralize the sulfuric acid until the aqueous solution is alkaline. Steam is then passed again in as rapidly as possible until all the quinoline and unchanged aniline have distilled. The distillate is acidified with concentrated sulfuric acid until the oily material is dissolved absolutely. The solution is cooled to about $5℃$ and a saturated solution of sodium nitrite is added until one drop of solution change the starch-potassium iodide paper to blue. The mixture is then warmed on a steam bath for 15 minutes or until active evolution of gas ceases. After cooling, the mixture is basified with 30% sodium hydroxide solution and is then distilled with steam. Oil phase is separated from the distillate and water phase is extracted with ether twice (25ml each time). Collect the oil phase and extraction and dried over sodium hydroxide overnight. After recycling ether, the residue is then distilled and collect the fraction which boils at $234 \sim 238℃$ yielding $8 \sim 10g$. (Lit. bp $238℃$; $114℃/17mmHg$).

Experimental instruction

Notes

1. In the Skraup synthesis of quinoline the principal difficulty has always been the violence with which the reaction generally takes place, it gets beyond control in the majority of cases. By the addition of ferrous sulfate, which appears to function as an oxygen carrier, the reaction is avoided too violent.

2. In a number of experiments, the glycerol used contained an appreciable amount of water. Under these conditions, the yield of product is much lower. To get rid of water, the glycerol can be heated in evaporating dish at $180℃$ in the hood. After cooling to $100℃$, the glycerol is placed in desiccators with sulfuric acid as desiccant for further use.

3. It is important that the materials should be added in the correct order; should the sulfuric acid be added before the ferrous sulfate, the reaction may start at once.

4. It is also important to mix the materials well before applying heat; the aniline sulfate should have dissolved almost completely, and the ferrous sulfate should be distributed throughout the solution. To avoid danger of overheating, it is well to apply the flame away from the center of the flask where any solids would be liable to congregate.

5. When acidified or basified, the reaction solution should be cooled appreciably and stirred thoroughly. After that, determine the solution whether it is shown acidity or basicity.

6. It proceeds very slowly when the diazotization reaction is close to completion. 2 ~ 3 minutes later after sodium nitrite solution is added, it would be determined the existence of nitrous acid.

7. The properties of diazotization reaction and diazonium salt are applied in this experiment to get rid of the aniline in the quinoline product. Following shows the procedure of the reaction.

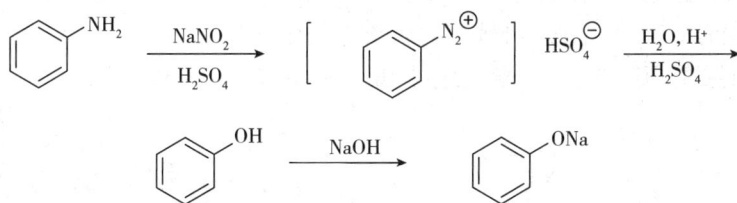

8. It is suggested that vacuum distillation is applied and collect the fraction at 110 ~ 114℃/14mmHg, 118 ~ 120℃/20mmHg or 130 ~ 132℃/40mmHg. The product is colorless, transparent liquid.

9. The percentage yields have been based on the amount of aniline taken. It would probably be more legitimate to base the calculation on the amounts of aniline taken and of nitrobenzene not recovered, since undoubtedly the latter is reduced to aniline during the course of the reaction.

Exercises

1. Steam distillation is used for three times in this experiment, please answer the following questions：

（1）Are there any aniline and quinoline in the distillate of the first steam distillation? Why?

（2）Why should the 30% sodium hydroxide be added to neutralize the acid produced by the reaction until the aqueous solution is alkaline before the second or third steam distillation?

（3）What is the convenient way to check if there is aniline in the distillate of the second steam distillation?

2. What are the expected products if using *p*-methylaniline or *o*-methylaniline rather than aniline in the Skraup synthesis? How to choose nitro compound?

3. Explain the main factors which influence the quality and yield of the product.

实验二十　二苯羟乙酸的制备

【目的要求】

　　了解　用生物化学反应催化剂合成安息香的原理和方法；安息香的氧化和二苯羟乙酸

重排反应的原理、方法，并熟悉用多步反应进行合成的方法。

【实验原理及方法】

（一）二苯羟乙酮的制备——辅酶催化合成安息香

1. 反应式

$$2 \ \text{PhCHO} \xrightarrow[60\sim75\,℃]{VB_1} \text{Ph-CO-CH(OH)-Ph}$$

二苯羟乙酮（安息香）

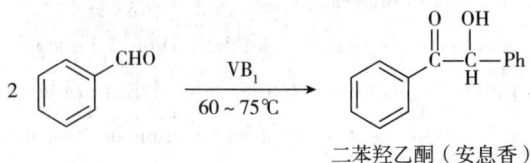

两分子苯甲醛在氰化钠（钾）的作用下，缩合生成二苯羟乙酮（安息香）的反应称为安息香缩合反应。由于氰化物是剧毒品，使用不当会有危险，本实验用维生素 B_1 盐酸盐代替氰化物进行催化。该反应条件温和，无毒，产率较高。

有生物活性的维生素 B_1 是一种辅酶，属于生物化学反应催化剂，其化学名称为硫胺素或噻胺，它的主要作用是使 α - 酮酸脱羧和形成偶姻（α - 羟基酮）。维生素 B_1 的结构式是：

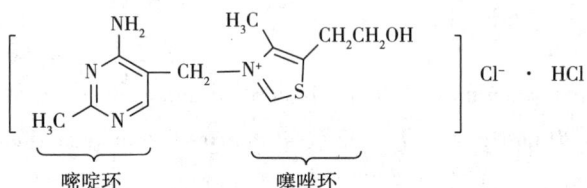

在反应中，维生素 B_1 的噻唑环上的氮和硫的邻位氢具有酸性，在碱作用下被夺去成为氮杂环卡宾，形成反应中心，其机制如下：

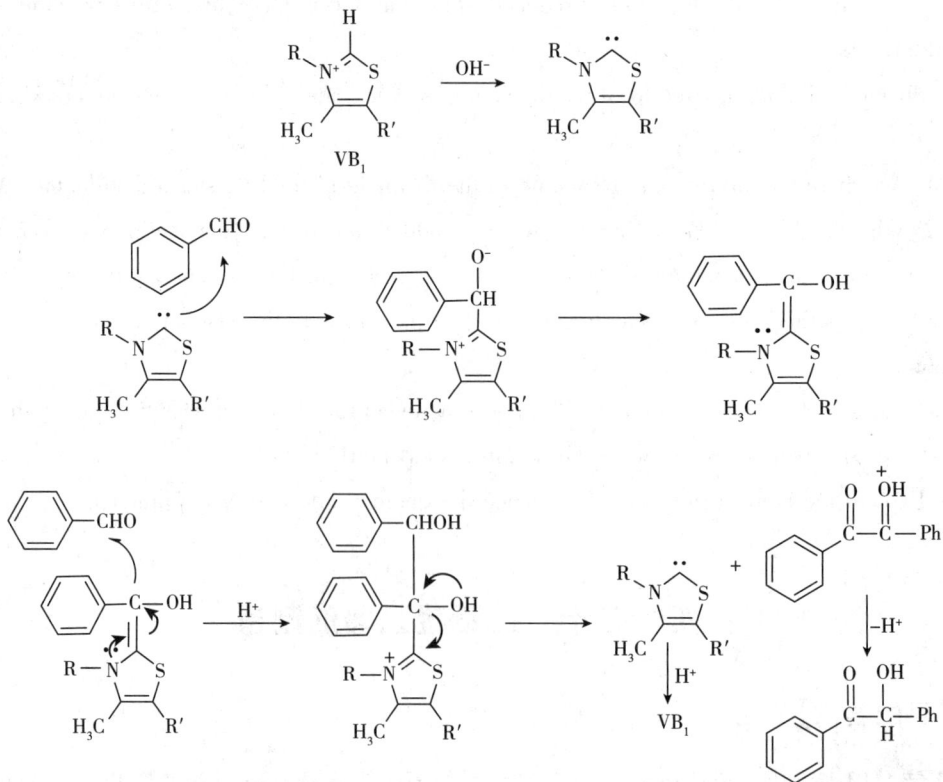

2. 原料与试剂

苯甲醛	10ml（0.09mol）
维生素 B_1	1.8g
95%乙醇	15ml
10%氢氧化钠	5ml

3. 步骤 在100ml的锥形瓶中加入1.8g VB_1、6ml蒸馏水和15ml 95%乙醇，用塞子塞上瓶口，放在冰盐浴中冷却。用试管取5ml 10%氢氧化钠溶液，也放在冰浴中冷却。10分钟后，将冷透的氢氧化钠溶液加入到冰盐浴冷却的 VB_1 溶液中，并立即再加入10ml新蒸过的苯甲醛，充分摇动使反应物混合均匀。然后在锥形瓶上装上回流冷凝管，加几粒沸石放在温水浴中加热反应。水浴温度控制在60~75℃之间，勿使反应剧烈沸腾。反应混合物呈桔黄或桔红色均相溶液。约80~90分钟后撤去水浴，将反应混合物逐渐冷至室温。析出浅黄色结晶，再用冰水浴冷却使其结晶完全。抽滤，用50ml冷水分两次洗涤结晶。称重，用80%乙醇进行重结晶。如产物呈黄色，可加少量活性炭脱色。纯产物为白色针状结晶。产品约4~5g，mp 134~136℃。文献值：mp 133~134℃。

（二）二苯乙二酮的制备

1. 反应式

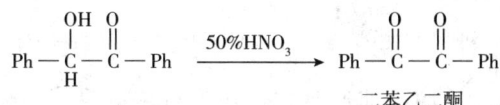

2. 原料与试剂

二苯羟乙酮	4g（0.019mol）
50%硝酸	8ml
95%乙醇	

3. 步骤 将二苯羟乙酮4g和50%硝酸8ml加到50ml圆底烧瓶中，装上回流冷凝管，水浴加热至上下层基本澄清，约需1.5小时。趁热将反应物倒入15ml水中，抽滤，以水洗至中性，置空气中干燥。粗产品用95%乙醇重结晶（每克产品约需3~4ml乙醇）。产品约2.5~3g，mp 92~94℃。文献值：mp 95~96℃。

（三）二苯羟乙酸的制备——二苯羟乙酸重排

1. 反应式

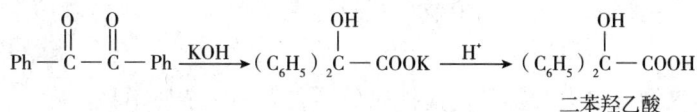

2. 原料与试剂

二苯乙二酮	2g（0.0095ml）
氢氧化钾	5g
95%乙醇	5ml
浓盐酸	3ml
无水乙醇	

3. 步骤 在 50ml 锥形瓶中，溶解 5g 氢氧化钾于 5ml 水中，然后加入 5ml 95% 乙醇。混合均匀后，加入 2g 二苯乙二酮。振荡锥形瓶，溶液呈深紫色。待固体全部溶解后，安装回流冷凝管，水浴上煮沸 15 分钟。加热过程中即有固体析出。冷却，冰水浴中放置 1 小时后，抽滤，用少量无水乙醇洗涤固体，得白色二苯羟乙酸钾盐。

将上述酸的钾盐溶于 60ml 水中，若有不溶物，过滤除去。然后将 3ml 浓盐酸与 20ml 水配成的盐酸溶液加入其中，即有白色结晶析出。经放置冷却后，抽滤，结晶用冷水洗几次，干燥。产品约 1.8g，mp 147~149℃。用苯重结晶（每克产品约需苯 6ml 左右）后，产品 mp 148~149℃。文献值：mp 151℃。

【实验指导】

（一）预习要求

1. 复习安息香缩合反应的机制。

2. 了解维生素 B_1 在安息香缩合反应中的催化机制及在反应中的注意事项。

3. 了解二苯羟乙酸重排的历程及实验方法。

4. 复习固体化合物的分离提纯方法。

（二）注意事项

1. 维生素 B_1 在酸性条件下是稳定的，但易吸水，在水溶液中易被空气氧化而失效。遇光和 Cu、Fe、Mn 等金属离子均可加速氧化。在氢氧化钠溶液中噻唑环易开环失效。因此 VB_1 溶液和 NaOH 溶液在反应前必须用冰水充分冷透，否则 VB_1 在碱性条件下会分解，这是本实验成败的关键。

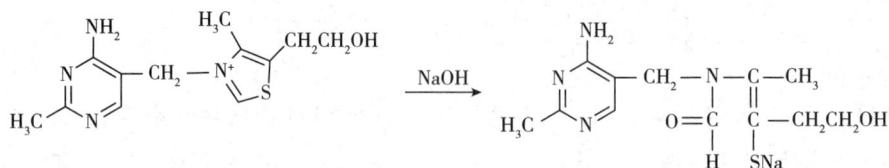

2. 反应过程中，溶液在开始时不必沸腾，反应后期可以适当升高温度至缓慢沸腾（80~90℃）。

3. 如果反应混合物中出现油层，应重新加热使其变成均相，再慢慢冷却，重新结晶。必要时可用玻棒磨擦锥形瓶内壁，促使其结晶。

4. 制备二苯乙二酮时，如终点不易观察可用斐林溶液检查。斐林溶液可被 α-羟基酮还原。

5. 反应物趁热倒入水中时要迅速搅拌以免结成大块使杂质不易洗净。

6. 重排亦可用 5g 氢氧化钠进行。操作与氢氧化钾相同，只是回流加热和冷却后不出现钠盐结晶。可将反应物倒进 100ml 水中，过滤除去不溶物后用浓盐酸酸化至刚果红试纸变蓝，即有产品析出。以下操作与氢氧化钾相同。

（三）思考题

1. 写出安息香缩合反应在氰化钾作用下的反应历程。

2. 什么结构类型的醛能进行安息香缩合反应？

3. 写出二苯羟乙酸重排的可能机制。

Experiment 20　Preparation of Benzilic Acid

I. Preparation of benzoin

Experimental principle

The synthesis of benzilic acid (5,5-diphenykhydantoin) is carried out in three steps. In the first reaction, in the presence of cyanide ion, benzaldehyde will undergo a unique self-condensation reaction, called the benzoin condensation, to yield a α-hydroxy ketone called benzoin. In this experiment, we shall use the benzoin condensation to synthesize benzoin.

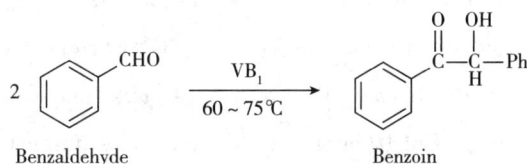

The complete mechanism for this reaction is shown below:

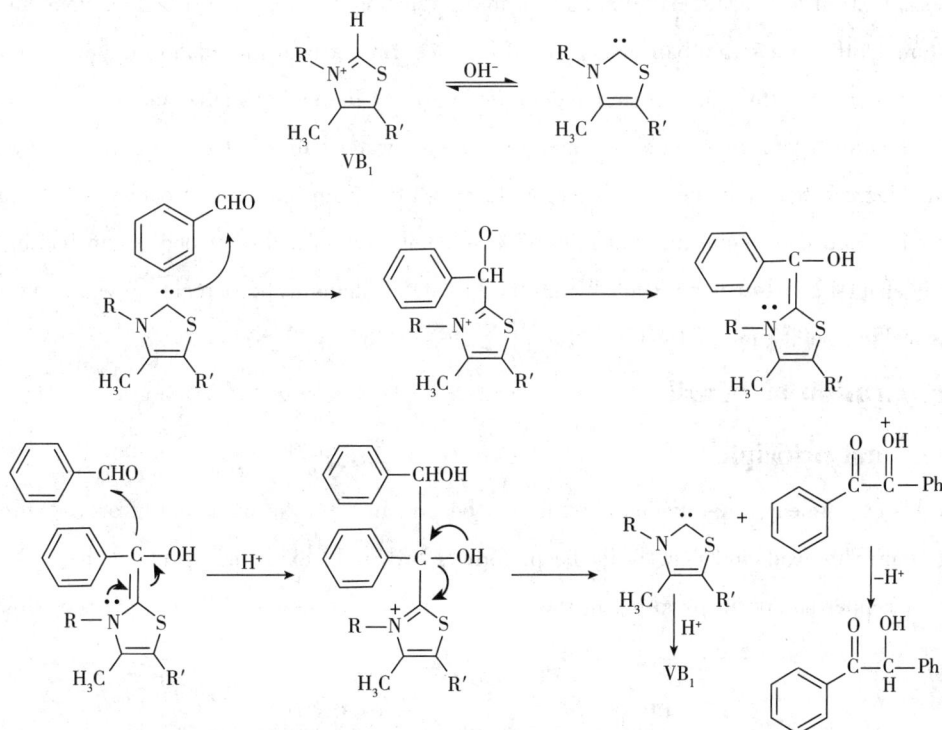

Sodium cyanide is extremely hazardous and toxic, when it is used in improper way. In this experiment, we apply thiamine in replacement of cyanide as catalyst. Under the mild, nontoxic conditions, the yield is good enough for preparation of benzoin.

Thiamine is the coenzyme for a number of enzyme-catalyzed reactions, including the formation of α-hydroxy ketone from benzaldehyde.

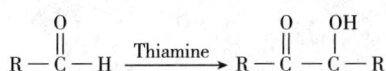

Breslow used the benzoin condensation as a model for the mechanism of thiamine coenzyme action. In Breslow's proposed mechanism, a thiazolium salt anion is formed under mildly basic conditions. The thiazolium anion acts like the cyanide anion.

Experimental procedures

1. Materials and reagents

benzaldehyde	10ml (0.09mol)
thiamine hydrochloride	1.8g
95% ethanol	15ml
10% sodium hydroxide	5ml

2. Procedures

To 1.8g of thiamine hydrochloride dissolved in a 100ml Erlenmeyer flask adds 15ml of 95% ethanol. Stopper the flask and then cool the solution by swirling the flask in an ice-water bath. Meanwhile, place 5ml of 10% sodium hydroxide in a glass tube. Cool this solution in the ice bath also. Then, over a period of about 10 minutes, add the cold sodium hydroxide solution to the thiamine solution.

Measure 20ml of benzaldehyde and add it to the reaction mixture. Add a boiling stone and heat the mixture gently on a steam bath for about 90 minutes. Do not heat the mixture under vigorous reflux. Allow the mixture to cool to room temperature, and then induce crystallization of the benzoin (it may already have begun) by cooling the mixture in an ice-water bath. Collect the product by vacuum filtration using a Büchner funnel. Wash the product with two 50ml portions of cold water. Weigh the crude product and then recrystallize it from 95% ethanol. The solubility of benzoin in boiling 95% ethanol is about 12 to 14g per 100ml. Weigh the product. Calculate the percentage yield, and determine its melting point (mp 134~136℃).

II. Preparation of benzil

Experimental principle

In this experiment, a α-diketone, benzil, will be prepared by the oxidation of an α-hydroxyketone, benzoin. This oxidation may easily be performed with mild oxidizing agents such as Fehling's solution or copper sulfate in pyridine. In this experiment, the oxidation will be performed with nitric acid.

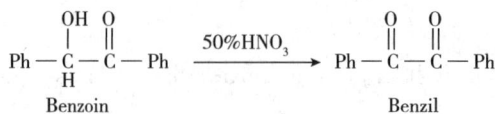

$$\underset{\text{Benzoin}}{\text{Ph}-\underset{\underset{\text{H}}{|}}{\overset{\overset{\text{OH}}{|}}{\text{C}}}-\overset{\overset{\text{O}}{\|}}{\text{C}}-\text{Ph}} \xrightarrow{50\%\text{HNO}_3} \underset{\text{Benzil}}{\text{Ph}-\overset{\overset{\text{O}}{\|}}{\text{C}}-\overset{\overset{\text{O}}{\|}}{\text{C}}-\text{Ph}}$$

Experimental procedures

1. Materials and reagents

benzoin	4g (0.019mol)
50% nitric acid	8ml
95% ethanol	

2. Procedures

Place 4g of benzoin in a 50ml round-bottomed flask with 50% nitric acid. Fit the flask with a reflux condenser. Heat on a steam bath with shaking, until reactants have dissolved. After reactants have dissolved, reflux 1.5 hours. Pour the reaction mixture into 15ml of ice water with stirring. Cool reaction mixture in an ice bath for 5 ~ 10 minutes. Collect the yellow crystals by vacuum filtration. Wash the crystals with cold water. Dry the product in the air overnight. Crystallize the benzil from 95% ethanol to yield about 2.5 ~ 3g, mp 92 ~ 94℃. (Lit. mp 95 ~ 96℃).

III. Preparation of benzilic acid

Experimental principle

In this experiment, benzilic acid will be prepared via the rearrangement of the α-diketone, benzil. The reaction proceeds in the following way:

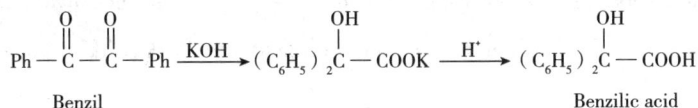

$$Ph - \overset{\overset{O}{\|}}{C} - \overset{\overset{O}{\|}}{C} - Ph \xrightarrow{KOH} (C_6H_5)_2\overset{\overset{OH}{|}}{C} - COOK \xrightarrow{H^+} (C_6H_5)_2\overset{\overset{OH}{|}}{C} - COOH$$

Benzil   Benzilic acid

Experimental procedures

1. Materials and reagents

benzil	2g (0.0095mol)
potassium hydroxide	5g
95% ethanol	5ml
hydrochloric acid	3ml
absolute ethanol	

2. Procedures

Dissolve 5g of potassium hydroxide in 5ml of water in a 50ml Erlenmeyer flask. Then add 5ml of 95% ethanol to the solution. After mixing thoroughly, dissolve 2g of benzil. The mixture turns to black-purple. Attach a reflux condenser to the flask. Reflux the mixture on a steam bath for 15 minutes. During this period, some of solid formed. Cool the mixture in an ice-bath for 1 hour. Collect the crystals by vacuum filtration and wash the crystals with cold absolute ethanol to give white potassium benzilate.

Dissolve the potassium benzilate in 60ml of water. Remove precipitated impurities be vacuum filtration. Add the solution of 3ml of concentrated hydrochloric acid in 20ml of water to the filtrate to give white crystals. Cool the mixture for a moment, then collect the crystals of benzilic acid by vacuum filtration and wash with cold water. Dry the crystals to give 1.8g of crude product, mp 147 ~ 149℃. Crystallize the product from benzene, mp 148 ~ 149℃. (Lit. mp 151℃).

Experimental instruction

Notes

1. Sodium cyanide is extremely dangerous. Do not handle if you have open wounds. Wear disposable gloves if available. Wash hands after handling. Do not get acid in the reaction mixture. Carry

out the reaction in a hood.

2. Thiamine hydrochloride is a heat and base sensitive reagent. It should be stored in a refrigerator when not in use. Since it may decompose on heating, you should take care to cool the reaction mixture thoroughly and not to heat the mixture to vigorously.

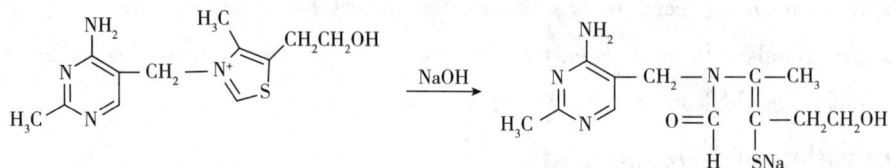

3. The benzaldehyde used for this experiment must be free of benzoic acid. Benzaldehyde is oxidized easily in air, and crystals of benzoic acid are often visible of reagent, it must be redistilled.

4. If the product separates as oil, reheat the mixture until it is once again homogeneous, and thenallow it to cool more slowly than before. Scratching of the flask with a glass rod may be required.

5. Vigorous evolution of nitrogen gas occurs and solution turns green when reactants dissolve.

6. Benzilic acid is a powerful anticonvulsant and must be handle with care.

Exercises

1. Review the mechanism of benzoin condensation.

2. Why is sodium hydroxide added to the solution of thiamine hydrochloride?

3. Using the information given in the essay that precedes this experiment, formulate a complete mechanism for the thiamine-catalyzed conversion of benzaldehyde to benzoin.

4. How do you think the appropriate enzyme would have affected the reaction yield?

5. What modifications of conditions would be appropriate if the enzyme were to be used?

6. Write down the mechanism of rearrangement of benzilic acid.

实验二十一　环己酮肟的贝克曼重排

【目的要求】

学习用贝克曼重排反应制备己内酰胺的原理及操作方法。

【实验原理】

反应式

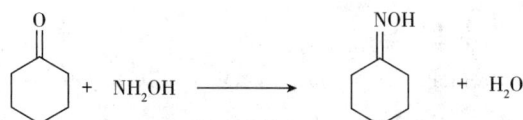

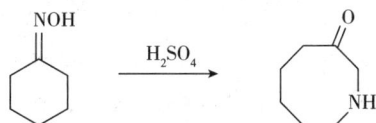

脂肪酮和芳香酮都可以和羟胺作用生成肟。肟在酸性催化剂如五氯化磷、硫酸或苯磺酰氯等作用下，发生分子重排生成酰胺，这个反应称为贝克曼（Beckmann）重排。

本实验就是用环己酮肟在硫酸存在下经贝克曼重排反应制备己内酰胺。

【实验步骤】

1. 原料与试剂

环己酮　　　　7g（0.07mol）

羟胺盐酸盐　　7g

结晶乙酸钠　　10g

70% 硫酸　　　10ml

氨水　　　　　18ml

2. 步骤

（1）环己酮肟的制备　在250ml锥形瓶中，加入7g羟胺盐酸盐和10g结晶乙酸钠，然后加30ml水溶解。用热水浴加热溶液至35～40℃。分批加入7.5ml环己酮，边加边振荡，即有固体析出。加完后，用橡皮塞塞紧瓶口，激烈振荡，白色粉状结晶析出表明反应完全。冷却后，抽滤，用少量水洗涤。抽干，于空气中晾干，得白色环己酮肟结晶，产量8g，mp 89～90℃。

（2）环己酮肟重排制备己内酰胺　称取5g干燥环己酮（0.044mol），加5ml 70%硫酸溶解备用。然后在装有搅拌器、温度计和滴液漏斗的三颈瓶中放3ml 70%硫酸。将环己酮肟溶液放入滴液漏斗，原容器用2ml 70%硫酸洗涤，洗涤液并入滴液漏斗。将三颈瓶内液体加热至130～135℃，缓缓搅拌。保持瓶内液体温度在130～135℃的情况下，将环己酮肟溶液缓缓滴入三颈瓶中，大约20分钟滴完。滴加完毕后继续搅拌5分钟，移去火源，瓶内温度降至80℃后，再用冰盐水冷却三颈瓶至0～5℃。冷却搅拌下滴加浓氨水至 pH = 8（大约需18ml）。在此过程中瓶内温度应低于20℃，大约需40分钟。反应混合物转移至中，三颈瓶用10ml水洗涤，洗涤液并入分液漏斗。用三氯甲烷萃取3次，每次8ml。三氯甲烷萃取液用无水硫酸镁干燥，放置澄清后滤入克氏蒸馏瓶中。先常压蒸馏回收三氯甲烷，残余物进行减压蒸馏。收集 bp 137～140℃/12mmHg 馏分，馏出物很快固化为无色晶体，产量4～5g。mp 69～70℃（文献值：mp 68～70℃）。

【实验指导】

（一）预习要求

1. 复习贝克曼重排反应的机制。

2. 复习进行减压蒸馏操作时的注意事项。

（二）注意事项

1. 如环己酮肟呈白色小球珠，表明反应尚未完全，须继续强烈振荡，约5～10分钟。也可采用下列加料方式：先将羟胺盐酸盐溶于 30ml 水中，加入 7.5ml 环己酮；再用 15ml 水溶解 10g 结晶乙酸钠。将乙酸钠溶液滴加到上述溶液中，边加边振荡便得粉末状环己酮肟产物。

2. 产品最好先在滤纸上挤压，然后再置空气中晾干，否则不易干。

3. 用 70%、85% 硫酸和浓硫酸分别控温在 130℃、120℃ 和 100℃ 时，产率依次为 78%、70% 和 50%，以用 70% 硫酸产率最高。

4. 用 70% 硫酸反应，滴加环己酮肟时若控制温度在 125~130℃，则重排反应进行不完全，产物中含有未反应的原料，产率也较低。若温度过高，可能导致产物聚合。故重排温度以 130~135℃ 为宜。

5. 用浓氨水中和结束后有白色硫酸铵固体析出，加入 10ml 水可洗下烧瓶中残余物并溶解此固体。

6. 也可收集 127~133℃/7mmHg 或 140~144℃/14mmHg 馏分。

7. 减压蒸馏时，为防止己内酰胺在冷凝管中凝结，最好不用冷凝管，即将蒸馏瓶直接与接液管相连接。

（三）思考题

1. 制备环己酮肟时，为什么要加乙酸钠？

2. 如产物中夹有未反应的少量原料环己酮肟，如何除去？

3. 用氨水中和时，为什么要把温度控制在 20℃ 以下？

4. 说明做好本实验的关键。

Experiment 21　Beckmann Rearrangement of Cyclohexanone Oxime

Experimental principle

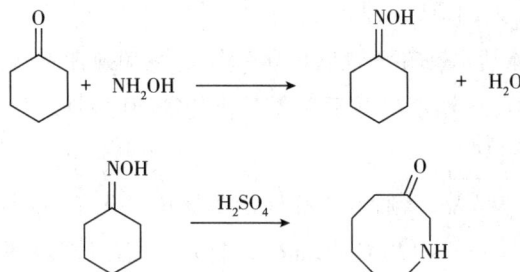

Oximes are prepared by the reaction of aliphatic or aromatic ketones with hydroxylamine hydrochloride. Oximes can be rearranged to form amides in the presence of some acid catalysts, for example: phosphorus pentachloride, sulfuric acid or benzenesulfonyl chloride. This reaction is called as Beckmann Rearrangement. In this experiment, ε-caprolactam is prepared from Beckmann rearrangement of cyclohexanone oxime catalyzed by sulfuric acid.

Experimental procedures

1. Materials and reagents

cyclohexanone　　　　　　　　7g（0.07mol）

hydroxylamine hydrochloride   7g

crystal sodium acetate   10g

70% sulfuric acid   10ml

ammonia   18ml

2. Procedures

Preparation of cyclohexanone oxime

In a 250ml of Erlenmeyer flask, are placed an aqueous solution of 7g of hydroxylamine hydrochloride and 10g of crystal sodium acetate in 30ml of water. The flask is heated to 35 ~ 40℃ with water bath. Then 7. 5ml of cyclohexanone is added in portions with shaking. Some of solids precipitate. After addition, plug the flask with rubber stopper and then shake the flask vigorously until the white powder cyclohexanone oxime is obtained. After cooling, collect the product by vacuum filtration and wash it with small amount of water. Dry the product in the air to give about 8g of the white cyclohexanone. mp 89 ~ 90℃.

Preparation of ε-caprolactam from rearrangement of cyclohexanone oxime

In a 100ml of three-necked, round-bottomed flask fitted with a mechanical stirrer, a thermometer and an additional funnel, is placed 3ml of 70% sulfuric acid. The flask is heated to 130 ~ 135℃ with a low flame. The stirrer is started slowly and a mixture of 5g of dried cyclohexanone oxime in 7ml of 70% sulfuric acid is added dropwise while the temperature is held at 130 ~ 135℃. This addition requires about 20 minutes. The stirring is continued for additional 5 minutes after the addition. The burner is taken off. The flask is surrounded in an ice-salt bath after the temperature is dropped to 80℃. Concentrated ammonia is slowly added with stirring to the reaction mixture to pH = 8. This addition requires about 20 minutes and the temperature is kept below 20℃. The mixture is transferred into separatory funnel and the flask is washed with water. Combine the water and reaction mixture and extract with chloroform three times (8ml each). Dry them over anhydrous magnesium sulfate. The chloroform solution and ε-caprolactam are transferred to a Claisen flask for distillation. The chloroform is removed under ordinary pressure and the residue is distilled under reduced pressure collecting the distillate at 137 ~ 140℃/12mmHg. The product is solidified as colorless crystal. The yield is about 4 ~ 5g, mp 69 ~ 70℃. (Lit. mp 68 ~ 70℃).

Experimental instruction

Notes

1. The reaction is incomplete if little white ball appears. It is necessary to shake violently for about 5 ~ 10min. It might take the following order to add materials: first dissolvehydroxylamine hydrochloride in 30ml water, then add 7. 5ml cyclohexanone; dissolve 10g crystal sodium acetate in 15ml water. Add the solution of sodium acetate to the above mixture with shaking; the powder cyclohexanone oxime is obtained.

2. It is better to press the product in the filter paper first, and then dry it in the air, otherwise it is difficult to be dried.

3. The yield is 78% , 70% and 50% respectively if 70% , 85% and concentrated sulfuric

acid is used under 130℃,120℃ and 100℃,among them,the yield is highest with 70% sulfuric acid.

4. The rearrangement reaction proceeds incompletely if the temperature is controlled between 125~135℃ with 70% sulfuric acid,so the yield is very low. If the temperature is higher,it would result in polymer of the product,therefore,the convenient temperature of arrangement is between 130~135℃

5. Whiteammonium sulfate is precipitated after concentrated ammonia water is used to neutralize the acid. Add 10ml water to wash the residue and dissolve the solid in the flask.

6. Collect 127~133℃/7mmHg fraction or 140~144℃/14mmHg fraction.

7. It is better not to use condenser in the vacuum distillation to prevent ε-caprolactam from condensing in it. Connect the distilling flask with the adapter directly.

Exercise

1. Why shouldsodium caproate be added in preparing cyclohexanone oxime

2. How is a little of unreacted cyclohexanone oxime removed from the crude product after the reaction has been completed?

3. Why should the temperature be controlled under 20℃ whenammonia water is used to adjust the pH?

4. Indicate the key points to do this experiment well.

实验二十二 7,7-二氯双环[4,1,0]庚烷的制备——相转移法

【目的要求】

1. 学习用相转移法制备7,7-二氯双环[4,1,0]庚烷的原理及操作方法。
2. 学习二氯卡宾的性质及其在合成中的应用。

【实验原理】

反应式

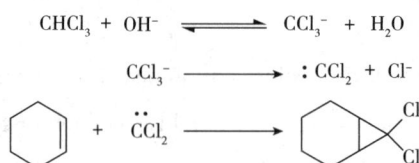

$$CHCl_3 + OH^- \rightleftharpoons CCl_3^- + H_2O$$

$$CCl_3^- \longrightarrow :CCl_2 + Cl^-$$

二氯卡宾是一种不稳定的活泼中间体,若:CCl_2产生后停留在水相中,则由于与水作用而不能有效地被环己烯所捕获,得到的加成物产率很低,仅为5%。假如在相转移催化剂(例如 TEBA)存在下进行反应,产率可达40%~60%。因为相转移催化剂在水和某些有机溶剂(如二氯甲烷)中都有溶解。因此,三氯甲烷在50%氢氧化钠的作用下,在水相中生成的CCl_3^-阴离子很快地转入有机相,生成:CCl_2。:CCl_2在有机溶剂中立即与环己烯发生

加成。所以采用相转移方法，操作简便，收率高。

【实验步骤】

1. 原料与试剂

环己烯	10.1g（0.12mol）
三氯甲烷	24.3ml（0.3mol）
TEBA	1g
50% NaOH	34g
石油醚（bp 30~60℃）	

2. 步骤 在250ml四颈瓶上装置机械搅拌器、回流冷凝器、恒压滴液漏斗和温度计，加入8.2g环己烯、24.3ml三氯甲烷和1g TEBA。在恒压滴液漏斗中放置34g 50%氢氧化钠溶液。将反应瓶置于水浴中，剧烈搅拌下滴入氢氧化钠溶液（滴加时保持瓶内温度40~45℃，大约15~20分钟滴完）。滴加完后在45~55℃下继续搅拌反应2小时。反应完毕，反应混合物冷却至室温后加水100ml，将混合液倒入分液漏斗中并分出油层；水层用石油醚提取两次，每次15ml。合并油层和石油醚提取液，水洗2~3次直至中性。有机层用无水硫酸钠干燥。滤去干燥剂，在水浴上蒸馏回收溶剂后，再进行减压蒸馏，收集83~85℃/24mmHg的馏分，产品为无色透明液体，产量10~14g。文献值：bp 197~198℃。

【实验指导】

（一）预习要求

1. 复习碳烯的结构、性质及反应。

2. 复习相转移催化反应的原理。

（二）注意事项

1. 环己烯要新蒸过的。

2. 三乙基苄基氯化铵（TEBA）的制备如下：

反应式：$C_6H_5CH_2Cl + (C_2H_5)_3N \longrightarrow C_6H_5CH_2N^+ (C_2H_5)_3Cl^-$

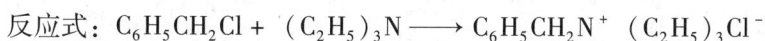

原料与试剂：氯化苄、三乙胺、1,2-二氯乙烷。

实验操作：在装有搅拌器和回流冷凝管的250ml三口瓶中，加入5.5ml氯化苄、7ml三乙胺和19ml 1,2-二氯乙烷。回流搅拌1.5~2小时。将反应液冷却，析出结晶，过滤，用少量的1,2-二氯乙烷洗涤2次，烘干后放在干燥器中（在空气中易潮解）。产量10g。

3. 温度高时，二氯卡宾易发生其他副反应，故须保持反应温度在40~50℃。

4. 回流过程中有固体析出，不影响搅拌。

5. 若油层不明显，可直接用石油醚提取。

6. 也可收集80~82℃/16mmHg，或95~97℃/35mmHg或102~104℃/50mmHg的馏分。

（三）思考题

1. 为什么本实验在水存在下，二氯卡宾可以和烯烃发生加成反应？

2. 常用的相转移催化剂除了季铵盐外，还有哪些？举例说明。

Experiment 22　Preparation of 7, 7-Dichlorobicyclo [4. 1. 0] heptane

Experimental principle

$$CHCl_3 + OH^- \rightleftharpoons CCl_3^- + H_2O$$

$$CCl_3^- \longrightarrow :CCl_2 + Cl^-$$

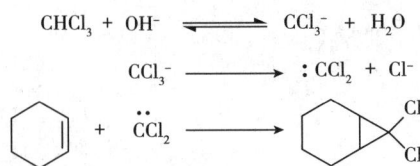

The first step in this reaction is the formation of the reactive intermediate dichlorocarbene. It is not stable when it still stays in water phase after formation because it can react with water. So the yield of additional product is very low, usually only about 5%. If the reaction is carrying through catalyzed by phase-transfer agents (for example TEBA), the yield obtained from such reaction is generally 40% ~ 60%. The catalytic action of $R_4N^+X^-$ arises from the fact that it is water-soluble and also soluble in organic solvents. If $R_4N^+X^-$ is dissolved in the aqueous phase of the two-phase reaction mixture, some of the salt also becomes dissolved in the organic layer. Dichlorocarbene can be obtained after anionic trichloromethane, which formed in water phase under reaction of chloroform with 50% sodium hydroxide, was transferred to organic layer. Dichlorocarbene react with cyclohexene immediately in organic solvents. This experiment performs easily and yield is good when phase-transfer catalysts are applied.

Experimental procedures

1. Materials and reagents

cyclohexene	10. 1g (0. 12mol)
chloroform	24. 3ml (0. 3mol)
TEBA	1g
50% sodium hydroxide	34g
petroleum ether	

2. Procedures

In a 250ml of four-necked, round-bottomed flask fitted with a good mechanical stirrer, an additional funnel, a thermometer, and a reflux condenser, are placed 10. 1g of cyclohexene, 24. 3ml (0. 3mol) of chloroform and 1g of TEBA. In the additional funnel is placed 34g of 50% sodium hydroxide. The flask is surrounded by a water bath and the stirrer is started. Sodium hydroxide is added at such a rate that the temperature is kept between 40 and 45℃. This addition requires about 15 ~ 20 minutes. The stirring is continued for two hours at about 45 ~ 55℃ after the base has been added. The reaction mixture is cooled to room temperature, and 100ml of water is added with stirring. The mixture is then transferred to a separatory funnel. The upper oil layer is separated and the water phase is extracted with petroleum ether twice (15ml each). Combine the organic layer and the ether extraction and dry over anhydrous magnesium sulfate. The organic solution is transferred to a flask for distillation. The petroleum ether is removed under ordinary pressure and the 7,7-Dichlorobicyclo[4. 1. 0]heptane is distilled under reduced pressure collecting the distillate at 83 ~ 85℃/ 24mmHg. The product is clear, colorless liquid and the yield is about 10 ~ 14g (Lit. bp 197 ~ 198℃).

Experimental instruction

Notes

1. The stirrer should be very efficient, as otherwise the reaction proceeds between two phases.

2. Cyclohexene must be redistilled before use.

3. TEBA is prepared as follow:

(1) Materials and reagents

Benzyl chloride	5. 5ml
Triethylamine	7ml
1,2-dichloroethane	19ml

(2) Procedures

In a 250ml of three-necked, round-bottomed flask fitted with a mechanical stirrer and a reflux condenser are placed 5. 5ml of benzyl chloride, 7ml of triethylamine and 19ml of 1,2-dichloroethane. The stirrer is started and the solution is refluxed for 1. 5 ~ 2 hours. Allow the mixture to cool to room temperature, and collect the product by vacuum filtration using a Büchner funnel. Wash the product with two 5ml portions of 1,2-dichloroethane. Store the product in a desiccator after drying. The yield is about 10g.

4. The temperature should be maintained between 40 ~ 45℃, otherwise some of other adverse reactions will happen if the temperature is higher. Because the reaction is exothermic.

5. During this period, some of solid formed. The stirring keeps continuously.

6. The reaction mixture can be extracted with petroleum ether directly if the two phases are not clear separately.

7. The distillate can also be collect at 80 ~ 82℃/16mmHg, 95 ~ 97℃/35mmHg or 102 ~ 104℃/50mmHg.

Exercises

1. Why could dichlorocarbene react with alkene in the presence of water?

2. Please give some examples of phase transfer catalysts used frequently in addition to quaternary ammonium salt.

实验二十三　二苯甲酮的制备

【目的要求】

1. 学习付瑞德尔－克拉夫茨（Friedel-Crafts）反应在合成中的应用及偕二卤代物水解成酮的反应。

2. 学习二苯甲酮的合成方法。

【实验原理】

反应式

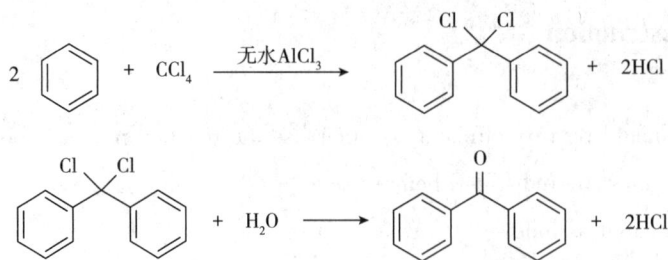

本实验用无水三氯化铝作催化剂。由于三氯化铝遇水和潮气会分解失效，故反应中所有的仪器和试剂都应是干燥和无水的，装置中凡是开口的地方，均应装干燥管。在本实验的两步反应中都有氯化氢气体放出，故要安装气体吸收装置。

付瑞德尔－克拉夫茨反应是一个放热反应，但它有一个诱导期，所以在操作时要注意温度的变化。

【实验步骤】

1. 原料与试剂

无水苯	12ml（0.13mol）
四氯化碳	30ml（0.195mol）
无水三氯化铝	9g（0.067mol）
无水硫酸镁	

2. 步骤

在 250ml 三颈瓶上，分别安装搅拌器、冷凝管和 Y 形管。冷凝管上端装氯化钙干燥管，后者再接氯化氢气体吸收装置。Y 形管上分别安装滴液漏斗和温度计。

迅速称取 9g 无水三氯化铝，放入三颈瓶中，再加入 20ml 干燥四氯化碳。三颈瓶用冰水浴冷却到 10～15℃，维持瓶内温度在 5～10℃ 之间（约 15 分钟），在搅拌下滴入 12ml 无水苯和 10ml 四氯化碳的混合液。滴加完后，在 10℃ 左右继续搅拌 1 小时。然后仍将三颈瓶浸入冰水浴，在搅拌下慢慢滴加 100ml 水，滴加完后改成蒸馏装置，在水浴上尽量蒸去过量的四氯化碳。再在石棉网上加热半小时，以除去残留的四氯化碳，并使二氯二苯甲烷水解完全。分出上层粗产物，水层用苯（约 20ml）萃取一次，合并粗产物与苯萃取液后用无水硫酸镁干燥。先在常压下蒸去苯，当温度升至 90℃ 左右时停止加热，稍冷后再进行减压蒸馏。收集 187～190℃/15mmHg 的馏分。产物冷却后固化，产量 9～10g，mp 47～48℃。文献值：mp 48.1℃（α 型）；bp 306℃。

【实验指导】

（一）预习要求

1. 复习付瑞德尔－克拉夫茨烷基化反应，了解其反应机制。

2. 复习醛酮的制备方法及卤代烃的性质。

3. 复习无水操作的要求。

4. 了解无水三氯化铝的使用方法。

（二）注意事项

1. 仪器必须充分干燥，否则影响反应顺利进行。

2. 无水三氯化铝的质量是实验成败的关键之一。研细、称量、投料都要迅速，避免长时间暴露在空气中。

3. 将四氯化碳重蒸一次，并弃去最初 10% 的馏分。无水苯的干燥方法与四氯化碳相同。

4. 温度低于 5℃ 时，反应缓慢；高于 10℃ 时则有焦油状物产生。反应液颜色的加深及氯化氢的产生，表明反应开始。在反应过程中逐渐有棕色固体出现，那是二氯二苯甲烷和三氯化铝形成的络盐 $(C_6H_5)_2CCl_2 \cdot AlCl_3$。

5. 加水后，络盐将水解，深颜色褪去可得清净的两层液体。

$$(C_6H_5)_2CCl_2 \cdot AlCl_3 + H_2O \longrightarrow (C_6H_5)_2CCl_2 + AlCl_3 (H_2O)$$

6. 可回收约 20ml 四氯化碳，其中含少量苯。

7. 也可用水蒸气蒸馏的方法带出剩余的四氯化碳，并使二氯二苯甲烷水解成二苯甲酮。

8. 冷却后有时不易立即得到结晶，这是由于形成低熔点（mp 26℃）β 型二苯甲酮之故。也可用石油醚（bp 60~90℃）进行重结晶，代替减压蒸馏。

（三）思考题

1. 水和潮气对本实验有何影响？在仪器装置和操作中应注意哪些事项？

2. 本实验中为什么是四氯化碳过量而不是苯过量？如苯过量有什么结果？

3. 在烷基化和酰基化反应中，三氯化铝的用量有何不同，为什么？

4. 指出如何由 Friedel-Crafts 反应制备下列化合物？

（1）二苯甲烷；（2）苄基苯基酮；（3）对硝基二苯酮。

Experiment 23　Preparation of Benzophenone

Experimental principle

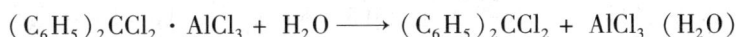

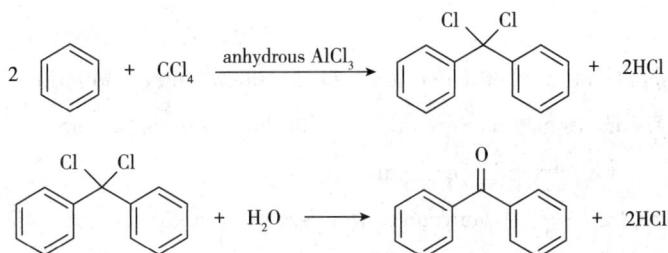

This reaction iscatalyzed by anhydrous aluminum chloride. All the apparatus and reagents in the reaction should be dry and anhydrous because aluminum chloride will invalidate by decomposition if it encounters water or moisture. So it is desirable to introduce a drying tube between the condenser and the trap. The evolution of hydrogen chloride take place in this experiment, it is needed to fit with a gas absorption trap.

Experimental procedures

1. Materials and reagents

anhydrous benzene　　　　　　12ml（0.13mol）

carbon tetrachloride	30ml (0.195mol)
anhydrous aluminum chloride	9g (0.067mol)
magnesium sulfate	

2. Procedures

In a 250ml of three-necked, round-bottomed flask fitted with a good mechanical stirrer, a separatory funnel, a thermometer, and a reflux condenser connected with a trap for absorbing the hydrogen chloride evolved, are placed 9g of anhydrous aluminum chloride and 20ml of dry carbon tetrachloride. The flask is surrounded by an ice bath. The stirrer is started and when the temperature of carbon tetrachloride has dropped to 10 ~ 15℃, a mixture of 12ml of anhydrous benzene and 10ml of carbon tetrachloride is added at such a rate that the temperature is kept between 5 ~ 10℃. The reaction begins immediately as is indicated by the evolution of hydrogen chloride and a rising temperature. This addition requires about 15 minutes. The stirring is continued for another one hour after the benzene-carbon tetrachloride solution has been added, while the temperature is held at about 10℃. The reaction mixture is still kept in an ice bath, and 10ml of water is slowly added with stirring. After addition, the equipment is changed to distillation. The mixture is then first heated on a steam bath to remove most of the excess of carbon tetrachloride, and then the mixture is distilled with heating to carry over the remaining carbon tetrachloride, and to hydrolysis the benzophenone dichloride to benzophenone. The upper benzophenone layer is then separated from the aqueous layer and the latter is extracted with about 20ml of benzene. Combine the benzene solution and the benzophenone and dry them over anhydrous magnesium sulfate. The benzene solution and benzophenone are transferred to a flask for distillation. The benzene is removed under ordinary pressure and the benzophenone is distilled under reduced pressure collecting the distillate at 187 ~ 190℃/15mmHg. The product is solidified and the yield is about 9 ~ 10g, mp 47 ~ 48℃. Lit. mp 48.1℃.

Experimental instruction

Notes

1. The stirrer should be very efficient, as otherwise the aluminum chloride tends to cake on the sides of the flask. This makes cooling very difficult and thus increase the time necessary for the addition of the benzene-carbon tetrachloride mixture.

2. Gas absorption trap. ——A convenient trap is necessary for the absorption of hydrogen chloride. In the reaction involving compounds sensitive to water it is desirable to introduce a drying tube between the condenser and the trap in order to absorb any moisture which might diffuse up from the trap.

3. A good grade of technical anhydrous aluminum chloride was used to obtain the results given in the procedure. The yield decreases considerably when the quality of this reagent is not good.

4. No difference in yield is noticed in using the ordinary of 'pure' grade carbon tetrachloride and the sulfur-free c. p. grade. It is easily dried by distilling the commercial product and rejecting the first 10 percent of the distillate.

5. It is necessary to allow the reaction to start before packing in an ice-salt mixture. If the tem-

perature is too low (below 10℃) the reaction does not start. After the reaction has started, the cooling should be as efficient as possible so that the mixture of benzene and carbon tetrachloride may be added in the minimum amount of time. If the temperature drops below 5℃ the reaction is too slow. If the temperature goes above 10℃ there is increasing formation of tarry matter and lowering of the yield.

6. The yield is 5 to 10 percent lower if the ordinary technical grade of benzene is used. The benzene is dried in the same manner as the carbon tetrachloride.

7. There is considerable tendency for the benzophenone to foam over during the early part of the distillation under reduced pressure and care must be taken to prevent this.

Exercises

1. How is this experiment influenced by water and moisture? Which notes should we pay attention to in the apparatus and operation?

2. Why should carbon tetrachloride rather than benzene be excessive? What is the consequence if benzene is excessive?

3. What are the different quantities of aluminum chloride in the alkylation and acylation? Why?

4. How to prepare the following compounds with Friedel-Crafts?

(1) Diphenylmethane; (2) Benzyl phenyl methanone; (3) Bis-(*p*-nitrophenyl) methanone.

实验二十四　樟脑的还原反应

【目的要求】

1. **掌握**　用 $NaBH_4$ 还原樟脑的原理及操作方法。

2. **了解**　薄层层析在合成反应中的应用。

【实验原理】

用硼氢化钠还原樟脑得到冰片和异冰片 2 个非对映异构体。由于立体选择性较高，所得产物以异冰片为主。冰片和异冰片具有不同的物理性质，两者极性不同。

反应式

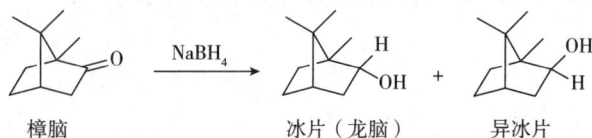

樟脑　　　　　　　　　　冰片（龙脑）　　　异冰片

【实验步骤】

1. 原料与试剂

樟脑	1g	(6.6mmol)
硼氢化钠	0.6g	(16.0mmol)
甲醇	10ml	
乙醚	25ml	

无水硫酸钠或无水硫酸镁

2. 步骤

（1）樟脑的还原　在25ml锥形瓶中将1g樟脑溶于10ml甲醇，室温下小心分批加入0.6g硼氢化钠，一边振摇一边加硼氢化钠。必要时可用冰水浴控制反应温度。当所有硼氢化钠加完后，将反应混合物加热回流至硼氢化钠消失。将反应混合物冷却到室温，搅拌下将反应液倒入20g冰水中，待冰全部熔化后，抽滤，收集白色固体，滤饼洗涤数次，晾干。将固体转移至100ml干净的锥形瓶中，加入25ml乙醚溶解固体，随后加入6~7刮刀无水硫酸钠或无水硫酸镁。干燥5分钟后将溶液（除去干燥剂）转移至预先称好重的烧杯或锥形瓶中。在通风橱中蒸馏除去溶剂得到白色固体，并用无水乙醇重结晶。产量约为0.6g，mp 212℃。

（2）产物的鉴别　取一片5cm×15cm的薄层板，分别用冰片、异冰片、樟脑和樟脑还原产物的乙醚溶液点样，置于层析缸中展开。取出层析板，待薄层上尚残留少许展开剂时，立即用另一块与薄层板同样大小并均匀地涂上浓硫酸的玻璃板覆盖在薄层板上，即可显色。对比4个点的R_f值，可证明樟脑已被还原成冰片和异冰片。也可用溴化钾压片做产物的红外光谱。

【实验指导】

（一）预习要求

1. 复习还原剂$NaBH_4$的反应原理及应用范围。

2. 复习$NaBH_4$还原羰基的立体化学。

（二）注意事项

1. $NaBH_4$吸水后易变质，放出氢气，故开封后的试剂需置干燥器内保存。

2. 薄层板的制法是：取5g硅胶与13ml 0.5%~1%的羧甲基纤维素钠水溶液，在研钵中调匀，铺在清洁干燥的玻璃片上，薄层的厚度约0.25mm。室温晾干后，在110℃烘箱内活化半小时，取出放冷后置干燥器内备用。

3. 以三氯甲烷-苯（2∶1，*V/V*）为展开剂。

（三）思考题

1. 测定产物熔点时应注意什么？

2. 除薄层层析外，还可用其他什么方法来区别和鉴别冰片和异冰片。

3. 原冰片酮用$NaBH_4$还原时，你预计得到的主要产物是什么？

原冰片酮

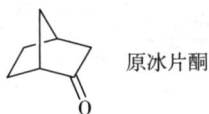

Experiment 24　The Reduction of camphor

Experimental principle

Camphor will be reduced to a mixture of borneol and isoborneol which are diastereoisomers by the action of sodium borohydride. Because of the high stereoselectivity, the main product is isoborneol. Borneol and isoborneol have different physical property and polarity.

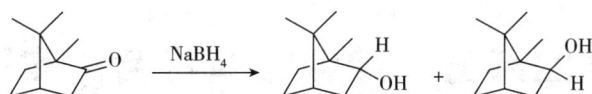

Experimental procedures

1. Materials and reagents

camphor	1g（6.6mmol）
sodium borogydride	0.6g（16.0mmol）
methanol	10ml
ether	25ml

anhydrous sodium or magnesium sulfate.

2. Procedures

To the camphor（1.0g）in the 25ml Erlenmeyer flask, add methanol（10ml）. Stir with a glass rod or microspatula until the solid has dissolved. In portions, cautiously and intermittently add 0.6g of sodium borohydride to the solution at room temperature. If necessary, cool the Erlenmeyer flask in an ice bath to control the temperature of the reaction mixture. When all the borohydride is added, heat the contents of the flask to reflux until all the sodium borohydride has dissolved.

Allow the reaction mixture to cool to room temperature, and then carefully add to ice water （20ml）while stirring. Collect the white solid which forms by filtering through a Büchner funnel, and suction-dry it for several minutes while you clean and dry the 100ml Erlenmeyer flask. Transfer the solid back to the clean flask, and add 25ml of ether to dissolve the solid followed by 6~7 microspatulafuls of anhydrous sodium or magnesium sulfate. After about 5 minutes of drying, transfer the solution（leaving behind the drying agent）to a previously weighed beaker or Erlenmeyer flask. Evaporate the solvent off in the hood to obtain the product as a white solid. Recrystallize the crude product from aqueous ethanol. The yield of the product is about 0.9g.

Weigh the product and calculate the percentage yield. Determine the melting point（literature mp：isoborneol 212℃）in a sealed capillary tube and record the IR spectrum as a KBr pellet.

Experimental instruction

Notes

1. Sodium borohydride liberates hydrogen upon reaction with water；soit should be kept it in a drying condition.

2. Ether is highly flammable, so keep itaway from fire.

Exercises

1. What should we pay attention to while determining the melting point of the product?

2. What kind of method we can use todistinguish and identify borneol and isoborneol except to using IR spectroscopy?

3. What is the main product in the reaction of sodium borohydridewith *ortho*-camphor?

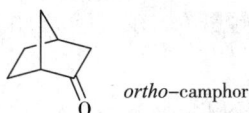

ortho-camphor

第四部分 综合性有机合成实验

Part IV Comprehensive Organic Synthetic Experiments

实验二十五 亚苄基乙酰苯的制备及其与溴的反应

【目的要求】

1. **掌握** 通过交叉羟醛缩合反应制备亚苄基乙酰苯的原理及操作方法。
2. **了解** 薄层层析在合成反应中的应用。
3. 验证亚苄基乙酰苯与溴加成的立体化学。

【实验原理】

反应式

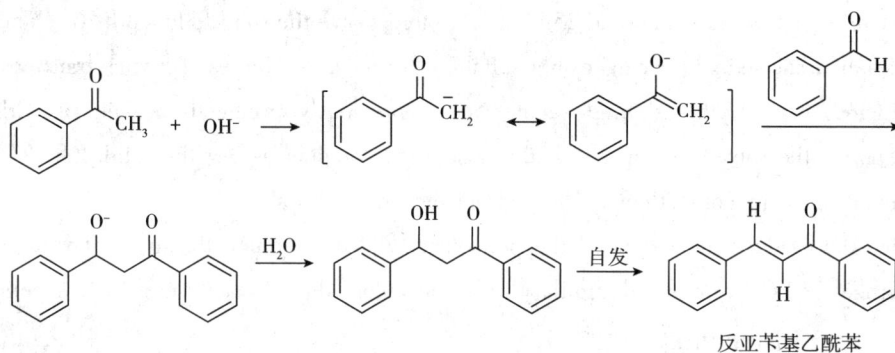

反亚苄基乙酰苯

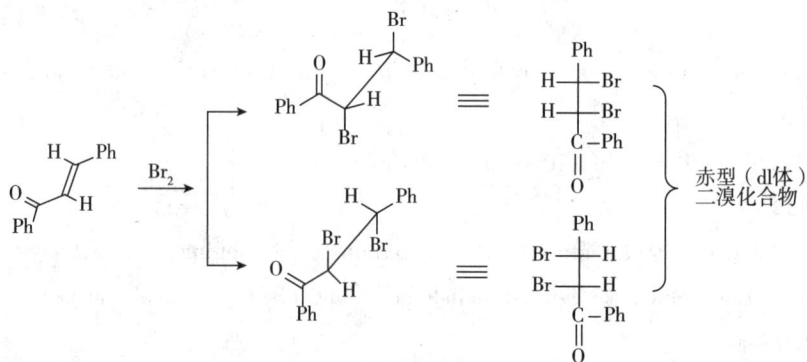

赤型（dl体）
二溴化合物

具有 α–H 的羰基化合物可发生羟醛缩合反应。苯甲醛与苯乙酮在稀氢氧化钠溶液存在下通过交叉羟醛缩合反应生成"羟醛"。在实验条件下"羟醛"自发脱水生成较稳定的反亚苄基乙酰苯。

反亚苄基乙酰苯与溴的加成产物以赤型二溴化物为主。

【实验步骤】

1. 原料与试剂

苯乙酮	6g（0.05mol）
苯甲醛	5.3g（0.05mol）
10%氢氧化钠溶液	25ml
95%乙醇	
溴的四氯化碳溶液	

2. 步骤

（1）反亚苄基乙酰苯的制备　在装有搅拌的100ml三颈瓶中加入6g（5.8ml）苯乙酮、20ml 95%乙醇及25ml 10%NaOH溶液。室温搅拌下加入等摩尔的苯甲醛（5.3g，5ml）。室温（25℃）搅拌约1.5小时，有黄色油状物出现，冰水浴冷却后有固体析出。继续冷却使结晶完全，抽滤，冷水洗涤，再用少许冷却过的95%乙醇洗涤。粗品用95%乙醇重结晶，得浅黄结晶5.5g，mp 58～59℃。文献值：mp 59℃。

反应过程可通过薄层色谱（TLC）法跟踪。

展开剂：石油醚：乙酸乙酯=3∶1

吸附剂：硅胶GF254

展开距离：10cm

显色方法：紫外光

此外，可对重结晶后的产物进行红外光谱分析。

（2）反式亚苄基乙酰苯与溴的加成反应——赤型二溴化物的形成　将1g干燥的反亚苄基乙酰苯溶于4ml四氯化碳中，冰水浴冷却下，一面振摇一面滴加4ml溴的四氯化碳溶液。将反应混合物放置室温5～10分钟，过滤收集结晶，用少量冷的95%乙醇洗涤2次，干燥，mp 155～157℃。文献值：mp 159～160℃。

【实验指导】

（一）预习要求

1. 复习（交叉）羟醛缩合反应的原理、反应条件及应用。

2. 了解投料方式对交叉羟醛缩合反应结果的影响。

3. 复习双键形成及其加成反应的立体化学。

（二）注意事项

1. 溴的四氯化碳溶液是按1g溴溶于6ml四氯化碳的比例配成。

2. 苯乙酮凝固点17～20℃，温度较低时固化，使用前应温热融化。量筒中残留的苯乙酮可用少量95%乙醇转移至反应瓶中。

3. 如无固体析出，可用玻璃棒或刮刀摩擦瓶壁，或加入少许亚苄基乙酰苯晶种引发结晶。亚苄基乙酰苯对皮肤有刺激作用，切勿与皮肤接触。

4. 每克干粗品加入4～5ml溶剂。

5. 苏型二溴化物 mp 123～124℃。

（三）思考题

1. 为什么本实验主产物是亚苄基乙酰苯而不是苯乙酮的自身缩合或苯甲醛的 Cannizzaro 反应产物？

2. 写出下列羰基化合物与碱反应所得的主要产物：

（1）丙醛、甲醛、稀氢氧化钠。

（2）苯甲醛、浓氢氧化钾。

（3）丙酮、苯甲醛（2mol）、稀氢氧化钠。

（4）苯甲醛、乙酸乙酯、乙醇钠。

3. 试解释本实验形成反式亚苄基乙酰苯及赤型二溴化物构型产物的原因。

4. 本实验所得赤型二溴化合物是否有旋光性？

Experiment 25　Preparation of Benzalacetophenone and Its Reaction With Bromine

Experimental principle

The carbonyl compound which have α-H can react by aldol condensation. The benzaldehyde reacts with acetophenone in dilute alkali solution by aldol condensation to produce 'aldol'. At experimental condition 'aldol' can dehydrate spontaneously to give stable *trans*-benzalacetophenone. The main additional product of *trans*-benzalacetophenone with bromine is erythro dibromide.

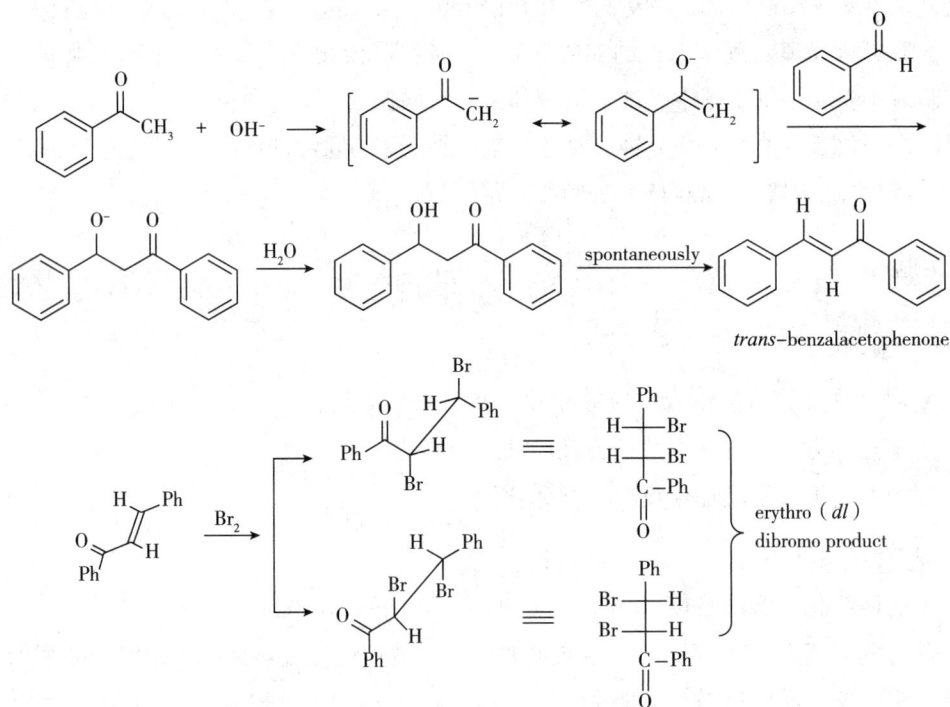

Experimental procedures

1. Materials and reagents

acetophenone　　　　　　6g（0.05mol）

benzaldehyde　　　　　　5.3g（0.05mol）

10% sodium hydroxide   25ml

95% alcohol

bromine in carbon tetrachloride solution

2. Procedures

（1）Preparation of *trans*-benzalacetophenone

A solution of 6g（5.8ml）acetophenone,15ml 95 percent alcohol and 25ml 10 percent sodium hydroxide are introduced into 100ml three-neck flasks,supplied with an effective stirrer. The stirrer started,an equal mole of benzaldehyde（5.3g,5ml）is then added at once. Stir the mixture at room temperature（25℃）for one and a half hour. Yellow oiled material appears. Some solid product separate out after it is cooled in a freezing bath to make the crystallization absolute filter,washed with water,then washed by some 95 percent alcohol,which previously cooled. The crude product is purified by recrystallization with 95 percent alcohol,give light yellow material 5.5g,mp 58～59℃.

The reaction can be monitored by TLC analysis.

eluents:petroleum：ethyl acetate ＝3：1（volume）

adsorbents:silica gel （GF254）

developing distance:10cm

visualization methods:a low-intensity ultraviolet lamp

In addition,the product after recrystallizationcan be analyzed by IR.

（2）The additional reaction of *trans*-benzalacetophenone with Bromine — the formation of erythro dibromide product

Dissolve 1g dried *trans*-benzalacetophenone in 4ml of carbon tetrachloride,cool the solution in an ice bath and put 4ml drops of bromine in carbon tetrachloride with shaking. Lay up the reacting mixture at room temperature for 5～10 minutes,filter,wash 2 times with some cold 95 percent alcohol,dry it,mp 155～157℃（lit. mp 159～160℃）.

Experimental instruction

Notes

1. The freezing point of acetophenone is 17～20℃,which can be solidified at low temperature, so it should be warmed and thawed before using. The remained acetophenone in volumetric cylinder can be removed by some 95% alcohol to reacting bottle.

2. If no solid substance separate out,you can clash the wall of bottle by glass stick or scraper, or put some benzalacetophenone crystal strain to produce crystallization.

3. The amount of recrystallization solvent is 4～5 times of dried crude product.

4. Be careful！ The benzalacetophenone may stimulate the skin,it can't be touch with skin.

5. The bromine in carbon tetrachloride is proportioned by dissolving 1g bromine in 6ml carbon tetrachloride.

6. The melting point of threo product is 123～124℃.

Exercises

1. Why is the mixed aldol condensation,which produces benzalacetophenone,the main reaction that occurs in this experiment rather than the two possible side reactions,self-condensation of aceto-

phenoneor Cannizzaro reaction of benzaldehyde?

2. Write down the equations to show the major products from reaction of the following carbonyl compounds with bases:

(1) propylaldehyde, formaldehyde, dilute sodium hydroxide.

(2) benzaldehyde, concentrated potassium hydroxide.

(3) acetone, benzaldehyde (2mol), dilute sodium hydroxide.

(4) benzaldehyde, ethyl acetate, sodium ethoxide in ethanol.

3. Suggest reasons for the fact that the *trans* isomer of benzalacetophenone and erythro dibromide predominates in the reaction mixture from the aldol condensation and additional reaction respectively.

4. Does the erythro dibromide product have optical activity?

实验二十六　降血脂药吉非罗齐中间体 3 - (2, 5 - 二甲基苯氧基) -1 -氯丙烷的制备 及反应过程跟踪

【目的要求】

1. **掌握**　制备 3 - (2, 5 - 二甲基苯氧基) -1 - 氯丙烷的原理及操作方法。

2. **了解**　薄层层析在合成反应中的应用。

【实验原理】

在 NaOH 存在下，2, 5 - 二甲基苯酚形成酚钠后与 1 - 氯 - 3 - 溴丙烷发生亲核取代反应，得 2,5 - 二甲基苯基 - 3 - 氯丙基醚。由于在反应条件下，反应物 2,5 - 二甲基苯酚钠与 1 - 氯 - 3 - 溴丙烷分别位于水相和有机相，故反应时间长，收率低。在相转移催化剂 (PTC，如 TEBA) 存在下，反应时间缩短，收率提高 30% 以上。

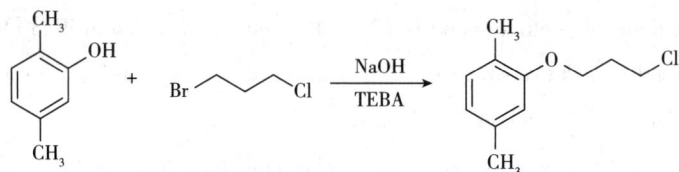

【实验步骤】

1. 原料与试剂

2,5 - 二甲基苯酚	3.8g (0.031mol)
1 - 氯 - 3 - 溴丙烷	7.9g (0.05mol)
1.6mol/L NaOH	30ml
TEBA	0.2g
乙醚	
饱和氯化钠溶液	

无水硫酸镁

苯

石油醚（bp 60～90℃）

2. 步骤 在 100ml 四颈瓶中加入 3.8g（0.031mol）2，5－二甲基苯酚，7.9g（0.05mol）1－氯－3－溴丙烷，0.2g TEBA，加热，维持 90～94℃快速搅拌下滴加 1.6N NaOH，约 1 小时滴完（滴加 1.6N NaOH 约 30ml）。滴完后维持 100℃快速搅拌至近中性（pH 6～7，约搅拌 4 小时），冷至室温，分液，水层用乙醚（15ml，10ml×2）萃取，合并有机层，饱和氯化钠洗涤，无水硫酸镁干燥。普通蒸馏回收乙醚后减压蒸馏，收集 108～110℃/266Pa 的馏分，得亮黄色液体 4.7g，收率 77.7%。

反应过程可通过薄层色谱（TLC）法跟踪。

展开剂：苯∶石油醚＝1∶1

吸附剂：硅胶 GF254

展开距离：10cm

显色方法：紫外光

【实验指导】

（一）预习要求

1. 复习 Williamson 醚制备法的反应原理及应用范围。

2. 复习相转移催化反应的原理。

（二）注意事项

1. 因该反应为相转移催化反应，故应维持较快的搅拌速度。

2. 如果 pH 偏小，应补滴加少量 NaOH。

3. 在实验条件下，2，5－二甲基苯酚钠与 1－氯－3－溴丙烷反应除了得到产物 3－（2，5－二甲基苯氧基）－1－氯丙烷外，还有少量 3－（2，5－二甲基苯氧基）－1－溴丙烷生成，其沸点为 124～132℃/266Pa。

（三）思考题

1. 2，5－二甲基苯酚钠与 1－氯－3－溴丙烷反应为什么要加相转移催化剂？

2. 写出（CH$_3$）$_3$C－O－C$_2$H$_5$ 的 Williamson 合成法。

3. 为什么只有少量 3－（2，5－二甲基苯氧基）－1－溴丙烷生成？

4. 为什么应维持较快的搅拌速度？

Experiment 26　Synthesis of 3-（2，5-Xylyloxyl）propyl Chloride and Monitoration of Reaction Process

Experimental principle

3-(2,5-xylyloxyl) propyl chloride was synthesized from 2,5-dimethylphenol reacting with 1-bromo-3-chloropropane in the presence of sodium hydroxide. Because 2,5-dimethylphenol and 1-

bromo-3-chloropropane exist respectively in organic phase and aqueous phase, the time of reaction is long and the yield is low. If the reaction is catalyzed by phase-transfer catalyst (PTC, for example TEBA), the time of reaction is shortened and the yield is increased by 30% or more.

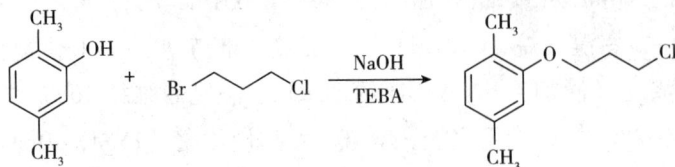

Experimental procedures

1. Materials and reagents

2,5-dimethylphenol	3.8g(0.031mol)
1-bromo-3-chloropropane	7.9g(0.05mol)
1.6mol/L sodium hydroxide	30ml
TEBA	0.2 g
ethyl ether	
saturated sodium chloride solution	
anhydrous magnesium sulfate	
benzene	
petroleum(bp 60~90℃)	

2. Procedures

In a 100ml four-necked round-bottomed flask provided with a mechanical stirrer, thermometer, dropping funnel, and reflux condenser are placed 3.8g(0.031mol)2,5-dimethylphenol, 7.9g (0.05mol)1-bromo-3-chloropropane, 0.2 g TEBA. The mixture is stirred vigorously and 30ml of 1.6N sodium hydroxide is added from a dropping funnel at such a rate that the whole is added in about one hour, while the temperature is maintained between 90~94℃. Stirring is continued at about 100℃ for another four hours until the pH is 6~7. Cool the mixture to room temperature, transfer the mixture to a separatory funnel, and separate the organic liquid from the aqueous layer. Extract the aqueous layer with diethyl ether(15ml, 10ml×2), combine the organic liquid and the extract liquor, wish it with 10ml of saturated aqueous sodium chloride, and separate the layers carefully. After dried over anhydrous magnesium sulfate, the ether is removed as completely as possible and the residual is distilled under reduced pressure collecting the distillate at 108~110℃/266Pa. The product is light yellow liquid and the yield is about 4.7g (77.7 percent of the theoretical amount).

The reaction can be monitored by TLC analysis.

eluents: benzene : petroleum = 1 : 1(volume)

adsorbents: silica gel (GF254)

developing distance: 10cm

visualization methods: a low-intensity ultraviolet lamp

Experimental instruction

Notes

1. Because the reaction is carrying through catalyzed by phase-transfer catalyst, it is necessary to stir vigorously.

2. If it is not, add extra base.

3. In addition to 3-(2,5-xylyloxyl) propyl chloride is obtained, 3-(2,5-xylyloxyl) propyl bromine, bp 124～132℃/266Pa, may be produced.

Exercises

1. Why should 2, 5-dimethylphenol react with 1-bromo-3-chloropropane in the presence of phase-transfer catalyst?

2. Suggest methods for preparing the following ethers via Williamson syntheses.

(1) $CH_3CH_2OCH_2CH_3$; (2) $CH_3CH_2OCH(CH_3)_2$; (3) $CH_3CH_2CH_2CH_2OCH_2CH_2CH_3$.

3. Why does only little 3-(2,5-xylyloxyl) propyl bromine be produced?

4. Why is it necessary to stir vigorously?

实验二十七　1-苯基-2-甲基-2-硝基丙醇的制备及反应过程跟踪

【目的要求】

1. **掌握**　制备1-苯基-2-甲基-2-硝基丙醇的的原理及操作方法。
2. **了解**　薄层层析在合成反应中的应用。

【实验原理】

硝基具有强吸电子作用，这就导致了α-氢原子有一定酸性。2-硝基丙烷与甲醇钠作用，形成碳负离子，该碳负离子由于电荷分散而稳定，其共振结构式为：

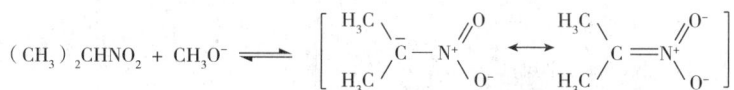

$$(CH_3)_2CHNO_2 + CH_3O^- \rightleftharpoons \left[\underset{H_3C}{\overset{H_3C}{>}}\overset{}{\underset{|}{C}} - \overset{O}{\underset{O^-}{N^+}} \longleftrightarrow \underset{H_3C}{\overset{H_3C}{>}}C = \overset{O}{\underset{O^-}{N^+}} \right]$$

接着，碳负离子进攻苯甲醛羰基，发生缩合反应，得到1-苯基-2-甲基-2-硝基丙醇。未反应的原料苯甲醛可用15%亚硫酸氢钠洗涤除去，可通过薄层色谱分析跟踪反应过程并对产品纯度进行初步检测。

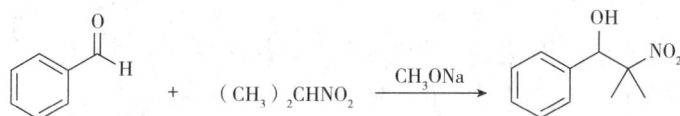

【实验步骤】

1. 原料与试剂

苯甲醛　　　　10.6g（0.1mol）

2-硝基丙烷　　9.4g（0.105mol）

金属钠　　　　　　0.5g（0.022mol）

无水甲醇　　　　　35ml

醋酸

乙醚

15%亚硫酸氢钠溶液

无水硫酸钠

石油醚（bp 60～90℃）

2. 步骤　在 100ml 圆底瓶中加入 35ml 无水甲醇，搅拌下逐渐加入 0.5g（0.022mol）切成薄片的金属钠，搅拌片刻直至钠消失。加入 9.4g（0.105mol）2 – 硝基丙烷，10.6g（0.1mol）新蒸馏的苯甲醛，室温搅拌 24 小时，得浅黄色液体，取少量点样。反应液用醋酸酸化至 pH 6～7（耗用醋酸约 2ml）。蒸去甲醇，将残留物溶于 30ml 乙醚及 15ml 水的混合液中，分液，水层用乙醚（10ml×2）萃取，合并有机层，10ml 水洗涤，15%亚硫酸氢钠溶液洗至原料苯甲醛消失（约需用亚硫酸氢钠溶液 50ml，分四次剧烈振摇洗涤，薄层色谱分析检查），再用 10ml 水洗涤，无水硫酸钠干燥。过滤，蒸去乙醚后室温放置，析出固体，抽滤，少量石油醚（bp 60～90℃）洗涤，烘干，得无色固体 6～7g，mp 66～69℃。

反应过程可通过薄层色谱（TLC）法跟踪。

展开剂：三氯甲烷

吸附剂：硅胶 GF254

展开距离：10cm

显色方法：紫外光

【实验指导】

（一）预习要求

1. 复习碳负离子的结构、性质及反应。

2. 复习金属钠的使用方法及注意事项。

3. 复习无水操作的要求。

4. 了解磁力搅拌器的使用方法。

（二）注意事项

1. 反应必须在无水条件下进行。

2. 应分批加入金属钠，以防温度过高使甲醇溢出（或在圆底瓶口置冷凝管）。甲醇钠制备后应立即使用。

3. 反应完毕后须用亚硫酸氢钠溶液将苯甲醛全部洗去，用薄层色谱分析检查追踪残留的苯甲醛。如洗涤四次后发现仍有苯甲醛存在，应继续洗涤。

4. 如产品熔点较低，可用正庚烷重结晶。

（三）思考题

1. 为什么与硝基相连碳上的氢有酸性？

2. 为什么反应必须在无水条件下进行？

3. 为什么亚硫酸氢钠溶液能洗涤除去原料苯甲醛？

Experiment 27　Preparation of 1-Phenyl-2-methyl-2-nitropropanol and Monitoration of Reaction Process

Experimental principle

The nitro group (—NO$_2$) withdraw electrons and cause α-hydrogen to be somewhat acidic. 2-nitropropane reacts with sodium methoxide to produce the carbanion. The resulting carbanion is stabilized by resonance as shown by the following reaction:

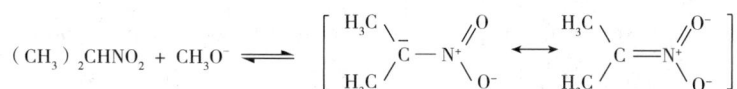

As a consequence nitro compounds undergo condensation with aldehydes that contain no α-hydrogen.

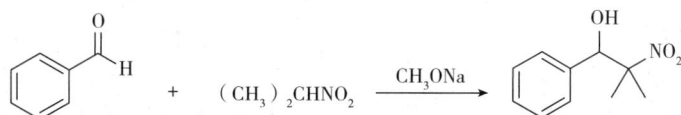

Experimental procedures

1. Materials and reagents

benzaldehyde　　　　10. 6g (10mmol)

2-nitropropane　　　　9. 4g (10. 5mmol)

Na　　　　　　　　　0. 5g (2. 2mmol)

anhydrous methanol　35ml

acetic acid

ethyl ether

15% aqueous sodium bisulfite solution

anhydrous sodium sulfate

petroleum(bp 60 ~ 90℃)

2. Procedures

To a solution prepared from 0. 5g (2. 2mmol) sodium and 35ml of anhydrous methanol was added 9. 4g (10. 5mmol) of 2-nitropropane and 10. 6g (10mmol) of freshly distilled benzaldehyde. After 24h at room temperature, the yellow solution was acidified with acetic acid and the methanol was distilled. The residue was dissolved in a mixture of water(15ml) and ethyl ether(30ml). The water layer was extracted with two 10ml portions of ethyl ether. The combined ether layer was washed with 10ml of water, extracted with four 10ml portions of 15% aqueous sodium bisulfite solution to remove the unreacted benzaldehyde, again washed with 10ml of water and was dried over anhydrous sodium sulfate.

The ester was distilled. Allow the material to stand in an ice-water bath and then collect the crystals with suction. Wash the product with a small amount of petroleum(60 ~ 90℃) and spread it on a clean watchglass to dry. Give the nitro alcohol as yellow crystals, mp 66 ~ 69℃, yield of 37%.

The reaction can be monitored by TLC analysis.

eluents: chloroform

adsorbents: silica gel (GF254)

developing distance: 10cm

visualization methods: a low-intensity ultraviolet lamp

Experimental instruction

Notes

1. It is essential that the reaction be free from water.

2. In order to avoid methanol escaping the sodium should be added in portions. As soon as the sodium methoxide solution has been prepared the next step had better be performed.

3. The ether layer is washed with sodium bisulfate solution until no unreacted benzaldehyde can be monitored by TLC.

4. If the melting point of the product is lower than that of expecting the product may be recrystallized by heptane.

Exercises

1. Why is the hydrogen on the carbon adjacent to thenitro acidic?

2. Why is it essential that the reaction be free from water?

3. Why can the unreacted benzaldehyde be removed by washing with aqueous sodium bisulfate solution?

第五部分 设计性有机合成实验

Part V Designing Organic Synthetic Experiment

实验二十八 肉桂酸的制备

【目的要求】

1. **掌握** 薄层层析色谱（TLC）法监测反应进程，确定反应终点。

2. 学习查阅文献资料，设计肉桂酸的合成路线，以提高学生独立思考和解决问题的能力。

3. 通过分析文献资料，综合所学知识，确定肉桂酸的合成方法及具体反应条件。

【文献查阅】

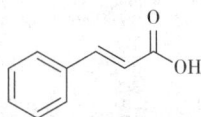

中文名称：肉桂酸；英文名称：cinnamic acid；CAS 号：140 - 10 - 3

要求学会系统查阅文献的方法，查阅内容包括以下内容。

1. 中文文献 掌握中国学术期刊网（CNKI，http：//acad. cnki. net/）的检索，通过关键词"肉桂酸""制备""合成"等进行检索，获取肉桂酸的合成方法文献。

2. 外文文献 掌握美国化学文摘 CA（网络版）SciFinder Web（https：//scifinder. cas. org/）的结构式检索，通过结构式检索获取肉桂酸最新合成方法的文献。

【合成方案的分析、讨论与确定】

本次实验要求每个学生在开展具体实验之前，4 个同学为一组，进行文献调研，检索国内外制备肉桂酸的方法及最新进展，在阅读文献的基础上进行以下内容。

1. 获得至少 5 种肉桂酸的制备方法（采用不同反应原料进行合成方可视为不同方法），并获得相应合成方法的原始文献。

2. 写出相应的反应式，思考并掌握相应反应机制。

3. 对比上述检索到的合成方法，从原料、试剂、催化剂的价格、反应时间、反应温度、反应收率、可操作性、试剂毒性等多个角度进行分析，对各方法进行优缺点评述，并最终确定 1～2 种不同于下述示例的优选合成方法。

4. 思考并分析具体的合成方案：包括反应物、反应温度、大概的反应时间、后处理及纯化方法、实验装置等。

5. 4 个同学为一组，将上述检索及分析过程在实验课堂上与老师进行讨论，确定最终的实验方案。（注：每组可推荐一位同学主讲，但其他同学也要参与到讨论之中）

6. 经过课堂讨论，确定 1 种优选的合成方法，书写预习报告、准备开展具体合成实验。

【实验内容】

1. 实验分组 将学生分为 8 个小组，其中 1 组按照示例方法进行，另外 7 组采用不同的反应条件进行实验。

2. 设计合成方案 根据所学的有关知识及文献资料，可从以下几个方面设计每一小组的合成方案。

（1）反应物的投料比例。

（2）催化剂用量。

（3）反应温度。

（4）反应时间。

（5）反应后处理方法。

3. TLC 监测反应进程 每隔 30 分钟监测一次反应进展情况。展开剂体系：石油醚：乙酸乙酯：醋酸 =4：1：0.05。点样：反应液、反应物、肉桂酸对照物，以及相应的合点。结果：在紫外灯 254 nm 下观察硅胶薄层色谱板上的斑点情况，根据反应物、产物的相对比例，确定是否可以终止反应。

4. 小组实验结果对比分析 从反应时间、反应收率、反应成本等角度，分析对比 8 组实验结果，最终确定实验最优方法。

【示例：采用 Perkin 反应制备肉桂酸】

1. 实验原理

利用 Perkin 反应，将芳醛与酸酐混合在相应的羧酸盐存在下加热，可以制得 α,β – 不饱和酸。例：

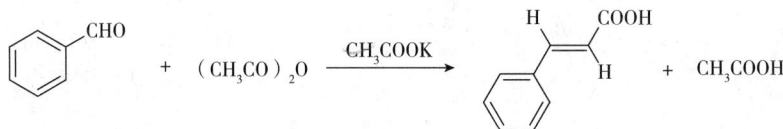

本实验按照 Kalnin 所提出的方法，用碳酸钾代替 Perkin 反应中的醋酸钾，反应时间短，产率高。

2. 实验步骤

（1）原料与试剂

苯甲醛	3.15g（3ml，0.03mol）
醋酸酐	8.64g（8ml，0.084mol）
无水碳酸钾	4.2g
10% 氢氧化钠溶液	20ml
浓盐酸	
20% 乙醇	

（2）实验操作 在 200ml 圆底烧瓶中放入 3ml（3.15g，0.03mol）新蒸馏过的苯甲醛、

8ml（8.64g，0.084mol）新蒸馏过的醋酐及研细的4.2g无水碳酸钾，在油浴中加热回流30分钟。由于有二氧化碳放出，初期有泡沫产生。

待反应物冷却后，加入20ml水，将瓶中生成的固体尽量捣碎，用水蒸气蒸馏出未反应完的苯甲醛。再将烧瓶冷却，加入10%氢氧化钠溶液20ml，以保证所有的肉桂酸成钠盐而溶解，抽滤，将滤液倾入250ml烧杯中，冷却至室温，在搅拌下用浓盐酸酸化至刚果红试纸变蓝。冷却，抽滤，用少量冷水洗涤沉淀。抽干，让粗产品在空气中晾干，产量约3g（产率65%~70%）。粗产品用20%乙醇溶液重结晶。纯肉桂酸 mp 133℃。

【实验指导】

（一）预习要求

1. 复习 Perkin 反应的原理和在合成中的应用。
2. 复习水蒸汽蒸馏和重结晶。

（二）注意事项

1. 本反应所需苯甲醛和醋酐要重新蒸馏。
2. 碳酸钾须在120℃烘干1小时后放在干燥器内存放待用。
3. 肉桂酸有顺、反异构体，通常以反式存在，其熔点为133℃。

（三）思考题

1. 为什么要用新蒸馏的苯甲醛和醋酐？
2. 苯甲醛和丙酸酐在无水丙酸钾的存在下，相互作用后得到什么产物？
3. 为什么可以用碳酸钾代替 Perkin 反应中的醋酸钾？

Experiment 28　Preparation of Cinnamic Acid

Experimental purpose

1. Learn how to carry out the literature research and to design the synthetic route for cinnamic acid；to improve students' ability to think independently and solve problems.

2. With the full consideration of the literature analysis and the synthetic knowledge learned，the synthetic method and specific reaction conditions for cinnamic acid should be determined.

3. Master the TLC method to monitor the reaction process and determine the end point.

Literature search

Chinese name：肉桂酸；English name：cinnamic acid；CAS No. 140 – 10 – 3

It is required to learn how to systematically perform the literature research. The contents of the literature research include：

1. Chinese Literature：master the search of China National Knowledge Infrastructure（CNKI，http://acad. cnki. net/），using the key words "cinnamic acid" "preparation" "synthesis" and other keywords to obtain the literatures of the synthetic methods for cinnamic acid.

2. Foreign Literature：master the structural search using SciFinder Web（https://scifinder. cas. org/）of Chemical Abstract CA（Network Edition），and obtain the latest synthetic methods of

cinnamic acid by structural search.

Analysis, discussion and establishment of synthetic routes

This experiment requires each student to conduct a literature research before carrying out a specific experiment. Four students are asked to search the synthetic methods and latest progress worldwide for synthesizing cinnamic acid. On the basis of reading the literature:

1. Obtain at least five preparation methods of cinnamic acid, and obtain the original literature of the corresponding synthesis methods.

2. Write out the corresponding reaction scheme, think about and master the corresponding reaction mechanism.

3. By comparing the synthetic methods retrieved above, the advantages and disadvantages of each method are analyzed from the aspects of raw materials, reagents, catalyst price, reaction time, reaction temperature, reaction yield, operability and reagent toxicity. Finally, one or two preferred synthetic methods different from the following examples are determined.

4. Consideration and analysis of specific synthetic schemes with the consideration of reactants, reaction temperature, approximate reaction time, post-treatment and purification methods, experimental devices, and so on.

5. Four students are divided into a group. The retrieval and analysis process should be discussed with the teacher in the experimental class to determine the final experimental scheme. (Note: Each group may recommend one student to give a lecture, but other students should also participate in the discussion.

6. After discussion in class, the students should determine an optimum synthesis method, write the preview report, and prepare for the specific synthesis experiments.

Experimental arrangement

1. Experimental grouping

The students are divided into eight groups, one of which is conducted according to the example method, and the other seven groups conduct the experiments under different reaction conditions.

2. The design of synthesis route

According to the relevant knowledge and literature, the synthesis route of each group can be designed from the following aspects:

(1) Ratio of reactants.

(2) Catalyst dosage.

(3) Reaction temperature.

(4) Reaction time.

(5) Reaction post-treatment method.

3. Monitoration of the reaction process by TLC

The reaction progress should be monitored every 30 minutes. Eluents: petroleum ether : ethyl acetate : acetic acid = 4 : 1 : 0.05. Sample loading: reaction liquid, reactant, cinnamic acid as reference, and corresponding conjunction point. Results: The spots on TLC plate were observed at 254nm under ultraviolet lamp, and the reaction could be terminated according to the relative proportion of reactants and products.

4. Contrastive analysis of group experiment results

From the point of view of reaction time, yield and cost, eight groups of experimental results should be analyzed and compared, and the optimal method of experiment can be finally determined.

Examples: preparation of cinnamic acid by Perkin reaction

Experimental principle

According to Perkin Reaction, heat the mixture of aromatic aldehyde and acetic anhydride with the existence of the relative metallic salt of a carboxylic acid, and get α, β-unsaturated acid. For example:

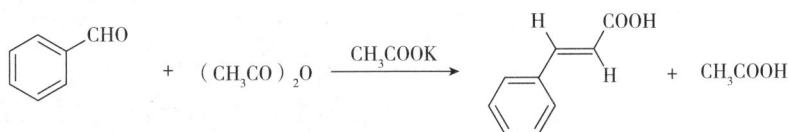

However, in this experiment, we use the method put forward by Kalnin, using Potassium carbonate instead ofpotassium acetate, because the time or reaction is short and the percentage yield is better.

Experimental procedures

1. Materials and reagents

benzaldehyde	3. 15g (3ml, 0. 03mol)
acetic anhydride	8. 64g (8ml, 0. 084mol)
anhydrous potassium carbonate	4. 2g
10% sodium hydroxide solution	20ml
hydrochloric acid	
20% alcohol	

2. Procedures

In a 200ml round-bottom flask, place 3ml (3. 15g, 0. 03mol) of benzaldehyde newly distillated, 8ml (8. 64g, 0. 084mol) of acetic anhydride newly distillated and 7. 4g of anhydrous potassium carbonate which has been made into powder. Heat them in an oil bath and reflux the mixture for 0. 5h. As there is some carbon dioxide escaping, bubbles can be found in the beginning.

Pour 20ml of water after cooling the contents of the flask for some time. The solid formed in the flask is to be made into pieces as much as possible. Then distillate off benzaldehyde left with steam distillation. Cool the flask again; pour 20ml of 10% sodium hydroxide solution to make sure that all the cinnamic acid be changed into sodium salt and dissolve in the water. Use vacuum filtration and pour the filtrate into a 250ml beaker, then cool it to room temperature. Add successive small portions of hydrochloric acid, while stirring the mixture, until the Congo red pH paper turns blue. Cool it and collect the crystals with suction. Wash the product with a small amount of cold water, and spread it on a clean watchglass to dry. The yield is about 3g (percentage yield 65% ~70%). Then the rude product should be recrystallized with 20% alcohol. The melting point of pure cinnamic acid is 133℃.

Experimental instruction

Notes

1. It is essential that benzaldehyde and acetic anhydride be newly distillated.

2. Anhydrous potassium carbonate should be dried at 120℃ for 1h.

Exercises

1. Why is it essential that benzaldehyde and acetic anhydride be newly distillated?

2. What product will be obtained when benzaldehyde reacts with anhydrous propionic anhydride in the presence of potassium propionate?

3. Why may potassium acetate be instead by potassium carbonate?

附　　录

一、工具书及实验参考书的初步介绍

（一）有机化学常用工具书

1.《有机化合物辞典》（第 6 版，1995 年）

Dictionary of Organic Compounds. 6th ed. 1995. I. Heilbron 主编，初版于 1934 年，目前本书第 6 版已有光盘版问世。这套辞典列出了有机化合物的化学结构、物理常数、化学性质及其衍生物等，并附有制备的文献资料和美国化学文摘社登记号。全套书共 9 卷，收录常见有机化合物近 3 万余条，加衍生物达 6 万余条。其中 1~6 卷为正文，按化合物名称的英文字母顺序排列，7~9 卷分别为化合物名称索引（Name Index）、分子式索引（Molecular Formula Index）及化学文摘登录号索引（Chemical Abstracts Service Registry Number Index），。该辞典第 3 版有中译本，即《汉译海氏有机化合物辞典》，由科学出版社出版。

2.《默克索引》（第 15 版，2013 年）

The Merk Index. 15th ed. 2013. 这是美国 Merck 公司出版的一部有机化合物、药物大辞典，共收集了 1 万多种化合物的性质、结构式、组成元素百分比、毒性数据、标题化合物的衍生物。对重要的中间体及药品提供较新的制备文献。本版书后附有 3 个索引：①治疗分类与生物活性索引（Therapeutic Category and Biological Activity Index）；②分子式索引（Formula Index）；③名称交替索引（Cross Index of Names）。可以从一个化合物的不同药品名称找到它的化学名。目前已停止发售光盘版，仅提供纸质版和网络版。

3.《化学和物理手册》（简称理化手册，第 97 版，2016 年）

Hand book of Chemistry and Physics. 97th ed. 2016. 理化手册是一本关于物理、化学资料的参考工具书，内容广泛齐全，收集了物理、化学方面最新的重要资料，有关的名词概念、定义、公式、数据、符号等。并列有相当数量的数学用表和数学公式。原为霍奇门（Homgman）主编创刊于 1913 年，第 45 版起改由 Weast 主编，是美国化学橡胶公司（Chemical Rubbers Co. 简称 CRC）出版。基本上是每年增补一次，每次都有大量新的参考资料增补进去，亦删去一些已经过时的资料。在第 44 版以前分装两册，上册包括数学用表和物理常数表，下册包括普通化学用表和其他理化数据。从第 45 版以后合并为一册，内容合并为 6 大部分。目前有网络版以供查阅。

（1）Section A　内容包括数学表的用法，数学用表，数学公式等。

（2）Section B　元素与无机化合物。

（3）Section C　有机化合物。这部分内容是全书的重点，也是药学工作者较常用的部分。

（4）Section D　普通化学。包括恒沸混合物、热力学常数、缓冲溶液的 pH 等。

（5）Section E　普通物理常数。内容主要是物理特性方面的各种常数、系数等数据。如热导系数、温度、介电常数、超导性折射率等。

（6）Section F　其他。包括许多重要的定义（Definitions）、公式（Formulas）、略语（Abbreviations）、符号（Symbols）、单位（Units）和命名法（Nomenclature）等。

4.《化工辞典》（第 5 版，2014 年）

前四版由王箴主编，第五版由欧阳平凯主编，这是一部综合性化学化工辞书，收集化学工业中的原料、材料、中间体、产品、生产方法、化工过程、化工机械和化工仪表自动化等方面词目以及有关的化学基本术语词目万余条。列有化合物分子式、结构式、物理常数和化学性质，对化合物制备和用途均有介绍。全书按汉字笔画排列，并附汉语拼音检字索引。

（二）实验参考书

1. Vogel's Textbook of practical Organic Chemistry. 5th ed. Vogel. 2003.

2.《有机化学实验与指导》罗一鸣主编，中南大学出版社，2019 年。

3. Experimental Organic Chemistry. 6th ed. John C. Gilbert, Stephen F. Martin, 2014.

4.《基础有机化学实验》武汉大学化学与分子科学学院实验中心编，科学出版社，2014 年。

5.《有机合成实验室手册（原著第 22 版）》（德国）Klaus Schwetlick 等，化学工业出版社，2010 年。

6.《有机化学实验（第 4 版）》吉卯祉等编，科学出版社，2019 年。

7.《有机化学实验（第三版）》北京大学化学与分子工程学院有机化学研究所编，北京大学出版社，2015 年。

二、试剂的配制

1. 1% 硝酸银 - 醇溶液

取 2g $AgNO_3$，溶于 10ml 蒸馏水中，再加乙醇稀释到 100ml。

2. 10% 硝酸银溶液

取 17g $AgNO_3$ 溶解在 100ml 蒸馏水中。

3. 饱和溴水

溶解 15g KBr 于 100ml 蒸馏水中，加入 10g 溴，振荡即成。

4. 碘 - 碘化钾溶液

将 20g 碘化钾溶于 100ml 蒸馏水中，然后加入 10g 研细的碘粉，搅拌使其全溶成深红色溶液，保存于棕色瓶中。

5. 0.1% 碘溶液

取 0.1g 碘和 0.2g 碘化钾于同一烧瓶中，先加适量蒸馏水使其全溶，再用蒸馏水稀释至 100ml。

6. 品红试剂

在 100ml 热水中溶解 0.2g 品红盐酸盐（也称盐基品红）。放置冷却后，加入 2g 亚硫酸氢钠和 2ml 浓盐酸，再用蒸馏水稀释至 200ml。

7. 2，4 - 二硝基苯肼试液

取 2，4 - 二硝基苯肼 2g，溶于 10ml 浓硫酸中，然后一边搅拌，一边将此溶液加到 14ml 水及 50ml 95% 乙醇中。剧烈搅拌，滤去不溶解的固体即得所需溶液。

8. β–萘酚溶液

将 5g β–萘酚溶于 50ml 5% 氢氧化钠溶液中。

9. 斐林试剂

斐林试剂是由斐林试剂甲和斐林试剂乙组成，使用时将两者等体积混合。

斐林试剂甲：将 3.5g 含有 5 分子结晶水的硫酸铜（$CuSO_4 \cdot 5H_2O$）溶于 100ml 水中得到淡蓝色的斐林试剂甲。

斐林试剂乙：将 17g 4 分子结晶水的酒石酸钾钠溶于 20ml 热水中，然后加入含有 5g 氢氧化钠的水溶液 20ml，稀释至 100ml 即得无色清亮的斐林试剂乙。

10. 苯肼试剂

称取 2 份重量的苯肼盐酸盐和 3 份重量的无水乙酸钠混合均匀，于研钵中研磨成粉末即得盐酸苯肼–乙酸钠混合物，贮存于棕色试剂瓶中。苯肼盐酸盐与乙酸钠经复分解反应生成苯肼乙酸盐，后者是弱酸强碱盐，在水溶液中强烈水解，生成的苯肼和糖作用成脎。游离苯肼难溶于水所以不能直接使用苯肼。

取苯肼盐酸盐 5g，加入水 160ml，微热助溶，再加入活性炭 0.5g，脱色，过滤，在滤液中加入乙酸钠结晶 9g，搅拌、溶解后贮存于棕色瓶中。

11. 卢卡氏试剂

将 34g 无水氯化锌在蒸发皿中强烈熔融，不断用玻璃棒搅动，使之凝固成小块。稍冷后，放在干燥器中冷至室温，取出溶于 23ml 浓盐酸中（相对密度 1.187），搅拌，同时把容器放在冰水浴中冷却，以防氯化氢逸出。此溶剂一般是临用时配制。

12. 溴–四氯化碳溶液

取 100ml 四氯化碳溶液，加入 5ml 溴，振摇溶液呈红色，贮于棕色瓶内备用。

13. 亚硫酸氢钠溶液

取 12ml 40% 亚硫酸氢钠溶液，加 3ml 无水乙醇混合，滤去析出的少量亚硫酸氢钠结晶，所得清液贮存待用。此溶液不稳定，易氧化和分解，因此一般是临用时配制。

14. 盐酸羟胺甲醇溶液

取盐酸羟胺 69g，溶于 1000ml 甲醇中。